Current Clinical Strategies

Family Medicine

Year 2002 Edition

Paul D. Chan, MD
Christopher R. Winkle, MD
Peter J. Winkle, MD

Current Clinical Strategies Publishing

www.ccspublishing.com/ccs

Digital Book and Updates

Purchasers of this book can download the Palm, Pocket PC, Windows CE, Windows or Macintosh version and updates at the Current Clinical Strategies Publishing web site: www.ccspublishing.com/ccs

Current Clinical Strategies Publishing
27071 Cabot Road
Laguna Hills, California 92653
Phone: 800-331-8227; 949-348-8404
Fax: 800-965-9420; 949-348-8405
Internet: www.ccspublishing.com/ccs
E-mail: info@ccspublishing.com

Printed in USA   ISBN 1929622-14-7

Table of Contents

Complications of Pregnancy 259

References 290

Commonly Used Formulas 291

Drug Levels of Commonly Used Medications 292

INTERNAL MEDICINE

Cardiology

Advanced Cardiac Life Support

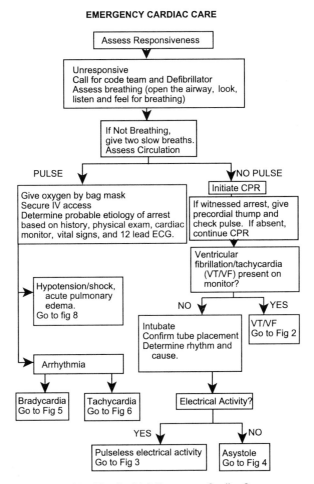

EMERGENCY CARDIAC CARE

Assess Responsiveness

Unresponsive
Call for code team and Defibrillator
Assess breathing (open the airway, look, listen and feel for breathing)

If Not Breathing, give two slow breaths. Assess Circulation

PULSE

Give oxygen by bag mask
Secure IV access
Determine probable etiology of arrest based on history, physical exam, cardiac monitor, vital signs, and 12 lead ECG.

Hypotension/shock, acute pulmonary edema.
Go to fig 8

Arrhythmia

Bradycardia
Go to Fig 5

Tachycardia
Go to Fig 6

NO PULSE

Initiate CPR

If witnessed arrest, give precordial thump and check pulse. If absent, continue CPR

Ventricular fibrillation/tachycardia (VT/VF) present on monitor?

NO

YES

Intubate
Confirm tube placement
Determine rhythm and cause.

VT/VF
Go to Fig 2

Electrical Activity?

YES

NO

Pulseless electrical activity
Go to Fig 3

Asystole
Go to Fig 4

Fig 1 - Algorithm for Adult Emergency Cardiac Care

VENTRICULAR FIBRILLATION AND PULSELESS VENTRICULAR TACHYCARDIA

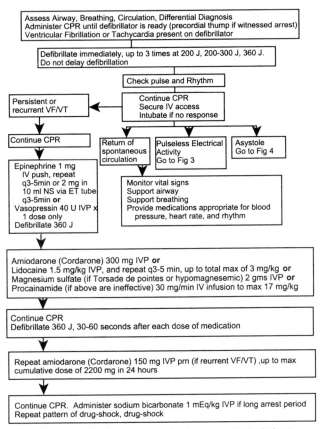

Note: Epinephrine, lidocaine, atropine may be given via endotracheal tube at
2-2.5 times the IV dose. Dilute in 10 cc of saline.
After each intravenous dose, give 20-30 mL bolus of IV fluid and elevate
extremity.

Fig 2 - Ventricular Fibrillation and Pulseless Ventricular Tachycardia

PULSELESS ELECTRICAL ACTIVITY

Pulseless Electrical Activity Includes:
      Electromechanical dissociation (EMD)
      Pseudo-EMD
      Idioventricular rhythms
      Ventricular escape rhythms
      Bradyasystolic rhythms
      Postdefibrillation idioventricular rhythms

Initiate CPR, secure IV access, intubate, assess pulse.

Determine differential diagnosis and treat underlying cause:
  Hypoxia (ventilate)
  Hypovolemia (infuse volume)
  Pericardial tamponade (performpericardiocentesis)
  Tension pneumothorax (perform needle decompression)
  Pulmonary embolism (thrombectomy, thrombolytics)
  Drug overdose with tricyclics, digoxin, beta, or calcium blockers
  Hyperkalemia or hypokalemia
  Acidosis (give bicarbonate)
  Myocardial infarction (thrombolytics)
  Hypothemia (active rewarming)

Epinephrine 1.0 mg IV bolus q3-5 min, or high dose
  epinephrine 0.1 mg/kg IV push q3-5 min; may give via
  ET tube.
Continue CPR

If bradycardia (<60 beats/min), give atroprine 1 mg IV, q3-5
  min, up to total of 0.04 mg/kg
Consider bicarbonate, 1 mEq/kg IV (1-2 amp, 44 mEq/amp),
  if hyperkalemia or other indications.

Fig 3 - Pulseless Electrical Activity

ASYSTOLE

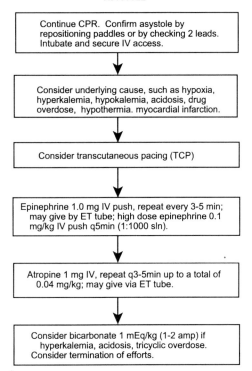

Continue CPR. Confirm asystole by repositioning paddles or by checking 2 leads. Intubate and secure IV access.

Consider underlying cause, such as hypoxia, hyperkalemia, hypokalemia, acidosis, drug overdose, hypothermia. myocardial infarction.

Consider transcutaneous pacing (TCP)

Epinephrine 1.0 mg IV push, repeat every 3-5 min; may give by ET tube; high dose epinephrine 0.1 mg/kg IV push q5min (1:1000 sln).

Atropine 1 mg IV, repeat q3-5min up to a total of 0.04 mg/kg; may give via ET tube.

Consider bicarbonate 1 mEq/kg (1-2 amp) if hyperkalemia, acidosis, tricyclic overdose. Consider termination of efforts.

Fig 4 - Asystole

BRADYCARDIA

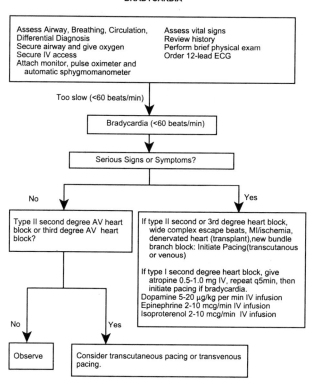

Assess Airway, Breathing, Circulation,
Differential Diagnosis
Secure airway and give oxygen
Secure IV access
Attach monitor, pulse oximeter and
automatic sphygmomanometer

Assess vital signs
Review history
Perform brief physical exam
Order 12-lead ECG

Too slow (<60 beats/min)

Bradycardia (<60 beats/min)

Serious Signs or Symptoms?

No

Yes

Type II second degree AV heart
block or third degree AV heart
block?

If type II second or 3rd degree heart block,
wide complex escape beats, MI/ischemia,
denervated heart (transplant),new bundle
branch block: Initiate Pacing(transcutaneous
or venous)

If type I second degree heart block, give
atropine 0.5-1.0 mg IV, repeat q5min, then
initiate pacing if bradycardia.
Dopamine 5-20 µg/kg per min IV infusion
Epinephrine 2-10 mcg/min IV infusion
Isoproterenol 2-10 mcg/min IV infusion

No

Yes

Observe

Consider transcutaneous pacing or transvenous
pacing.

Fig 5 - Bradycardia (with patient not in cardiac arrest).

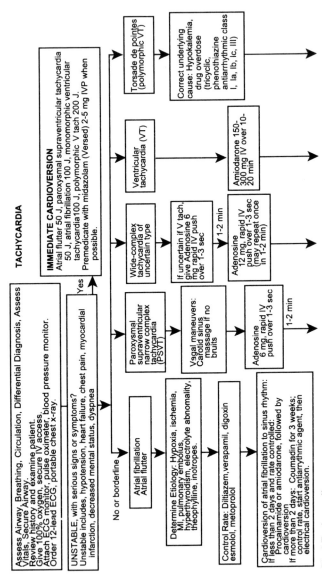

TACHYCARDIA

Assess Airway, Breathing, Circulation, Differential Diagnosis, Assess Vitals, Secure Airway.
Review history and examine patient.
Give 100% oxygen, secure IV access.
Attach ECG monitor, pulse oximeter, blood pressure monitor.
Order 12-lead ECG, portable chest x-ray.

UNSTABLE, with serious signs or symptoms?
Unstable includes, hypotension, heart failure, chest pain, myocardial infarction, decreased mental status, dyspnea

Yes

IMMEDIATE CARDIOVERSION
Atrial flutter 50 J, paroxysmal supraventricular tachycardia 50 J, atrial fibrillation 100 J, monomorphic ventricular tachycardia100 J, polymorphic V tach 200 J.
Premedicate with midazolam (Versed) 2-5 mg IVP when possible.

No or borderline

Atrial fibrillation / Atrial flutter

Determine Etiology: Hypoxia, ischemia, MI, pulmonary embolus, hyperthyroidism, electrolyte abnormality, theophylline, inotropes.

Control Rate: Diltiazem, verapamil, digoxin esmolol, metoprolol

Cardioversion of atrial fibrillation to sinus rhythm: If less than 2 days and rate controlled: Procainamide or amiodarone, followed by cardioversion.
If more than 2 days: Coumadin for 3 weeks; control rate, start antiarrhythmic agent, then electrical cardioversion.

Paroxysmal supraventricular narrow complex tachycardia (PSVT)

Vsgal maneuvers: Carotid sinus massage if no bruits

Adenosine 6 mg. rapid IV push over 1-3 sec

1-2 min

Wide-complex tachycardia of uncertain type

If uncertain if V tach, give Adenosine 6 mg rapid IV push over 1-3 sec

1-2 min

Adenosine 12 mg, rapid IV push over 1-3 sec (may repeat once in 1-2 min)

Ventricular tachycardia (VT)

Amiodarone 150-300 mg IV over 10-20 min

Torsade de pointes (polymorphic VT)

Correct underlying cause: Hypokalemia, drug overdose (tricyclic, phenothiazine antiarrhythmic class I, Ia, Ib, Ic, III)

Fig 6 Tachycardia

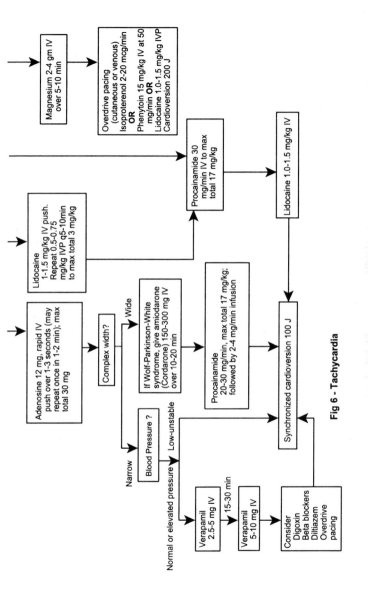

Fig 6 - Tachycardia

Magnesium 2-4 gm IV over 5-10 min

Overdrive pacing (cutaneous or venous) Isoproterenol 2-20 mcg/min **OR** Phenytoin 15 mg/kg IV at 50 mg/min **OR** Lidocaine 1.0-1.5 mg/kg IVP Cardioversion 200 J

Procainamide 30 mg/min IV to max total 17 mg/kg

Lidocaine 1.0-1.5 mg/kg IV

Lidocaine 1-1.5 mg/kg IV push. Repeat 0.5-0.75 mg/kg IVP q5-10min to max total 3 mg/kg

Adenosine 12 mg, rapid IV push over 1-3 seconds (may repeat once in 1-2 min); max total 30 mg

Complex width?

Wide

If Wolf-Parkinson-White syndrome, give amiodarone (Cordarone) 150-300 mg IV over 10-20 min

Procainamide 20-30 mg/min, max total 17 mg/kg; followed by 2-4 mg/min infusion

Narrow

Blood Pressure ?

Low-unstable

Synchronized cardioversion 100 J

Normal or elevated pressure

Verapamil 2.5-5 mg IV

15-30 min

Verapamil 5-10 mg IV

Consider Digoxin Beta blockers Diltiazem Overdrive pacing

STABLE TACHYCARDIA

Stable tachycardia with serious signs and symptoms related to the tachycardia. Patient not in cardiac arrest.

If ventricular rate is >150 beats/min, prepare for immediate cardioversion.
Treatment of Stable Patients is based on Arrhythmia Type:

Ventricular Tachycardia:
Procainamide (Pronestyl) 30 mg/min IV, up to a total max of 17 mg/kg, or
Amiodarone (Cordarone) 150-300 mg IV over 10-20 min, or
Lidocaine 0.75 mg/kg. Procainamide is contraindicated if ejection fraction is <40%.

Paroxysmal Supraventricular Tachycardia: Carotid sinus pressure (if bruits absent), then adenosine 6 mg rapid IVP, followed by 12 mg rapid IVP x 2 doses to max total 30 mg. If no response, verapamil 2.5-5.0 mg IVP; may repeat dose with 5-10 mg IVP if adequate blood pressure; or Esmolol 500 mcg/kg IV over 1 min, then 50 mcg/kg/min IV infusion, and titrate up to 200 mcg/kg/min IV infusion.

Atrial Fibrillation/Flutter:
Ejection fraction ≥40%: Diltiazem (Cardizem) 0.25 mg/kg IV over 2 min; may repeat 0.35 mg/kg IV over 2 min prn x 1 to control rate. Then give procainamide (Pronestyl) 30 mg/min IV infusion, up to a total max of 17 mg/kg
Ejection fraction <40%: Digoxin 0.5 mg IVP, then 0.25 mg IVP q4h x 2 to control rate. Then give amiodarone (Cordarone) 150-300 mg IV over 10-20 min.

Check oxygen saturation, suction device, intubation equipment. Secure IV access

Premedicate whenever possible with Midazolam (Versed) 2-5 mg IVP or sodium pentothal 2 mg/kg rapid IVP

Synchronized cardioversion
Atrialflutter	50 J
PSVT	50 J
Atrial	100 J
Monomorphic V-tach	100 J
Polymorphic V tach	200 J

Fig 7 - Stable Tachycardia (not in cardiac arrest)

HYPOTENSION, SHOCK, AND ACUTE PULMONARY EDEMA

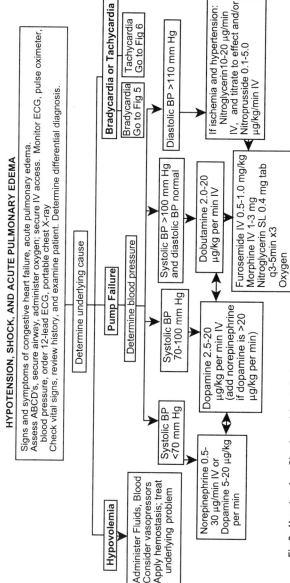

Signs and symptoms of congestive heart failure, acute pulmonary edema.
Assess ABCD's, secure airway, administer oxygen; secure IV access. Monitor ECG, pulse oximeter, blood pressure, order 12-lead ECG, portable chest X-ray
Check vital signs, review history, and examine patient. Determine differential diagnosis.

Determine underlying cause

Hypovolemia

Administer Fluids, Blood
Consider vasopressors
Apply hemostasis; treat underlying problem

Pump Failure

Determine blood pressure

Systolic BP <70 mm Hg

Norepinephrine 0.5-30 µg/min IV or Dopamine 5-20 µg/kg per min

Systolic BP 70-100 mm Hg

Dopamine 2.5-20 µg/kg per min IV (add norepinephrine if dopamine is >20 µg/kg per min)

Systolic BP >100 mm Hg and diastolic BP normal

Dobutamine 2.0-20 µg/kg per min IV

Bradycardia or Tachycardia

Bradycardia Go to Fig 5

Tachycardia Go to Fig 6

Diastolic BP >110 mm Hg

If ischemia and hypertension: Nitroglycerin10-20 µg/min IV, and titrate to effect and/or Nitroprusside 0.1-5.0 µg/kg/min IV

Furosemide IV 0.5-1.0 mg/kg
Morphine IV 1-3 mg
Nitroglycerin SL 0.4 mg tab q3-5min x3
Oxygen

Fig 8 - Hypotension, Shock, and Acute Pulmonary Edema

Medical Documentation

History and Physical Examination

Identifying Data: Patient's name; age, race, sex. List the patient's significant medical problems. Name of informant (patient, relative).

Chief Compliant: Reason given by patient for seeking medical care and the duration of the symptom.

History of Present Illness (HPI): Describe the course of the patient's illness, including when it began, character of the symptoms, location where the symptoms began; aggravating or alleviating factors; pertinent positives and negatives. Describe past illnesses or surgeries, and past diagnostic testing.

Past Medical History (PMH): Past diseases, surgeries, hospitalizations; medical problems; history of diabetes, hypertension, peptic ulcer disease, asthma, myocardial infarction, cancer. In children include birth history, prenatal history, immunizations, and type of feedings.

Medications:

Allergies: Penicillin, codeine?

Family History: Medical problems in family, including the patient's disorder. Asthma, coronary artery disease, heart failure, cancer, tuberculosis.

Social History: Alcohol, smoking, drug usage. Marital status, employment situation. Level of education.

Review of Systems (ROS):

General: Weight gain or loss, loss of appetite, fever, chills, fatigue, night sweats.

Skin: Rashes, skin discolorations.

Head: Headaches, dizziness, masses, seizures.

Eyes: Visual changes, eye pain.

Ears: Tinnitus, vertigo, hearing loss.

Nose: Nose bleeds, discharge, sinus diseases.

Mouth and Throat: Dental disease, hoarseness, throat pain.

Respiratory: Cough, shortness of breath, sputum (color).

Cardiovascular: Chest pain, orthopnea, paroxysmal nocturnal dyspnea; dyspnea on exertion, claudication, edema, valvular disease.

Gastrointestinal: Dysphagia, abdominal pain, nausea, vomiting, hematemesis, diarrhea, constipation, melena (black tarry stools), hematochezia (bright red blood per rectum).

Genitourinary: Dysuria, frequency, hesitancy, hematuria, discharge.

Gynecological: Gravida/para, abortions, last menstrual period (frequency, duration), age of menarche, menopause; dysmenorrhea, contraception, vaginal bleeding, breast masses.

Endocrine: Polyuria, polydipsia, skin or hair changes, heat intolerance.

Musculoskeletal: Joint pain or swelling, arthritis, myalgias.

Skin and Lymphatics: Easy bruising, lymphadenopathy.

Neuropsychiatric: Weakness, seizures, memory changes, depression.

Physical Examination

General appearance: Note whether the patient looks "ill," well, or malnourished.

Vital Signs: Temperature, heart rate, respirations, blood pressure.

Skin: Rashes, scars, moles, capillary refill (in seconds).

Lymph Nodes: Cervical, supraclavicular, axillary, inguinal nodes; size, tenderness.

Head: Bruising, masses. Check fontanels in pediatric patients.

Eyes: Pupils equal round and react to light and accommodation (PERRLA); extra ocular movements intact (EOMI), and visual fields. Funduscopy (papilledema, arteriovenous nicking, hemorrhages, exudates); scleral icterus, ptosis.

Ears: Acuity, tympanic membranes (dull, shiny, intact, injected, bulging).

Mouth and Throat: Mucus membrane color and moisture; oral lesions, dentition, pharynx, tonsils.

Neck: Jugular venous distention (JVD) at a 45 degree incline, thyromegaly, lymphadenopathy, masses, bruits, abdominojugular reflux.

Chest: Equal expansion, tactile fremitus, percussion, auscultation, rhonchi, crackles, rubs, breath sounds, egophony, whispered pectoriloquy.

Heart: Point of maximal impulse (PMI), thrills (palpable turbulence); regular rate and rhythm (RRR), first and second heart sounds (S1, S2); gallops (S3, S4), murmurs (grade 1-6), pulses (graded 0-2+).

Breast: Dimpling, tenderness, masses, nipple discharge; axillary masses.

Abdomen: Contour (flat, scaphoid, obese, distended); scars, bowel sounds, bruits, tenderness, masses, liver span by percussion; hepatomegaly, splenomegaly; guarding, rebound, percussion note (tympanic), costovertebral angle tenderness (CVAT), suprapubic tenderness.

Genitourinary: Inguinal masses, hernias, scrotum, testicles, varicoceles.

Pelvic Examination: Vaginal mucosa, cervical discharge, uterine size, masses, adnexal masses, ovaries.

Extremities: Joint swelling, range of motion, edema (grade 1-4+); cyanosis, clubbing, edema (CCE); pulses (radial, ulnar, femoral, popliteal, posterior tibial, dorsalis pedis; simultaneous palpation of radial and femoral pulses).

Rectal Examination: Sphincter tone, masses, fissures; test for occult blood, prostate (nodules, tenderness, size).

Neurological: Mental status and affect; gait, strength (graded 0-5); touch sensation, pressure, pain, position and vibration; deep tendon reflexes (biceps, triceps, patellar, ankle; graded 0-4+); Romberg test (ability to stand erect with arms outstretched and eyes closed).

Cranial Nerve Examination:

    I: Smell

    II: Vision and visual fields

    III, IV, VI: Pupil responses to light, extraocular eye movements, ptosis

    V: Facial sensation, ability to open jaw against resistance, corneal reflex.

    VII: Close eyes tightly, smile, show teeth

    VIII: Hears watch tic; Weber test (lateralization of sound when tuning fork is placed on top of head); Rinne test (air conduction last longer than bone conduction when tuning fork is placed on mastoid process)

    IX, X: Palette moves in midline when patient says "ah," speech

    XI: Shoulder shrug and turns head against resistance

    XII: Stick out tongue in midline

Labs: Electrolytes (sodium, potassium, bicarbonate, chloride, BUN, creatinine), CBC (hemoglobin, hematocrit, WBC count, platelets, differential); x-rays, ECG, urine analysis (UA), liver function tests (LFTs).

Assessment (Impression): Assign a number to each problem and discuss separately. Discuss differential diagnosis and give reasons that support the working diagnosis; give reasons for excluding other diagnoses.

Plan: Describe therapeutic plan for each numbered problem, including testing, laboratory studies, medications, and antibiotics.

Admission Check List

1. **Call and request** old chart, ECG, and X-rays.
2. **Stat labs:** CBC, Chem 7, cardiac enzymes (myoglobin, troponin, CPK), INR, PTT, C&S, ABG, UA.
3. **Labs:** Toxicology screens and drug levels.
4. **Cultures:** Blood culture x 2, urine and sputum culture (before initiating antibiotics), sputum Gram stain, urinalysis.
5. **CXR, ECG**, diagnostic studies.
6. **Discuss case with resident, attending**, and family.

Progress Notes

Daily progress notes should summarize developments in a patient's hospital course, problems that remain active, plans to treat those problems, and arrangements for discharge. Progress notes should address every element of the problem list.

Progress Note

Date/time:
Subjective: Any problems and symptoms of the patient should be charted. Appetite, pain, headaches or insomnia may be included.
Objective:
General appearance.
Vitals, including highest temperature over past 24 hours. Fluid I/O (inputs and outputs), including oral, parenteral, urine, and stool volumes.
Physical exam, including chest and abdomen, with particular attention to active problems. Emphasize changes from previous physical exams.
Labs: Include new test results and circle abnormal values.
Current medications: List all medications and dosages.
Assessment and Plan: This section should be organized by problem. A separate assessment and plan should be written for each problem.

Procedure Note

A procedure note should be written in the chart when a procedure is performed. Procedure notes are brief operative notes.

Procedure Note

Date and time:
Procedure:
Indications:
Patient Consent: Document that the indications and risks were explained to the patient and that the patient consented: "The patient understands the risks of the procedure and consents in writing."
Lab tests: Relevant labs, such as the INR and CBC
Anesthesia: Local with 2% lidocaine
Description of Procedure: Briefly describe the procedure, including sterile prep, anesthesia method, patient position, devices used, anatomic location of procedure, and outcome.
Complications and Estimated Blood Loss (EBL):
Disposition: Describe how the patient tolerated the procedure.
Specimens: Describe any specimens obtained and labs tests which were ordered.

Discharge Note

The discharge note should be written in the patient's chart prior to discharge.

Discharge Note

Date/time:
Diagnoses:
Treatment: Briefly describe treatment provided during hospitalization, including surgical procedures and antibiotic therapy.
Studies Performed: Electrocardiograms, CT scans.
Discharge Medications:
Follow-up Arrangements:

Discharge Summary

Patient's Name and Medical Record Number:
Date of Admission:
Date of Discharge:
Admitting Diagnosis:
Discharge Diagnosis:
Attending or Ward Team Responsible for Patient:
Surgical Procedures, Diagnostic Tests, Invasive Procedures:
Brief History, Pertinent Physical Examination, and Laboratory Data: Describe the course of the patient's disease up until the time that the patient came to the hospital, including physical exam and laboratory data.
Hospital Course: Describe the course of the patient's illness while in the hospital, including evaluation, treatment, medications, and outcome of treatment.
Discharged Condition: Describe improvement or deterioration in the patient's condition, and describe present status of the patient.
Disposition: Describe the situation to which the patient will be discharged (home, nursing home), and indicate who will take care of patient.
Discharged Medications: List medications and instructions for patient on taking the medications.
Discharged Instructions and Follow-up Care: Date of return for follow-up care at clinic; diet, exercise.
Problem List: List all active and past problems.
Copies: Send copies to attending, clinic, consultants.

Prescription Writing

- Patient's name:
- Date:
- Drug name, dosage form, dose, route, frequency (include concentration for oral liquids or mg strength for oral solids): Amoxicillin 125mg/5mL 5 mL PO tid
- Quantity to dispense: mL for oral liquids, # of oral solids
- Refills: If appropriate
- Signature

Cardiovascular Disorders

Myocardial Infarction and Unstable Angina

1. **Admit to:** Coronary care unit
2. **Diagnosis:** Rule out myocardial infarction
3. **Condition:**
4. **Vital signs:** q1h. Call physician if pulse >90,<60; BP >150/90, <90/60; R>25, <12; T >38.5˚C.
5. **Activity:** Bed rest with bedside commode.
7. **Nursing:** Guaiac stools. If patient has chest pain, obtain 12-lead ECG and call physician.
8. **Diet:** Cardiac diet, 1-2 gm sodium, low fat, low cholesterol diet. No caffeine or temperature extremes.
9. **IV Fluids:** D5W at TKO
10. **Special Medications:**
    -Oxygen 2-4 L/min by NC.
    -Aspirin 325 mg PO, chew and swallow, then 160 mg PO qd **OR**
    -Clopidogrel (Plavix) 75 mg PO qd (if allergic to aspirin).
    -Nitroglycerine infusion 15 mcg IV bolus, then 10 mcg/min infusion (50 mg in 250-500 mL D5W, 100-200 mcg/mL). Titrate to control symptoms in 5-10 mcg/min steps, up to 200-300 mcg/min; maintain systolic BP >90 **OR**
    -Nitroglycerine SL, 0.4 mg (0.15-0.6 mg) SL q5min until pain free (up to 3 tabs) **OR**
    -Nitroglycerin spray (0.4 mg/aerosol spray)1-2 sprays under the tongue q 5min;
    MR x 2.
    -Heparin 70 U/kg IV push, then 15-17 U/kg/hr by continuous IV infusion for 48 hours to maintain aPTT of 50-70 seconds. Check aPTTq6h x 4, then qd. Repeat aPTT 6 hours after each heparin dosage change.

Glycoprotein II$_b$/III$_a$ Blockers for Acute Coronary Syndromes:
-**Eptifibatide (Integrilin)** 180mcg/kg IVP, then 2 mcg/kg/min for 72 hours.
-**Tirofiban (Aggrastat)** 0.4 mcg/kg/min for 30 min, then 0.1 mcg/kg/min for 48-108 hours.

Glycoprotein IIb/IIIa blockers for Use With Angioplasty:
-**Abciximab (ReoPro)** 0.25 mg/kg IVP, then 0.125 mcg/kg/min IV infusion for 12 hours.
-**Eptifibatide (Integrilin)** 180 mcg/kg IVP, then 2 mcg/kg/min for 20-24 hours.

Thrombolytic Therapy

Absolute Contraindications to Thrombolytics: Active internal bleeding, history of hemorrhagic stroke, head trauma, pregnancy, surgery within 2 wk, recent non-compressible vascular puncture, uncontrolled hypertension (>180/110 mmHg).

Relative Contraindications to Thrombolytics: Absence of ST-segment elevation, severe hypertension, cerebrovascular disease, recent surgery (within 2 weeks), cardiopulmonary resuscitation.

A. Alteplase (tPA, tissue plasminogen activator, Activase):
  1. 15 mg IV push over 2 min, followed by 0.75 mg/kg (max 50 mg) IV infusion over 30 min, followed by 0.5 mg/kg (max 35 mg) IV infusion over 60 min (max total dose 100 mg).
  2. **Labs:** INR/PTT, CBC, fibrinogen.

B. Reteplase (Retavase):
  1. 10 U IV push over 2 min; repeat second 10 U IV push after 30 min.
  2. **Labs:** INR, aPTT, CBC, fibrinogen.

C. Tenecteplase (TNKase):

<60 kg	30 mg IVP
60-69 kg	35 mg IVP
70-79 kg	40 mg IVP

    80-89 kg   45 mg IVP
    ≥90 kg   50 mg IVP

C. Streptokinase (Streptase):
1. 1.5 million IU in 100 mL NS IV over 60 min. Pretreat with diphenhydramine (Benadryl) 50 mg IV push **AND** Methylprednisolone (Soln-Medrol) 250 mg IV push.
2. Check fibrinogen level now and q6h for 24h until level >100 mg/dL.
3. No IM or arterial punctures, watch IV for bleeding.

Angiotensin Converting Enzyme Inhibitor:
-Lisinopril (Zestril, Prinivil) 2.5-5 mg PO qd; titrate to 10-20 mg qd.

Long-acting Nitrates:
-Nitroglycerin patch 0.2 mg/hr qd. Allow for nitrate-free period to prevent tachyphylaxis.
-Isosorbide dinitrate (Isordil) 10-60 mg PO tid [5,10,20, 30,40 mg] **OR**
-Isosorbide mononitrate (Imdur) 30-60 mg PO qd.

Beta-Blockers: Contraindicated in cardiogenic shock.
-Metoprolol (Lopressor) 5 mg IV q2-5min x 3 doses; then 25 mg PO q6h for 48h, then 100 mg PO q12h; keep HR <60/min, hold if systolic BP <100 mmHg **OR**
-Atenolol (Tenormin), 5 mg IV, repeated in 5 minutes, followed by 50-100 mg PO qd **OR**
-Esmolol hydrochloride (Brevibloc) 500 mcg/kg IV over 1 min, then 50 mcg/kg/min IV infusion, titrated to heart rate >60 bpm (max 300 mcg/kg/min).

11. **Symptomatic Medications:**
-Morphine sulfate 2-4 mg IV push prn chest pain.
-Acetaminophen (Tylenol) 325-650 mg PO q4-6h prn headache.
-Lorazepam (Ativan) 1-2 mg PO tid-qid prn anxiety
-Zolpidem (Ambien) 5-10 mg qhs prn insomnia.
-Docusate (Colace) 100 mg PO bid.
-Dimenhydrinate (Dramamine) 25-50 mg IV over 2-5 min q4-6h or 50 mg PO q4-6h prn nausea.
-Ranitidine (Zantac) 150 mg PO bid or 50 mg IV q8h.

12. **Extras:** ECG stat and in 12h and in AM, portable CXR, impedence cardiography, echocardiogram. Cardiology consult.

13. **Labs:** SMA7 and 12, magnesium. Cardiac enzymes: CPK-MB, troponin T, myoglobin STAT and q6h for 24h. CBC, INR/PTT, UA.

Congestive Heart Failure

1. **Admit to:**
2. **Diagnosis:** Congestive Heart Failure
3. **Condition:**
4. **Vital signs:** q1h. Call physician if P >120; BP >150/100 <80/60; T >38.5°C; R >25, <10.
5. **Activity:** Bed rest with bedside commode.
6. **Nursing:** Daily weights, measure inputs and outputs. Head-of-bed at 45 degrees, legs elevated.
7. **Diet:** 1-2 gm salt, cardiac diet.
8. **IV Fluids:** Heparin lock with flush q shift.
9. **Special Medications:**
-Oxygen 2-4 L/min by NC.

Diuretics:
-Furosemide 10-160 mg IV qd-bid or 20-80 mg PO qAM-bid [20,40,80 mg] **OR**
-Torsemide (Demadex) 10-40 mg IV or PO qd; max 200 mg/day [5, 10, 20, 100 mg] **OR**
-Bumetanide (Bumex) 0.5-1 mg IV q2-3h until response; then 0.5-1.0 mg IV q8-24h (max 10 mg/d); or 0.5-2.0 mg PO qAM.
-Metolazone (Zaroxolyn) 2.5-10 mg PO qd, max 20 mg/d; 30 min before loop

diuretic [2.5,5,10 mg].

ACE Inhibitors:
- Quinapril (Accupril) 5-10 mg PO qd x 1 dose, then 20-80 mg PO qd in 1 to 2 divided doses [5,10,20,40 mg] **OR**
- Lisinopril (Zestril, Prinivil) 5-40 mg PO qd [5,10,20,40 mg] **OR**
- Benazepril (Lotensin) 10-40 mg PO qd, max 80 mg/d [5,10,20,40 mg] **OR**
- Fosinopril (Monopril) 10-40 mg PO qd, max 80 mg/d [10,20 mg] **OR**
- Ramipril (Altace) 2.5-10 mg PO qd, max 20 mg/d [1.25,2.5,5,10 mg].
- Captopril (Capoten) 6.25-50 mg PO q8h [12.5, 25,50,100 mg] **OR**
- Enalapril (Vasotec) 1.25-5 mg slow IV push q6h or 2.5-20 mg PO bid [5,10,20 mg] **OR**
- Moexipril (Univasc) 7.5 mg PO qd x 1 dose, then 7.5-15 mg PO qd-bid [7.5, 15 mg tabs] **OR**
- Trandolapril (Mavik) 1 mg qd x 1 dose, then 2-4 mg qd [1, 2, 4 mg tabs].

Angiotensin-II Receptor Blockers:
- Irbesartan (Avapro) 150 mg qd, max 300 mg qd [75, 150, 300 mg].
- Losartan (Cozaar) 25-50 mg bid [25, 50 mg].
- Valsartan (Diovan) 80 mg qd; max 320 mg qd [80, 160 mg].
- Candesartan (Atacand) 8-16 mg qd-bid [4, 8, 16, 32 mg].
- Telmisartan (Micardis) 40-80 mg qd [40, 80 mg].

Beta-blockers:
- Carvedilol (Coreg) 1.625-3.125 mg PO bid, then slowly increase the dose every 2 weeks to target dose of 25-50 mg bid [tab 3.125, 6.25, 12.5, 25 mg] **OR**
- Metoprolol (Lopressor) start at 12.5 mg bid, then slowly increase to target dose of 100 mg bid [50, 100 mg].
- Bisoprolol (Zebeta) start at 1.25 mg qd, then slowly increase to target of 10 mg qd. [5,10 mg].

Digoxin: (Lanoxin) 0.125-0.5 mg PO or IV qd [0.125,0.25, 0.5 mg].

Inotropic Agents:
- Dobutamine (Dobutrex) 2.5-10 mcg/kg/min IV, max of 14 mcg/kg/min (500 mg in 250 mL D5W, 2 mcg/mL) **OR**
- Dopamine (Intropin) 3-15 mcg/kg/min IV (400 mg in 250 cc D5W, 1600 mcg/mL), titrate to CO >4, CI >2; systolic >90 **OR**
- Milrinone (Primacor) 0.375 mcg/kg/min IV infusion (40 mg in 200 mL NS, 0.2 mg/mL); titrate to 0.75 mgc/kg/min; arrhythmogenic; may cause hypotension

Potassium:
- KCL (Micro-K) 20-60 mEq PO qd.

10. Symptomatic Medications:
- Morphine sulfate 2-4 mg IV push prn dyspnea or anxiety.
- Heparin 5000 U SQ q12h.
- Docusate sodium 100-200 mg PO qhs.
- Ranitidine (Zantac)150 mg PO bid or 50 mg IV q8h.

11. Extras: CXR PA and LAT, ECG now and repeat if chest pain or palpitations, impedence cardiography, echocardiogram.

12. Labs: SMA 7&12, CBC; cardiac enzymes: CPK-MB, troponin T, myglobin STAT and q6h for 24h. Repeat SMA 7 in AM. UA.

Supraventricular Tachycardia

1. **Admit to:**
2. **Diagnosis:** PSVT
3. **Condition:**
4. **Vital signs:** q1h. Call physician if BP >160/90, <90/60; apical pulse >130, <50; R >25, <10; T >38.5°C
5. **Activity:** Bedrest with bedside commode.
6. **Nursing:**
7. **Diet:** Low fat, low cholesterol, no caffeine.
8. **IV Fluids:** D5W at TKO.

9. Special Medications:
Attempt vagal maneuvers (Valsalva maneuver and/or carotid sinus massage) before drug therapy:

Cardioversion (if unstable or refractory to drug therapy):
1. NPO for 6h, digoxin level must be less than 2.4 and potassium and magnesium must be normal.
2. Midazolam (Versed) 2-5 mg IV push.
3. If stable, cardiovert with synchronized 10-50 J, and increase by 50 J increments if necessary. If unstable, start with 75-100 J, then increase to 200 J and 360 J.

Pharmacologic Therapy of Supraventricular Tachycardia:
-Adenosine (Adenocard) 6 mg rapid IV over 1-2 sec, followed by saline flush, may repeat 12 mg IV after 2-3 min, up to max of 30 mg total **OR**
-Verapamil (Isoptin) 2.5-5 mg IV over 2-3min (may give calcium gluconate 1 gm IV over 3-6 min prior to verapamil); then 40-120 mg PO q8h [40, 80, 120 mg] or verapamil SR 120-240 mg PO qd [120, 180, 240 mg] **OR**
-Esmolol hydrochloride (Brevibloc) 500 mcg/kg IV over 1 min, then 50 mcg/kg/min IV infusion titrated to HR of <60 (max of 300 mcg/kg/min) **OR**
-Diltiazem (Cardizem) 0.25 mg/kg IV over 2-5 minutes **OR**
-Propranolol 1-5 mg (0.15 mg/kg) given IV in 1 mg aliquots; then propranolol-LA 60-320 mg PO qd [60, 80, 120, 160 mg] OR
-Digoxin 0.25 mg q4h as needed; up to 1.0-1.5 mg; then 0.125-0.25 mg PO qd.

10.Symptomatic Medications:
-Lorazepam (Ativan) 1-2 mg PO tid prn anxiety.

11.Extras: Portable CXR, ECG; repeat if chest pain. Cardiology consult.

12.Labs: CBC, SMA 7&12, Mg, thyroid panel. UA.

Ventricular Arrhythmias

1. Ventricular Fibrillation and Tachycardia:
-**If unstable (see ACLS protocol):** Defibrillate with unsynchronized 200 J, then 300 J.
-Oxygen 100% by mask.
-Lidocaine (Xylocaine) loading dose 75-100 mg IV, then 2-4 mg/min IV **OR**
-Bretylium (Bretylol) loading dose 5-10 mg/kg over 5-10 min, then 1-4 mg/min IV infusion.
-Amiodarone (Cordarone) 150 mg in 100 mL of D5W, IV infusion over 10 min, then 900 mg in 500 mL of D5W, at 1 mg/min for 6 hrs, then at 0.5 mg/min thereafter.
-**Also see "other antiarrhythmics" below**.

2. Torsades De Pointes Ventricular Tachycardia:
-Correct underlying cause and consider discontinuing quinidine, procainamide, disopyramide, moricizine, lidocaine, amiodarone, sotalol, cisapride, Ibutilide, phenothiazine, haloperidol, tricyclic and tetracyclic antidepressants, ketoconazole, itraconazole, bepridil, hypokalemia, and hypomagnesemia.
-Magnesium sulfate 1-4 gm in IV bolus over 5-15 min or infuse 3-20 mg/min for 7-48h until QT interval <440 msec.
-Isoproterenol (Isuprel), 2-20 mcg/min (2 mg in 500 mL D5W, 4 mcg/mL).
-Consider ventricular pacing and/or cardioversion.

3. Other Antiarrhythmics:
Class I:
-Moricizine (Ethmozine) 200-300 mg PO q8h, max 900 mg/d [200, 250, 300 mg].

Class Ia:
-Quinidine gluconate (Quinaglute) 324-648 mg PO q8-12h [324 mg].
-Procainamide (Procan, Procanbid)
IV: 15 mg/kg IV loading dose at 20 mg/min, followed by 2-4 mg/min continuous IV infusion.

PO: 500 mg (nonsustained release) PO q2h x 2 doses, then Procanbid 1-2 gm PO q12h [500, 1000 mg].
-Disopyramide (Nor-pace, Norpace CR) 100-300 mg PO q6-8h [100, 150, mg] or disopyramide CR 100-150 mg PO bid [100, 150 mg].

Class Ib:
-Lidocaine (Xylocaine) 75-100 mg IV, then 2-4 mg/min IV
-Mexiletine (Mexitil) 100-200 mg PO q8h, max 1200 mg/d [150, 200, 250 mg].
-Tocainide (Tonocard) loading 400-600 mg PO, then 400-600 mg PO q8-12h (1200-1800 mg/d) PO in divided doses q8-12h [400, 600 mg].
-Phenytoin (Dilantin), loading dose 100-300 mg IV given as 50 mg in NS over 10 min IV q5min, then 100 mg IV q5min prn.

Class Ic:
-Flecainide (Tambocor) 50-100 mg PO q12h, max 400 mg/d [50, 100, 150 mg].
-Propafenone (Rythmol) 150-300 mg PO q8h, max 1200 mg/d [150, 225, 300 mg].

Class II:
-Propranolol (Inderal) 1-3 mg IV in NS (max 0.15 mg/kg) or 20-80 mg PO tid-qid [10, 20, 40, 60, 80 mg]; propranolol-LA (Inderal-LA), 80-120 mg PO qd [60, 80, 120, 160 mg]
-Esmolol (Brevibloc) loading dose 500 mcg/kg over 1 min, then 50-200 mcg/kg/min IV infusion
-Atenolol (Tenormin) 50-100 mg/d PO [25, 50, 100 mg].
-Nadolol (Corgard) 40-100 mg PO qd-bid [20, 40, 80, 120, 160 mg].
-Metoprolol (Lopressor) 50-100 mg PO bid-tid [50, 100 mg], or metoprolol XL 50-200 mg PO qd [50, 100, 200 mg].

Class III:
-Amiodarone (Cordarone), PO loading 400-1200 mg/d in divided doses for 2-4 weeks, then 200-400 mg PO qd (5-10 mg/kg) [200 mg] or amiodarone (Cordarone) 150 mg in 100 mL of D5W, IV infusion over 10 min, then 900 mg in 500 mL of D5W, at 1 mg/min for 6 hrs, then at 0.5 mg/min thereafter.
-Bretylium (Bretylol) 5-10 mg/kg IV over 5-10 min, then maintenance of 1-4 mg/min IV or repeat boluses 5-10 mg/kg IV q6-8h; infusion of 1-4 mg/min IV.
-Sotalol (Betapace) 40-80 mg PO bid, max 320 mg/d in 2-3 divided doses [80, 160 mg].

4. **Extras:** CXR, ECG, Holter monitor, signal averaged ECG, cardiology consult.
5. **Labs:** SMA 7&12, Mg, calcium, CBC, drug levels. UA.

Hypertensive Emergency

1. **Admit to:**
2. **Diagnosis:** Hypertensive emergency
3. **Condition:**
4. **Vital signs:** q30min until BP controlled, then q4h.
5. **Activity:** Bed rest
6. **Nursing:** Intra-arterial BP monitoring, daily weights, inputs and outputs.
7. **Diet:** Clear liquids.
8. **IV Fluids:** D5W at TKO.
9. **Special Medications:**
-Nitroprusside sodium 0.25-10 mcg/kg/min IV (50 mg in 250 mL of D5W), titrate to desired BP
-Labetalol (Trandate, Normodyne) 20 mg IV bolus (0.25 mg/kg), then 20-80 mg boluses IV q10-15min titrated to desired BP. Infusion of 1.0-2.0 mg/min
-Fenoldopam (Corlopam) 0.01mcg/kg/min IV infusion. Adjust dose by 0.025-0.05 mcg/kg/min q15min to max 0.3 mcg/kg/min. [10 mg in 250 mL D5W].
-Nicardipine (Cardene IV) 5 mg/hr IV infusion, increase rate by 2.5 mg/hr every 15 min up to 15 mg/hr (25 mg in D5W 250 mL).
-Enalaprilat (Vasotec IV) 1.25- 5.0 mg IV q6h. Do not use in presence of AMI.
-Esmolol (Brevibloc) 500 mcg/kg/min IV infusion for 1 minute, then 50

mcg/kg/min; titrate by 50 mcg/kg/min increments to 300 mcg/kg/min (2.5 gm in D5W 250 mL).
  -Clonidine (Catapres), initial 0.1-0.2 mg PO followed by 0.05-0.1 mg per hour until DBP <115 (max total dose of 0.8 mg).
  -Phentolamine (pheochromocytoma), 5-10 mg IV, repeated as needed up to 20 mg.
  -Trimethaphan camsylate (Arfonad)(dissecting aneurysm) 2-4 mg/min IV infusion (500 mg in 500 mL of D5W).
10. Symptomatic Medications:
11. Extras: Portable CXR, ECG, impedence cardiography, echocardiogram.
12. Labs: CBC, SMA 7, UA with micro. TSH, free T4, 24h urine for metanephrines. Plasma catecholamines, urine drug screen.

Hypertension

I. **Initial Diagnostic Evaluation of Hypertension**
  A. **15 Lead electrocardiography** may document evidence of ischemic heart disease, rhythm and conduction disturbances, or left ventricular hypertrophy.
  B. **Screening labs** include a complete blood count, glucose, potassium, calcium, creatinine, BUN, uric acid, and fasting lipid panel.
  C. **Urinalysis.** Dipstick testing should include glucose, protein, and hemoglobin.
  D. Selected patients may require plasma renin activity, 24 hour urine catecholamines, or renal function testing (glomerular filtration rate and blood flow).
II. **Antihypertensive Drugs**
  A. **Thiazide Diuretics**
    1. **Hydrochlorothiazide (HCTZ, HydroDiuril)**, 12.5-25 mg qd [25 mg].
    2. **Chlorothiazide (Diuril)** 250 mg qd [250, 500 mg].
    3. **Thiazide/Potassium Sparing Diuretic Combinations**
      a. **Maxzide** (hydrochlorothiazide 50/triamterene 75 mg) 1 tab qd.
      b. **Moduretic** (hydrochlorothiazide 50 mg/amiloride 5 mg) 1 tab qd.
      c. **Dyazide** (hydrochlorothiazide 25 mg/triamterene 37.5) 1 cap qd.
  B. **Beta-Adrenergic Blockers**
    1. **Cardioselective Beta-Blockers**
      a. **Atenolol (Tenormin)** initial dose 50 mg qd, then 50-100 mg qd, max 200 mg/d [25, 50, 100 mg].
      b. **Metoprolol XL (Toprol XL)** 100-200 mg qd [50, 100, 200 mg tab ER].
      c. **Bisoprolol (Zebeta)** 2.5-10 mg qd; max 20 mg qd [5,10 mg].
    2. **Non-Cardioselective Beta-Blockers**
      a. **Propranolol LA (Inderal LA)**, 80-160 mg qd [60, 80, 120, 160 mg].
      b. **Nadolol (Corgard)** 40-80 mg qd, max 320 mg/d [20, 40, 80, 120, 160 mg].
      c. **Pindolol (Visken)** 5-20 mg qd, max 60 mg/d [5, 10 mg].
      d. **Carteolol (Cartrol)** 2.5-10 mg qd [2.5, 5 mg].
  C. **Angiotensin-Converting Enzyme (ACE) Inhibitors**
    1. **Ramipril (Altace)** 2.5-10 mg qd, max 20 mg/day [1.25, 2.5, 5, 10 mg].
    2. **Quinapril (Accupril)** 20-80 mg qd [5, 10, 20, 40 mg].
    3. **Lisinopril (Zestril, Prinivil)** 10-40 mg qd [2.5, 5, 10, 20, 40 mg].
    4. **Benazepril (Lotensin)** 10-40 mg qd, max 80 mg/day [5, 10, 20, 40 mg].
    5. **Fosinopril (Monopril)** 10-40 mg qd [10, 20 mg].
    6. **Enalapril (Vasotec)** 5-40 mg qd, max 40 mg/day [2.5, 5, 10, 20 mg].
    7. **Moexipril (Univasc)** 7.5-15 mg qd [7.5 mg].
  D. **Angiotensin Receptor Antagonists**
    1. **Losartan (Cozaar)** 25-50 mg bid [25, 50 mg].
    2. **Valsartan (Diovan)** 80-160 mg qd [80, 160 mg].
    3. **Irbesartan (Avapro)** 150 mg qd; max 300 mg qd [75, 150, 300 mg].
    4. **Candesartan (Atacand)** 8-16 mg qd-bid [4, 8, 16, 32 mg].

   5. **Telmisartan (Micardis)** 40-80 mg qd [40, 80 mg].
E. **Calcium Entry Blockers**
   1. **Diltiazem SR (Cardizem SR)** 60-120 mg bid [60, 90, 120 mg] or **Cardizem CD** 180-360 mg qd [120, 180, 240, 300 mg].
   2. **Nifedipine XL (Procardia-XL, Adalat-CC)** 30-90 mg qd [30, 60, 90 mg].
   3. **Verapamil SR (Calan SR, Covera-HS)** 120-240 mg qd [120, 180, 240 mg].
   4. **Amlodipine (Norvasc)** 2.5-10 mg qd [2.5, 5, 10 mg].
   5. **Felodipine (Plendil)** 5-10 mg qd [2.5, 5, 10 mg].

Syncope

1. **Admit to:** Monitored ward
2. **Diagnosis:** Syncope
3. **Condition:**
4. **Vital signs:** q1h, postural BP and pulse q12h. Call physician if BP >160/90, <90/60; P >120, <50; R>25, <10
5. **Activity:** Bed rest.
6. **Nursing:** Fingerstick glucose.
7. **Diet:** Regular
8. **IV Fluids:** Normal saline at TKO.
9. **Special medications:**
High-grade AV Block with Syncope:
   -Atropine 1 mg IV x 2.
   -Isoproterenol 0.5-1 mcg/min initially, then slowly titrate to 10 mcg/min IV infusion (1 mg in 250 mL NS).
   -Transthoracic pacing.
Drug-induced Syncope:
   -Discontinue vasodilators, centrally acting hypotensive agents, tranquilizers, antidepressants, and alcohol use.
Vasovagal Syncope:
   -Scopolamine 1.5 mg transdermal patch q3 days.
Postural Syncope:
   -Midodrine (ProAmatine) 2.5 mg PO tid, then increase to 5-10 mg PO tid [2.5, 5 mg]; contraindicated in coronary artery disease.
   -Fludrocortisone 0.1-1.0 mg PO qd.
10. **Extras:** CXR, ECG, 24h Holter monitor, electrophysiologic study, tilt test, CT/MRI, EEG, impedence cardiography, echocardiogram.
11. **Labs:** CBC, SMA 7&12, CK-MB, troponin T, Mg, calcium, drug levels. UA, urine drug screen.

Pulmonary Disorders

Asthma

1. **Admit to:**
2. **Diagnosis:** Exacerbation of asthma
3. **Condition:**
4. **Vital signs:** q6h. Call physician if P >140; R >30, <10; T >38.5°C; pulse oximeter <90%
5. **Activity:** Up as tolerated.
6. **Nursing:** Pulse oximeter, bedside peak flow rate before and after bronchodilator treatments.
7. **Diet:** Regular, no caffeine.
8. **IV Fluids:** D5 ½ NS at 125 cc/h.
9. **Special Medications:**
   -Oxygen 2 L/min by NC. Keep O_2 sat >90%.

Beta Agonists, Acute Treatment:
   -Albuterol (Ventolin) 0.5 mg and ipratropium (Atrovent) 0.5 mg in 2.5 mL NS q1-2h until peak flow meter ≥200-250 L/min and sat ≥90%, then q4h **OR**
   -Albuterol (Ventolin) MDI 3-8 puffs, then 2 puffs q3-6h prn, or powder 200 mcg/capsule inhaled qid.
   -Albuterol/Ipratropium (Combivent) 2-4 puffs qid.

Systemic Corticosteroids:
   -Methylprednisolone (Solu-Medrol) 60-125 mg IV q6h; then 30-60 mg PO qd. **OR**
   -Prednisone 20-60 mg PO qAM.

Aminophylline and Theophylline (second-line therapy):
   -Aminophylline load dose: 5.6 mg/kg **total** body weight in 100 mL D5W IV over 20min. Maintenance of 0.5-0.6 mg/kg **ideal** body weight/h (500 mg in 250 mL D5W); reduce if elderly, heart/liver failure (0.2-0.4 mg/kg/hr). Reduce load 50-75% if taking theophylline (1 mg/kg of aminophylline will raise levels 2 mcg/mL) **OR**
   -Theophylline IV solution loading dose 4.5 mg/kg **total** body weight, then 0.4-0.5 mg/kg **ideal** body weight/hr.
   -Theophylline (Theo-Dur) PO loading dose of 6 mg/kg, then maintenance of 100-400 mg PO bid-tid (3 mg/kg q8h); 80% of total daily IV aminophylline in 2-3 doses.

Inhaled Corticosteroids (adjunct therapy):
   -Beclomethasone (Beclovent) MDI 4-8 puffs bid, with spacer 5 min after bronchodilator, followed by gargling with water
   -Triamcinolone (Azmacort) MDI 2 puffs tid-qid or 4 puffs bid.
   -Flunisolide (AeroBid) MDI 2-4 puffs bid.
   -Fluticasone (Flovent) 2-4 puffs bid (44 or 110 mcg/puff); requires 1-2 weeks for full effect.

Maintenance Treatment:
   -Salmeterol (Serevent) 2 puffs bid; not effective for acute asthma because of delayed onset of action.
   -Pirbuterol (Maxair) MDI 2 puffs q4-6h prn.
   -Bitolterol (Tornalate) MDI 2-3 puffs q1-3min, then 2-3 puffs q4-8h prn.
   -Fenoterol (Berotec) MDI 3 puffs, then 2 bid-qid.
   -Ipratropium (Atrovent) MDI 2-3 puffs tid-qid.

Prevention and Prophylaxis:
   -Cromolyn (Intal) 2-4 puffs tid-qid.
   -Nedocromil (Tilade) 2-4 puffs bid-qid.
   -Montelukast (Singulair) 10 mg PO qd.
   -Zafirlukast (Accolate) 20 mg PO bid.
   -Zileuton (Zyflo) 600 mg PO qid.

Acute Bronchitis
   -Ampicillin/sulbactam (Unasyn) 1.5 gm IV q6h **OR**

-Ampicillin 0.5-1 gm IV q6h or 250-500 mg PO qid **OR**
-Cefuroxime (Zinacef) 750 mg IV q8h **OR**
-Cefuroxime axetil (Ceftin) 250-500 mg PO bid **OR**
-Trimethoprim/Sulfamethoxazole (Bactrim DS), 1 tab PO bid **OR**
-Levofloxacin (Levaquin) 500 mg PO/IV PO qd [250, 500 mg].
10. **Symptomatic Medications:**
   -Docusate sodium (Colace) 100 mg qhs.
   -Ranitidine (Zantac) 50 mg IV q8h or 150 mg PO bid.
11. **Extras:** Portable CXR, ECG, pulmonary function tests before and after bronchodilators; pulmonary rehabilitation; impedence cardiography, echocardiogram.
12. **Labs:** ABG, CBC with eosinophil count, SMA7. Theophylline level stat and after 24h of infusion. Sputum Gram stain, C&S.

Chronic Obstructive Pulmonary Disease

1. **Admit to:**
2. **Diagnosis:** Exacerbation of COPD
3. **Condition:**
4. **Vital signs:** q4h. Call physician if P >130; R >30, <10; T >38.5°C; O_2 Sat <90%.
5. **Activity:** Up as tolerated; bedside commode.
6. **Nursing:** Pulse oximeter. Measure peak flow with portable peak flow meter bid and chart with vital signs. No sedatives.
7. **Diet:** No added salt, no caffeine. Push fluids.
8. **IV Fluids:** D5 ½ NS with 20 mEq KCL/L at 125 cc/h.
9. **Special Medications:**
   -Oxygen 1-2 L/min by NC or 24-35% by Venturi mask, keep O_2 saturation 90-91%.
Beta-Agonists, Acute Treatment:
   -Albuterol (Ventolin) 0.5 mg and ipratropium (Atrovent) 0.5 mg in 2.5 mL NS q1-2h until peak flow meter ≥200-250 L/min, then q4h **OR**
   -Albuterol (Ventolin) MDI 2-4 puffs q4-6h.
   -Albuterol/Ipratropium (Combivent) 2-4 puffs qid.
Corticosteroids and Anticholinergics:
   -Methylprednisolone (Solu-Medrol) 60-125 mg IV q6h or 30-60 mg PO qd.
   Followed by:
   -Prednisone 20-60 mg PO qd.
   -Triamcinolone (Azmacort) MDI 2 puffs qid or 4 puffs bid.
   -Beclomethasone (Beclovent) MDI 4-8 puffs bid with spacer, followed by gargling with water **OR**
   -Flunisolide (AeroBid) MDI 2-4 puffs bid **OR**
   -Ipratropium (Atrovent) MDI 2 puffs tid-qid **OR**
   -Fluticasone (Flovent) 2-4 puffs bid (44 or 110 mcg/puff.
Aminophylline and Theophylline (second line therapy):
   -Aminophylline loading dose, 5.6 mg/kg **total** body weight over 20 min (if not already on theophylline); then 0.5-0.6 mg/kg **ideal** body weight/hr (500 mg in 250 mL of D5W); reduce if elderly, or heart or liver disease (0.2-0.4 mg/kg/hr). Reduce loading to 50-75% if already taking theophylline (1 mg/kg of aminophylline will raise levels by 2 mcg/mL) **OR**
   -Theophylline IV solution loading dose, 4.5 mg/kg **total** body weight, then 0.4-0.5 mg/kg **ideal** body weight/hr.
   -Theophylline long acting (Theo-Dur) 100-400 mg PO bid-tid (3 mg/kg q8h); 80% of daily IV aminophylline in 2-3 doses.
Acute Bronchitis
   -Ampicillin 1 gm IV q6h or 500 mg PO qid **OR**
   -Trimethoprim/sulfamethoxazole (Septra DS) 160/800 mg PO bid or 160/800 mg IV q12h (10-15 mL in 100 cc D5W tid) **OR**
   -Cefuroxime (Zinacef) 750 mg IV q8h **OR**
   -Ampicillin/sulbactam (Unasyn) 1.5 gm IV q6h **OR**

-Doxycycline (Vibra-tabs) 100 mg PO/IV bid
-Azithromycin (Zithromax) 500 mg x 1, then 250 mg PO qd x 4 or 500 mg IV q24h **OR**
-Clarithromycin (Biaxin) 250-500 mg PO bid **OR**
-Levofloxacin (Levaquin) 500 mg PO/IV qd [250, 500 mg] **OR**
-Sparfloxacin (Zagam) 400 mg PO x 1, then 200 mg PO qd [200 mg].

10. **Symptomatic Medications:**
-Docusate sodium (Colace) 100 mg PO qhs.
-Ranitidine (Zantac)150 mg PO bid or 50 mg IV q8h.

11. **Extras:** Portable CXR, PFT's with bronchodilators, ECG, impedence cardiography, echocardiogram.

12. **Labs:** ABG, CBC, SMA7, UA. Theophylline level stat and after 12-24h of infusion. Sputum Gram stain and C&S, alpha 1 antitrypsin level.

Hemoptysis

1. **Admit to:** Intensive care unit
2. **Diagnosis:** Hemoptysis
3. **Condition:**
4. **Vital signs:** q1-6h. Orthostatic BP and pulse bid. Call physician if BP >160/90, <90/60; P >130, <50; R>25, <10; T >38.5°C; O_2 sat <90%
5. **Activity:** Bed rest with bedside commode. Keep patient in lateral decubitus, Trendelenburg's position, bleeding side down.
6. **Nursing:** Quantify all sputum and expectorated blood, suction prn. O_2 at 100% by mask, pulse oximeter. Discontinue narcotics and sedatives. Have double lumen endotracheal tube available for use.
7. **Diet:**
8. **IV Fluids:** 1 L of NS wide open (≥6 gauge), then transfuse PRBC, Foley to gravity.
9. **Special Medications:**
-Transfuse 2-4 U PRBC wide open.
-Promethazine/codeine (Phenergan with codeine) 5 cc PO q4-6h prn cough. Contraindicated in massive hemoptysis.
-Consider empiric antibiotics if any suggestion that bronchitis or infection may be contributing to hemoptysis.
10. **Extras:** CXR PA, LAT, ECG, VQ scan, contrast CT, bronchoscopy. PPD, pulmonary and thoracic surgery consults.
11. **Labs:** Type and cross 2-4 U PRBC. ABG, CBC, platelets, SMA7 and 12, ESR. Anti-glomerular basement antibody, rheumatoid factor, complement, anti-nuclear cytoplasmic antibody. Sputum Gram stain, C&S, AFB, fungal culture, and cytology qAM for 3 days. UA, INR/PTT, von Willebrand Factor. Repeat CBC q6h.

Anaphylaxis

1. **Admit to:**
2. **Diagnosis:** Anaphylaxis
3. **Condition:**
4. **Vital signs:** q1h; Call physician if BP systolic >160, <90; diastolic. >90, <60; P >120, <50; R>25, <10; T >38.5°C
5. **Activity:** Bedrest
6. **Nursing:** O_2 at 6 L/min by NC or mask. Keep patient in Trendelenburg's position, No. 4 or 5 endotracheal tube at bedside.
7. **Diet:** NPO
8. **IV Fluids:** 2 IV lines. Normal saline or LR 1 L over 1-2h, then D5 ½ NS at 125 cc/h. Foley to closed drainage.
9. **Special Medications:**
Gastrointestinal Decontamination:
-Gastric lavage if indicated for recent oral ingestion.

-Activated charcoal 50-100 gm, followed by cathartic.
Bronchodilators:
-Epinephrine (1:1000) 0.3-0.5 mL SQ or IM q10min or 1-4 mcg/min IV **OR** in severe life threatening reactions, give 0.5 mg (5.0 mL of 1: 10,000 sln) IV q5-10min prn. Epinephrine, 0.3 mg of 1:1000 sln may be injected SQ at site of allergen injection **OR**
-Albuterol (Ventolin) 0.5%, 0.5 mL in 2.5 mL NS q30min by nebulizer prn **OR**
-Aerosolized 2% racemic epinephrine 0.5-0.75 mL.
Corticosteroids:
-Methylprednisolone (Solu-Medrol) 250 mg IV x 1, then 125 mg IV q6h **OR**
-Hydrocortisone sodium succinate 200 mg IV x 1, then 100 mg q6h, followed by oral prednisone 60 mg PO qd, tapered over 5 days.
Antihistamines:
-Diphenhydramine (Benadryl) 25-50 mg IV q4-6h **OR**
-Hydroxyzine (Vistaril) 25-50 mg IM or PO q2-4h.
-Famotidine (Pepcid) 20 mg IV q8h or 20 mg PO bid **OR**
-Ranitidine (Zantac) 150 mg IV or PO bid.
Pressors and other Agents:
-Norepinephrine (Levophed) 8-12 mcg/min IV, titrate to systolic 100 mmHg (8 mg in 500 mL D5W) **OR**
-Isoproterenol (Isuprel) 0.5-5 mcg/min IV **OR**
-Dopamine (Intropin) 5-20 mcg/kg/min IV.
10. Extras: Portable CXR, ECG, allergy/immunology consult.
11. Labs: CBC, SMA 7&12.

Pleural Effusion

1. **Admit to:**
2. **Diagnosis:** Pleural effusion
3. **Condition:**
4. **Vital signs:** q shift. Call physician if BP >160/90, <90/60; P>120, <50; R>25, <10; T >38.5°C
5. **Activity:**
6. **Diet:** Regular.
7. **IV Fluids:** D5W at TKO
8. **Extras:** CXR PA and LAT, repeat after thoracentesis; left and right lateral decubitus x-rays, ECG, ultrasound, PPD; pulmonary consult.
9. **Labs:** CBC, SMA 7&12, protein, albumin, amylase, ANA, ESR, INR/PTT, UA. Cryptococcal antigen, histoplasma antigen, fungal culture.
Thoracentesis:
   Tube 1: LDH, protein, amylase, triglyceride, glucose (10 mL).
   Tube 2: Gram stain, C&S, AFB, fungal C&S (20-60 mL, heparinized).
   Tube 3: Cell count and differential (5-10 mL, EDTA).
   Syringe: pH (2 mL collected anaerobically, heparinized on ice)
   Bag or Bottle: Cytology.

Hematologic Disorders

Anticoagulant Overdose

Unfractionated Heparin Overdose:
1. Discontinue heparin infusion.
2. Protamine sulfate, 1 mg IV for every 100 units of heparin infused in preceding hour, dilute in 25 mL fluid IV over 10 min (max 50 mg in 10 min period). Watch for signs of anaphylaxis, especially if patient has been on NPH insulin therapy.

Low Molecular Weight Heparin (Enoxaparin) Overdose:
-Protamine sulfate 1 mg IV for each 1 mg of enoxaparin given. Repeat protamine 0.5 mg IV for each 1 mg of enoxaparin, if bleeding continues after 2-4 hours. Measure factor Xa.

Warfarin (Coumadin) Overdose:
-Gastric lavage and activated charcoal if recent oral ingestion. Discontinue Coumadin and heparin, and monitor hematocrit q2h.

Partial Reversal:
-Vitamin K (Phytonadione), 0.5-1.0 mg IV/SQ. Check INR in 24 hours, and repeat vitamin K dose if INR remains elevated.

Minor Bleeds:
-Vitamin K (Phytonadione), 5-10 mg IV/SQ q12h, titrated to desired INR.

Serious Bleeds:
-Vitamin K (Phytonadione), 10-20 mg in 50-100 mL fluid IV over 30-60 min (check INR q6h until corrected) **AND**
-Fresh frozen plasma 2-4 units x 1.
-Type and cross match for 2 units of PRBC, and transfuse wide open.
-Cryoprecipitate 10 U x 1 if fibrinogen is less than100 mg/dL.

Labs: CBC, platelets, PTT, INR.

Deep Venous Thrombosis

1. **Admit to:**
2. **Diagnosis:** Deep vein thrombosis
3. **Condition:**
4. **Vital signs:** q shift. Call physician if BP systolic >160, <90 diastolic, >90, <60; P >120, <50; R>25, <10; T >38.5°C.
5. **Activity:** Bed rest with legs elevated.
6. **Nursing:** Guaiac stools, warm packs to leg prn; measure calf circumference qd; no intramuscular injections.
7. **Diet:** Regular
8. **IV Fluids:** D5W at TKO
9. **Special Medications:**
Anticoagulation:
-Heparin (unfractionated) IV bolus 5000-10,000 Units (100 U/kg) IVP, then 1000-1500 U/h IV infusion (20 U/kg/h) [25,000 U in 500 mL D5W (50 U/mL)]. Check PTT 6 hours after initial bolus; adjust q6h until PTT 1.5-2.0 times control (50-80 sec). Overlap heparin and warfarin (Coumadin) for at least 4 days and discontinue heparin when INR has been 2.0-3.0 for two consecutive days.
-Enoxaparin (Lovenox) 1 mg/kg SQ q12h. Overlap enoxaparin and warfarin as outlined above.
-Warfarin (Coumadin) 5-10 mg PO qd x 2-3 d; maintain INR 2.0-3.0. Coumadin is initiated on the first or second day only if the PTT is 1.5-2.0 times control [tab 1, 2, 2.5, 3, 4, 5, 6, 7.5, 10 mg].

10. Symptomatic Medications:
   -Propoxyphene/acetaminophen (Darvocet N100) 1-2 tab PO q3-4h prn pain
   OR
   -Hydrocodone/acetaminophen (Vicodin), 1-2 tab q4-6h PO prn pain.
   -Docusate sodium (Colace) 100 mg PO qhs.
   -Ranitidine (Zantac) 150 mg PO bid.
11. Extras: CXR PA and LAT, ECG; Doppler scan of legs, venography. V/Q scan. Lower extremity (venogram).
12. Labs: CBC, INR/PTT, SMA 7. Protein C, protein S, antithrombin III, anticardiolipin antibody. UA with dipstick for blood. PTT 6h after bolus and q4-6h until PTT 1.5-2.0 x control then qd. INR at initiation of warfarin and qd.

Pulmonary Embolism

1. **Admit to:**
2. **Diagnosis:** Pulmonary embolism
3. **Condition:**
4. **Vital signs:** q1-4h. Call physician if BP >160/90, <90/60; P >120, <50; R >30, <10; T >38.5°C; O_2 sat < 90%
5. **Activity:** Bedrest with bedside commode
6. **Nursing:** Pulse oximeter, guaiac stools, O_2 at 2 L by NC. Antiembolism stockings. No intramuscular injections.
7. **Diet:** Regular
8. **IV Fluids:** D5W at TKO.
9. **Special Medications:**
Anticoagulation:
   -Heparin IV bolus 5000-10,000 Units (100 U/kg) IVP, then 1000-1500 U/h IV infusion (20 U/kg/h) [25,000 U in 500 mL D5W (50 U/mL)]. Check PTT 6 hours after initial bolus; adjust q6h until PTT to 1.5-2 times control (60-80 sec). Overlap heparin and Coumadin for at least 4 days and discontinue heparin when INR has been 2.0-3.0 for two consecutive days.
   -Enoxaparin (Lovenox) 1 mg/kg sq q12h for 5 days for uncomplicated pulmonary embolism. Overlap warfarin as outlined above.
   -Warfarin (Coumadin) 5-10 mg PO qd for 2-3 d, then 2-5 mg PO qd. Maintain INR of 2.0-3.0. Coumadin is initiated on second day if the PTT is 1.5-2.0 times control. Check INR at initiation of warfarin and qd [tab 1, 2, 2.5, 3, 4, 5, 6, 7.5, 10 mg].
Thrombolytics (indicated if hemodynamic compromise):
   Baseline Labs: CBC, INR/PTT, fibrinogen q6h.
   Alteplase (recombinant tissue plasminogen activator, Activase): 100 mg IV infusion over 2 hours, followed by heparin infusion at 15 U/kg/h to maintain PTT 1.5-2.5 x control **OR**
   Streptokinase (Streptase): Pretreat with methylprednisolone 250 mg IV push and diphenhydramine (Benadryl) 50 mg IV push. Then give streptokinase, 250,000 units IV over 30 min, then 100,000 units/h for 24-72 hours. Initiate heparin infusion at 10 U/kg/hour; maintain PTT 1.5-2.5 x control.
10. Symptomatic Medications:
   -Meperidine (Demerol) 25-100 mg IV prn pain.
   -Docusate sodium (Colace) 100 mg PO qhs.
   -Ranitidine (Zantac) 150 mg PO bid.
11. Extras: CXR PA and LAT, ECG, VQ scan; chest CT scan, pulmonary angiography; Doppler scan of lower extremities, impedence cardiography.
12. Labs: CBC, INR/PTT, SMA7, ABG, cardiac enzymes. Protein C, protein S, antithrombin III, anticardiolipin antibody. UA . PTT 6 hours after bolus and q4-6h. INR at initiation of warfarin and qd.

Sickle Cell Crisis

1. **Admit to:**
2. **Diagnosis:** Sickle Cell Crisis
3. **Condition:**
4. **Vital signs:** q shift.
5. **Activity:** Bedrest
6. **Nursing:**
7. **Diet:** Regular diet, push oral fluids.
8. **IV Fluids:** D5 ½ NS at 100-125 mL/h.
9. **Special Medications:**
    -Oxygen 2 L/min by NC or 30-100% by mask.
    -Meperidine (Demerol) 50-150 mg IM/IV/SC q4-6h prn pain.
    -Hydroxyzine (Vistaril) 25-100 mg IM/IV/PO q3-4h prn pain.
    -Morphine sulfate 10 mg IV/IM/SC q2-4h prn pain **OR**
    -Ketorolac (Toradol) 30-60 mg IV/IM then 15-30 mg IV/IM q6h prn pain (maximum of 5 days).
    -Acetaminophen/codeine (Tylenol 3) 1-2 tabs PO q4-6h prn.
    -Folic acid 1 mg PO qd.
    -Penicillin V (prophylaxis), 250 mg PO qid [tabs 125,250,500 mg].
    -Prochlorperazine (Compazine) 5-10 mg PO or IM q6h prn nausea or vomiting.

Vaccination:
    -Pneumovax before discharge 0.5 cc IM x 1 dose.
    -Influenza vaccine (Fluogen) 0.5 cc IM once a year in the Fall.
10. **Extras:** CXR.
11. **Labs:** CBC, SMA 7, blood C&S, reticulocyte count, blood type and screen, parvovirus titers. UA.

40 Sickle Cell Crisis

Infectious Diseases

Meningitis

1. **Admit to:**
2. **Diagnosis:** Meningitis.
3. **Condition:**
4. **Vital signs:** q1h. Call physician if BP systolic >160/90, <90/60; P >120, <50; R>25, <10; T >39°C or less than 36°C
5. **Activity:** Bed rest with bedside commode.
6. **Nursing:** Respiratory isolation, inputs and outputs, lumbar puncture tray at bedside.
7. **Diet:** NPO
8. **IV Fluids:** D5 ½ NS at 125 cc/h with KCL 20 mEq/L.
9. **Special Medications:**
Empiric Therapy 15-50 years old:
    -Vancomycin 1 gm IV q12h **AND EITHER**
    -Ceftriaxone (Rocephin) 2 gm IV q12h (max 4 gm/d) **OR**
    Cefotaxime (Claforan) 2 gm IV q4h.
Empiric Therapy >50 years old, Alcoholic, Corticosteroids or Hematologic Malignancy or other Debilitating Condition:
    -Ampicillin 2 gm IV q4h **AND EITHER**
    -Cefotaxime (Claforan) 2 gm IV q6h **OR**
    Ceftriaxone (Rocephin) 2 gm IV q12h **OR**
    Ceftazidime (Fortaz) 2 gm IV q8h.
    -Use Vancomycin 1 mg IV q12h in place of ampicillin if drug-resistant pneumococcus is suspected.
10. **Symptomatic Medications:**
    -Acetaminophen (Tylenol) 650 mg PO/PR q4-6h prn temp >39°C.
11. **Extras:** CXR, ECG, PPD, CT scan.
12. **Labs:** CBC, SMA 7&12. Blood C&S x 2. UA with micro, urine C&S. Antibiotic levels peak and trough after 3rd dose, VDRL.
Lumbar Puncture:
    CSF Tube 1: Gram stain, C&S for bacteria (1-4 mL).
    CSF Tube 2: Glucose, protein (1-2 mL).
    CSF Tube 3: Cell count and differential (1-2 mL).
    CSF Tube 4: Latex agglutination or counterimmunoelectrophoresis antigen tests for S. pneumoniae, H. influenzae (type B), N. meningitides, E. coli, group B strep, VDRL, cryptococcal antigen, toxoplasma titers. India ink, fungal cultures, cryptococcal antigen, AFB (8-10 mL).

Infective Endocarditis

1. **Admit to:**
2. **Diagnosis:** Infective endocarditis
3. **Condition:**
4. **Vital signs:** q4h. Call physician if BP systolic >160/90, <90/60; P >120, <50; R>25, <10; T >38.5°C
5. **Activity:** Up ad lib
6. **Diet:** Regular
7. **IV Fluids:** Heparin lock with flush q shift.
8. **Special Medications:**
Subacute Bacterial Endocarditis Empiric Therapy:
    -Penicillin G 3-5 million U IV q4h or ampicillin 2 gm IV q4h **AND**
    Gentamicin 1-1.5/mg/kg IV q8h.
Acute Bacterial Endocarditis Empiric Therapy
    -Gentamicin 2 mg/kg IV; then 1-1.5 mg/kg IV q8h **AND**
    Nafcillin or oxacillin 2 gm IV q4h **OR**

Vancomycin 1 gm IV q12h (1 gm in 250 mL of D5W over 1h).
Streptococci viridans/bovis:
-Penicillin G 3-5 million U IV q4h for 4 weeks **OR**
Vancomycin 1 gm IV q12h for 4 weeks **AND**
Gentamicin 1 mg/kg q8h for first 2 weeks.
Enterococcus:
-Gentamicin 1 mg/kg IV q8h for 4-6 weeks **AND**
Ampicillin 2 gm IV q4h for 4-6 weeks **OR**
Vancomycin 1 gm IV q12h for 4-6 weeks.
Staphylococcus aureus (methicillin sensitive, native valve):
-Nafcillin or Oxacillin 2 gm IV q4h for 4-6 weeks **OR**
Vancomycin 1 gm IV q12h for 4-6 weeks **AND**
Gentamicin 1 mg/kg IV q8h for first 3-5 days.
Methicillin resistant Staphylococcus aureus (native valve):
-Vancomycin 1 gm IV q12h (1 gm in 250 mL D5W over 1h) for 4-6 weeks **AND**
Gentamicin 1 mg/kg IV q8h for 3-5 days.
Methicillin resistant Staph aureus or epidermidis (prosthetic valve):
-Vancomycin 1 gm IV q12h for 6 weeks **AND**
Rifampin 600 mg PO q8h for 6 weeks **AND**
Gentamicin 1 mg/kg IV q8h for 2 weeks.
Culture Negative Endocarditis:
-Penicillin G 3-5 million U IV q4h for 4-6 weeks **OR**
Ampicillin 2 gm IV q4h for 4-6 weeks **AND**
Gentamicin 1.5 mg/kg for 2 weeks (or nafcillin, 2 gm IV q4h, and gentamicin if Staph aureus suspected in drug abuser or prosthetic valve).
Fungal Endocarditis:
-Amphotericin B 0.5 mg/kg/d IV plus flucytosine (5-FC) 150 mg/kg/d PO.
9. Extras: CXR PA and LAT, echocardiogram, ECG.
11. Labs: CBC with differential, SMA 7&12. Blood C&S x 3-4 over 24h, serum cidal titers, minimum inhibitory concentration, minimum bactericidal concentration. Repeat C&S in 48h, then once a week. Antibiotic levels peak and trough at 3rd dose. UA, urine C&S.

Pneumonia

1. **Admit to:**
2. **Diagnosis:** Pneumonia
3. **Condition:**
4. **Vital signs:** q4-8h. Call physician if BP >160/90, <90/60; P >120, <50; R>25, <10; T >38.5°C or O_2 saturation <90%.
5. **Activity:**
6. **Nursing:** Pulse oximeter, inputs and outputs, nasotracheal suctioning prn, incentive spirometry.
7. **Diet:** Regular.
8. **IV Fluids:** IV D5 ½ NS at 125 cc/hr.
9. **Special Medications:**
-Oxygen by NC at 2-4 L/min, or 24-50% by Ventimask, or 100% by non-rebreather (reservoir) to maintain O_2 saturation >90%.
Moderately ill Patients Without Underlying Lung Disease from the Community:
-Cefuroxime (Zinacef) 0.75-1.5 gm IV q8h **OR**
Ampicillin/sulbactam (Unasyn) 1.5 gm IV q6h **AND EITHER**
-Erythromycin 500 mg IV/PO q6h **OR**
Clarithromycin (Biaxin) 500 mg PO bid **OR**
Azithromycin (Zithromax) 500 mg PO x 1, then 250 mg PO qd x 4 **OR**
Doxycycline (Vibramycin) 100 mg IV/PO q12h.

Moderately ill Patients With Recent Hospitalization or Debilitated Nursing Home Patient:
-Ceftazidime (Fortaz) 1-2 gm IV q8h **OR**
Cefepime (Maxipime) 1-2 gm IV q12h **OR**
Cefoperazone (Cefobid) 1-2 gm IV q8h **AND EITHER**
Gentamicin 1.5-2 mg/kg IV, then 1.0-1.5 mg/kg IV q8h or 7 mg/kg in 50 mL of D5W over 60 min IV q24h **OR**
Ciprofloxacin (Cipro) 400 mg IV q12h or 500 mg PO q12h **OR**
Levofloxacin (Levaquin) 500 mg IV/PO qd.

Critically ill Patients:
-Initial treatment should consist of a macrolide with 2 antipseudomonal agents for synergistic activity:
-Erythromycin 0.5-1.0 gm IV q6h **AND EITHER**
-Ceftazidime 1-2 gm q8h **OR**
Piperacillin/tazobactam (Zosyn) 3.75-4.50 gm IV q6h **OR**
Ticarcillin/clavulanate (Timentin) 3.1 gm IV q6h **OR**
Imipenem/cilastatin (Primaxin) 0.5-1.0 gm IV q6h **AND EITHER**
-Levofloxacin (Levaquin) 500 mg IV q24h **OR**
Ciprofloxacin (Cipro) 400 mg IV q12h **OR**
Tobramycin 2.0 mg/kg IV, then 1.5 mg/kg IV q8h or 7 mg/kg IV q24h **OR**
Trovafloxacin (Trovan) 300 mg IV x 1, then 200 mg IV q24h.

Aspiration Pneumonia (community acquired):
-Clindamycin (Cleocin) 600-900 mg IV q8h (with or without gentamicin or 3rd gen cephalosporin) **OR**
-Ampicillin/sulbactam (Unasyn) 1.5-3 gm IV q6h (with or without gentamicin or 3rd gen cephalosporin)

Aspiration Pneumonia (nosocomial):
-Tobramycin 2 mg/kg IV then 1.5 mg/kg IV q8h or 7 mg/kg in 50 mLs of D5W over 60 min IV q24h **OR**
Ceftazidime (Fortaz) 1-2 gm IV q8h **AND EITHER**
-Clindamycin (Cleocin) 600-900 mg IV q8h **OR**
Ampicillin/sulbactam or ticarcillin/clavulanate, or piperacillin/tazobactam or imipenem/cilastatin (see above).

10. Symptomatic Medications:
-Acetaminophen (Tylenol) 650 mg 2 tab PO q4-6h prn temp >38˚C or pain.
-Docusate sodium (Colace) 100 mg PO qhs.
-Ranitidine (Zantac) 150 mg PO bid or 50 mg IV q8h.
-Heparin 5000 U SQ q12h.

11. Extras: CXR PA and LAT, ECG, PPD.

12. Labs: CBC with differential, SMA 7&12, ABG. Blood C&S x 2. Sputum Gram stain, C&S. Methenamine silver sputum stain (PCP); AFB smear/culture. Aminoglycoside levels peak and trough at 3rd dose. UA, urine culture.

Specific Therapy for Pneumonia

Pneumococcal Pneumonia:
-Ceftriaxone (Rocephin) 2 gm IV q12h **OR**
-Cefotaxime (Claforan) 2 gm IV q6h **OR**
-Erythromycin 500 mg IV q6h **OR**
-Vancomycin 1 gm IV q12h if drug resistance.

Staphylococcus aureus Pneumonia:
-Nafcillin 2 gm IV q4h **OR**
-Oxacillin 2 gm IV q4h.

Klebsiella pneumoniae Pneumonia:
-Gentamicin 1.5-2 mg/kg IV, then 1.0-1.5 mg/kg IV q8h or 7 mg/kg in 50 mL of D5W over 60 min IV q24h **AND**
Ceftizoxime (Cefizox) 1-2 gm IV q8h **OR**
Cefotaxime (Claforan) 1-2 gm IV q6h.
Methicillin-resistant staphylococcus aureus:
-Vancomycin 1 gm IV q12h.
Haemophilus influenzae:
-Ampicillin 1-2 gm IV q6h (beta-lactamase negative) **OR**
-Ampicillin/sulbactam (Unasyn) 1.5-3.0 gm q6h **OR**
-Cefuroxime (Zinacef) 1.5 gm IV q8h (beta-lactamase pos) **OR**
-Ceftizoxime (Cefizox) 1-2 gm IV q8h **OR**
-Ciprofloxacin (Cipro) 400 mg IV q12h **OR**
-Ofloxacin (Floxin) 400 mg IV q12h.
-Levofloxacin (Levaquin) 500 mg IV q24h.
Pseudomonas aeruginosa:
-Tobramycin 1.5-2.0 mg/kg IV, then 1.5-2.0 mg/kg IV q8h or 7 mg/kg in 50 mL of D5W over 60 min IV q24h **AND EITHER**
Piperacillin, Ticarcillin, Mezlocillin or Azlocillin 3 gm IV q4h **OR**
Ceftazidime 1-2 gm IV q8h.
Mycoplasma pneumoniae:
-Clarithromycin (Biaxin) 500 mg PO bid **OR**
-Azithromycin (Zithromax) 500 mg PO x 1, then 250 mg PO qd for 4 days **OR**
-Erythromycin 500 mg PO or IV q6h **OR**
-Doxycycline (Vibramycin) 100 mg PO/IV q12h **OR**
-Levofloxacin (Levaquin) 500 mg PO/IV q24h.
Legionella pneumoniae:
-Erythromycin 1.0 gm IV q6h **OR**
-Levofloxacin (Levaquin) 500 mg PO/IV q24h.
-Rifampin 600 mg PO qd may be added to erythromycin or levofloxacin.
Moraxella catarrhalis:
-Trimethoprim/sulfamethoxazole (Bactrim, Septra) one DS tab PO bid or 10 mL IV q12h **OR**
-Ampicillin/sulbactam (Unasyn) 1.5-3 gm IV q6h **OR**
-Cefuroxime (Zinacef) 0.75-1.5 gm IV q8h **OR**
-Erythromycin 500 mg IV q6h **OR**
-Levofloxacin (Levaquin) 500 mg PO/IV q24h.
Anaerobic Pneumonia:
-Penicillin G 2 MU IV q4h **OR**
-Clindamycin (Cleocin) 900 mg IV q8h **OR**
-Metronidazole (Flagyl) 500 mg IV q8h.

Pneumocystis Carinii Pneumonia

1. **Admit to:**
2. **Diagnosis:** PCP pneumonia
3. **Condition:**
4. **Vital signs:** q2-6h. Call physician if BP >160/90, <90/60; P >120, <50; R>25, <10; T >38.5°C; O_2 sat <90%
5. **Activity:**
6. **Nursing:** Pulse oximeter.
7. **Diet:** Regular, encourage fluids.
8. **IV Fluids:** D5 ½ NS at 100 cc/h.
9. **Special Medications:**
Pneumocystis Carinii Pneumonia:
-Oxygen at 2-4 L/min by NC or by mask.
-Trimethoprim/sulfamethoxazole (Bactrim, Septra) 15 mg of TMP/kg/day (20 mL in 250 mL of D5W IVPB q8h) for 21 days [inj: 80/400 mg per 5 mL].
-If severe PCP (PaO_2 <70 mmHg): add prednisone 40 mg PO bid for 5 days, then 40 mg qd for 5 days, then 20 mg once daily for 11 days **OR**

Methylprednisolone (Solu-Medrol) 30 mg IV q12h for 5 days, then 30 mg IV qd for 5 days, then 15 mg IV qd for 11 days.
-Pentamidine (Pentam) 4 mg/kg IV qd for 21 days, with prednisone as above. Pentamidine is an alternative if inadequate response or intolerant to TMP-SMX.

Pneumocystis Carinii Prophylaxis (previous PCP or CD4 <200, or constitutional symptoms):
-Trimethoprim/SMX DS (160/800 mg) PO qd **OR**
-Pentamidine, 300 mg in 6 mL sterile water via Respirgard II nebulizer over 20-30 min q4 weeks **OR**
-Dapsone (DDS) 50 mg PO bid or 100 mg twice a week; contraindicated in G-6-PD deficiency.

Antiretroviral Therapy:
  A. Combination therapy with 3 agents (two nucleoside analogs and a protease inhibitor) is recommended as initial therapy.
  B. **Nucleoside Analogs**
    1. Abacavir (Ziagen) 300 mg PO bid [300 mg, 20 mg/mL].
    2. Didanosine (Videx, ddI) 200 mg bid for patients >60 kg; or 125 mg bid for patients <60 kg.[chewable tabs: 25, 50, 100, 150 mg; pwd 100, 167, 250 mg packets].
    3. Lamivudine (Epivir, 3TC) 150 mg twice daily [150 mg].
    4. Stavudine (Zerit, D4T) 40 mg bid [15-mg, 20-mg, 30-mg and 40-mg capsules].
    5. Zalcitabine (Hivid, ddC) 0.75 mg tid [0.375, 0.75].
    6. Zidovudine (Retrovir, AZT) 200 mg tid (100, 200 mg caps, 50 mg/5 mL syrup).
  C. **Protease Inhibitors**
    1. Amprenavir (Agenerase) 1200 mg bid [50, 150 mg]
    2. Indinavir (Crixivan) 800 mg tid [200, 400 mg].
    3. Saquinavir (Invirase) 600 mg tid with a meal [cap 200 mg].
    4. Ritonavir (Norvir) 600 mg bid [100 mg, 80 mg/dL]
    5. Nelfinavir (Viracept) 750 mg PO tid [250 mg].
  D. **Non-Nucleoside Reverse Transcriptase Inhibitors**
    1. Nevirapine (Viramune) 200 mg qd for 2 weeks, then bid [200 mg].
    2. Delavirdine (U-90) 400 mg tid.
    3. Efavirenz (Sustiva) 600 mg PO qd [50, 100, 200 mg].

Postexposure HIV Prophylaxis
  A. The injury should be immediately washed and scrubbed with soap and water.
  B. Zidovudine 200 mg PO tid and lamivudine (3TC) 150 mg PO bid, plus indinavir (Crixivan) 800 mg PO tid for highest risk exposures. Treatment is continued for one month.

Zidovudine-Induced Neutropenia/Ganciclovir-Induced Leucopenia
-Recombinant human granulocyte colony-stimulating factor (G-CSF, Filgrastim, Neupogen) 1-2 mcg/kg SQ qd until absolute neutrophil count 500-1000; indicated only if the patient's endogenous erythropoietin level is low.

10. **Extras:** CXR PA and LAT.
11. **Labs:** ABG, CBC, SMA 7&12. Blood C&S x 2. Sputum for Gram stain, C&S, AFB. Giemsa immunofluorescence for Pneumocystis. CD4 count, HIV RNA, VDRL, serum cryptococcal antigen, UA.

Opportunistic Infections in HIV-Infected Patients

Oral Candidiasis:
-Fluconazole (Diflucan) acute: 100-200 mg PO qd **OR**
-Ketoconazole (Nizoral), acute: 400 mg PO qd **OR**
-Itraconazole (Sporanox) 200 mg PO qd **OR**
-Clotrimazole (Mycelex) troches 10 mg dissolved slowly in mouth 5 times/d.

Candida Esophagitis:
-Fluconazole (Diflucan) 200-400 mg PO qd for 14-21 days **OR**

-Ketoconazole (Nizoral) 200 mg PO bid.
-Itraconazole (Sporanox) 200 mg PO qd for 2 weeks.

Primary or Recurrent Mucocutaneous HSV
-Acyclovir (Zovirax), 200-400 mg 5 times a day for 10 days, or 5 mg/kg IV q8h **OR** in cases of acyclovir resistance, foscarnet, 40 mg/kg IV q8h for 21 days.

Herpes Simplex Encephalitis (or visceral disease):
-Acyclovir 10 mg/kg IV q8h for 10-21 days.

Herpes Varicella Zoster
-Acyclovir 10 mg/kg IV over 60 min q8h for 7-14 days **OR** 800 mg PO 5 times/d for 7-10 days **OR**
-Famciclovir (Famvir) 500 mg PO q8h for 7 days [500 mg] **OR**
-Valacyclovir (Valtrex) 1000 mg PO q8h for 7 days [500 mg] **OR**
-Foscarnet (Foscavir) 40 mg/kg IV q8h.

Cytomegalovirus Retinitis:
-Ganciclovir (Cytovene) 5 mg/kg IV (dilute in 100 mL D5W over 60 min) q12h for 14-21 days **OR**
-Foscarnet (Foscavir) 60 mg/kg IV q8h for 2-3 weeks **OR**
-Cidofovir (Vistide) 5 mg/kg IV over 60 min q week for 2 weeks. Administer probenecid, 2 g PO 3 hours prior to cidofovir, 1 g PO 2 hours after, and 1 g PO 8 hours after.

Suppressive Treatment for Cytomegalovirus Retinitis:
-Ganciclovir 5 mg/kg qd.
-Foscarnet (Foscavir) 90-120 mg IV qd **OR**
-Cidofovir (Vistide) 5 mg/kg IV over 60 min every 2 weeks with probenecid.

Acute Toxoplasmosis:
-Pyrimethamine 200 mg, then 50-75 mg qd, plus sulfadiazine 1.0-1.5 gm PO q6h, plus folinic acid 10 mg PO qd **OR**
-Atovaquone (Mepron) 750 mg PO tid.

Suppressive Treatment for Toxoplasmosis:
-Pyrimethamine 25-50 mg PO qd plus sulfadiazine 0.5-1.0 gm PO q6h plus folinic acid 5 mg PO qd **OR**
-Pyrimethamine 50 mg PO qd, plus clindamycin 300 mg PO qid, plus folinic acid 5 mg PO qd.

Cryptococcus Neoformans Meningitis:
-Amphotericin B 0.7-1.0 mg/kg/d IV; total dosage of 2 g, with or without 5-flucytosine 100 mg/kg PO qd in divided doses, followed by fluconazole (Diflucan) 400 mg PO qd or itraconazole (Sporanox) 200 mg PO bid 6-8 weeks
OR
-Fluconazole (Diflucan) 400-800 mg PO qd for 8-12 weeks

Suppressive Treatment of Cryptococcus:
-Fluconazole (Diflucan) 200 mg PO qd indefinitely.

Active Tuberculosis:
-Isoniazid (INH) 300 mg PO qd; and rifampin 600 mg PO qd; and pyrazinamide 15-25 mg/kg PO qd (500 mg bid-tid); and ethambutol 15-25 mg/kg PO qd (400 mg bid-tid).
-All four drugs are continued for 2 months; isoniazid and rifampin are continued for a period of at least 9 months and at least 6 months after the last negative cultures.
-Pyridoxine (Vitamin B6) 50 mg PO qd concurrent with INH.

Prophylaxis for Inactive Tuberculosis:
-Isoniazid 300 mg PO qd; and pyridoxine 50 mg PO qd for 12 months.

Disseminated Mycobacterium Avium Complex (MAC):
-Clarithromycin (Biaxin) 500 mg PO bid **AND**
Ethambutol 800-1000 mg qd; with or without rifabutin 450 mg qd.

Prophylaxis against MAC:
-Azithromycin (Zithromax) 1200 mg once a week.

Disseminated Coccidioidomycosis:
-Amphotericin B 0.5-0.8 mg/kg IV qd, to a total dose 2.0 gm **OR**
Fluconazole (Diflucan) 400-800 mg PO or IV qd.

Disseminated Histoplasmosis:
 -Amphotericin B 0.5-0.8 mg/kg IV qd, to a total dose 15 mg/kg **OR**
 -Fluconazole (Diflucan) 400 mg PO qd. **OR**
 -Itraconazole (Sporanox) 300 mg PO bid for 3 days, then 200 mg PO bid.
Suppressive Treatment for Histoplasmosis:
 -Fluconazole (Diflucan) 400 mg PO qd **OR**
 -Itraconazole (Sporanox) 200 mg PO bid.

Septic Arthritis

1. **Admit to:**
2. **Diagnosis:** Septic arthritis
3. **Condition:**
4. **Vital signs:** q shift
5. **Activity:** No weight bearing on infected joint. Up in chair as tolerated. Bedside commode with assistance.
6. **Nursing:** Warm compresses prn, keep joint immobilized. Passive range of motion exercises of the affected joint bid; otherwise, keep knee in resting splint.
7. **Diet:** Regular diet.
8. **IV Fluids:** Heparin lock
9. **Special Medications:**
Empiric Therapy for Adults without Gonorrhea Contact:
 -Nafcillin or <u>oxacillin</u> 2 gm IV q4h **AND**
  Ceftizoxime (Cefizox) 1 gm IV q8h or ceftazidime 1 gm IV q8h or <u>ciprofloxacin 400 mg IV q12h</u> if Gram stain indicates presence of Gram negative organisms.
Empiric Therapy for Adults with Gonorrhea:
 -Ceftriaxone (Rocephin) 1 gm IV q12h **OR**
 -Ceftizoxime (Cefizox) 1 gm IV q8h **OR**
 -Ciprofloxacin (Cipro) 400 mg IV q12h.
 -May complete course of therapy with cefuroxime axetil (Ceftin) 400 mg PO bid.
10. **Symptomatic Medications:**
 -Acetaminophen and codeine (Tylenol 3) 1-2 PO q4-6h prn pain.
 -Heparin 5000 U SQ bid.
11. **Extras:** X-ray views of joint (AP and lateral), CXR. Synovial fluid culture. Physical therapy consult for exercise program.
12. **Labs:** CBC, SMA 7&12, blood C&S x 2, VDRL, UA. Gonorrhea cultures of urethra, cervix, urine, throat, sputum, skin, rectum. Antibiotic levels. Blood cultures x 2 for gonorrhea.
Synovial fluid:
 Tube 1 - Glucose, protein, lactate, pH.
 Tube 2 - Gram stain, C&S.
 Tube 3 - Cell count.

Septic Shock

1. **Admit to:**
2. **Diagnosis:** Sepsis
3. **Condition:**
4. **Vital signs:** q1h; Call physician if BP >160/90, <90/60; P >120, <50; R>25, <10; T >38.5°C; urine output < 25 cc/hr for 4h, O_2 saturation <90%.
5. **Activity:** Bed rest.
6. **Nursing:** Inputs and outputs, pulse oximeter. Foley catheter to closed drainage.
7. **Diet:** NPO
8. **IV Fluids:** 1 liter of normal saline wide open, then D5 ½ NS at 125 cc/h

9. Special Medications:
-Oxygen at 2-5 L/min by NC or mask.
Antibiotic Therapy
   A. Initial treatment of life-threatening sepsis should include a third-generation cephalosporin (ceftazidime, cefotaxime, ceftizoxime or ceftriaxone), or piperacillin/tazobactam, or ticarcillin/clavulanic acid or imipenem, each with an aminoglycoside (gentamicin, tobramycin or amikacin).
   B. Intra-abdominal or pelvic infections, likely to involve anaerobes, should be treated with ampicillin, gentamicin and metronidazole; or either ticarcillin/clavulanic acid, ampicillin/sulbactam, piperacillin/tazobactam, imipenem, cefoxitin or cefotetan, each with an aminoglycoside.
   C. Febrile neutropenic patients with neutrophil counts <500/mm^3 should be treated with vancomycin and ceftazidime, or piperacillin/tazobactam and tobramycin or imipenem and tobramycin.
   D. Dosages for Antibiotics Used in Sepsis
      -Ampicillin 1-2 gm IV q4-6h.
      -Cefotaxime (Claforan) 2 gm q4-6h.
      -Ceftizoxime (Cefizox) 1-2 gm IV q8h.
      -Ceftriaxone (Rocephin) 1-2 gm IV q12h (max 4 gm/d).
      -Cefoxitin (Mefoxin) 1-2 gm q6h.
      -Cefotetan (Cefotan) 1-2 gm IV q12h.
      -Ceftazidime (Fortaz) 1-2 g IV q8h.
      -Ticarcillin/clavulanate (Timentin) 3.1 gm IV q4-6h (200-300 mg/kg/d).
      -Ampicillin/sulbactam (Unasyn) 1.5-3.0 gm IV q6h.
      -Piperacillin/tazobactam (Zosyn) 3.375-4.5 gm IV q6h.
      -Piperacillin or ticarcillin 3 gm IV q4-6h.
      -Imipenem/cilastatin (Primaxin) 1.0 gm IV q6h.
      -Meropenem (Merrem) 05-1.0 gm IV q8h.
      -Gentamicin, tobramycin 100-120 mg (1.5 mg/kg) IV, then 80 mg IV q8h (1 mg/kg) or 7 mg/kg in 50 mL of D5W over 60 min IV q24h.
      -Amikacin (Amikin) 7.5 mg/kg IV loading dose; then 5 mg/kg IV q8h.
      -Vancomycin 1 gm IV q12h.
      -Metronidazole (Flagyl) 500 mg (7.5 mg/kg) IV q6-8h.
      -Clindamycin 900 mg IV q8h.
      -Aztreonam (Azactam) 1-2 gm IV q6-8h; max 8 g/day.
Nosocomial sepsis with IV catheter or IV drug abuse
   -Nafcillin or oxacillin 2 gm IV q4h **OR**
   -Vancomycin 1 gm q12h (1 gm in 250 cc D5W over 60 min) **AND**
   Gentamicin or tobramycin as above **AND EITHER**
   Ceftazidime (Fortaz) or ceftizoxime 1-2 gm IV q8h **OR**
   Piperacillin, ticarcillin or mezlocillin 3 gm IV q4-6h.
Blood Pressure Support
   -Dopamine 4-20 mcg/kg/min (400 mg in 250 cc D5W, 1600 mcg/mL).
   -Norepinephrine 2-8 mcg/min IV infusion (8 mg in 250 mL D5W).
   -Albumin 25 gm IV (100 mL of 25% sln) **OR**
   -Hetastarch (Hespan) 500-1000 cc over 30-60 min (max 1500 cc/d).
   -Dobutamine 5 mcg/kg/min, and titrate to bp keep systolic BP >90 mmHg; max 10 mcg/kg/min.
10. Symptomatic Medications:
   -Acetaminophen (Tylenol) 650 mg PR q4-6h prn temp >39°C.
   -Ranitidine (Zantac) 50 mg IV q8h.
   -Heparin 5000 U SQ q12h.
11. Extras: CxR, KUB, ECG. Ultrasound, lumbar puncture.
12. Labs: CBC with differential, SMA 7&12, blood C&S x 3, T&C for 3-6 units PRBC, INR/PTT, drug levels peak and trough at 3rd dose. UA. Cultures of urine, sputum, wound, IV catheters, decubitus ulcers, pleural fluid.

Peritonitis

1. **Admit to:**
2. **Diagnosis:** Peritonitis
3. **Condition:**
4. **Vital signs:** q1-6h. Call physician if BP >160/90, <90/60; P >120, <50; R>25, <10; T >38.5°C.
5. **Activity:** Bed rest.
6. **Nursing:** Guaiac stools.
7. **Diet:** NPO
8. **IV Fluids:** D5 ½ NS at 125 cc/h.
9. **Special Medications:**

Primary Bacterial Peritonitis -- Spontaneous:

Option 1:
-Ampicillin 1-2 gm IV q 4-6h (vancomycin 1 gm IV q12h if penicillin allergic)
   AND EITHER
   Cefotaxime (Claforan) 1-2 gm IV q6h **OR**
   Ceftizoxime (Cefizox) 1-2 gm IV q8h **OR**
   Gentamicin or tobramycin 1.5 mg/kg IV, then 1 mg/kg q8h or 7 mg/kg in 50 mL of D5W over 60 min IV q24h.

Option 2:
-Ticarcillin/clavulanate (Timentin) 3.1 gm IV q6h **OR**
-Piperacillin/tazobactam (Zosyn) 3.375 gm IV q6h **OR**
-Imipenem/cilastatin (Primaxin) 0.5-1.0 gm IV q6h **OR**
-Meropenem (Merrem) 500-1000 mg IV q8h.

Secondary Bacterial Peritonitis -- Abdominal Perforation or Rupture:

Option 1:
-Ampicillin 1-2 gm IV q4-6h **AND**
   Gentamicin or tobramycin as above **AND**
   Metronidazole (Flagyl) 500 mg IV q8h **OR**
   Cefoxitin (Mefoxin) 1-2 gm IV q6h **OR**
   Cefotetan (Cefotan) 1-2 gm IV q12h.

Option 2:
-Ticarcillin/clavulanate (Timentin) 3.1 gm IV q4-6h (200-300 mg/kg/d) with an aminoglycoside as above **OR**
-Piperacillin/tazobactam (Zosyn) 3.375 gm IV q6h with an aminoglycoside as above **OR**
-Ampicillin/sulbactam (Unasyn) 1.5-3.0 gm IV q6h with aminoglycoside as above **OR**
-Imipenem/cilastatin (Primaxin) 0.5-1.0 gm IV q6-8h **OR**
-Meropenem (Merrem) 500-1000 mg IV q8h.

Fungal Peritonitis:
-Amphotericin B peritoneal dialysis, 2 mg/L of dialysis fluid over the first 24 hours, then 1.5 mg in each liter OR
-Fluconazole (Diflucan) 200 mg IV x 1, then 100 mg IV qd.

10. **Symptomatic Medications:**
-Ranitidine (Zantac) 50 mg IV q8h.
-Acetaminophen (Tylenol) 325 mg PO/PR q4-6h prn temp >38.5°C.
-Heparin 5000 U SQ q12h.

11. **Extras:** Plain film, upright abdomen, lateral decubitus, CXR PA and LAT; surgery consult; ECG, abdominal ultrasound. CT scan.
12. **Labs:** CBC with differential, SMA 7&12, amylase, lactate, INR/PTT, UA with micro, C&S; drug levels peak and trough 3rd dose.

Paracentesis Tube 1: Cell count and differential (1-2 mL, EDTA purple top tube)

Tube 2: Gram stain of sediment; inject 10-20 mL into anaerobic and aerobic culture bottle; AFB, fungal C&S (3-4 mL).

Tube 3: Glucose, protein, albumin, LDH, triglycerides, specific gravity, bilirubin, amylase (2-3 mL, red top tube).

Syringe: pH, lactate (3 mL).

Diverticulitis

1. **Admit to:**
2. **Diagnosis:** Diverticulitis
3. **Condition:**
4. **Vital signs:** qid. Call physician if BP systolic >160/90, <90/60; P >120, <50; R>25, <10; T >38.5°C
5. **Activity:** Up ad lib.
6. **Nursing:** Inputs and outputs.
7. **Diet:** NPO. Advance to clear liquids as tolerated.
8. **IV Fluids:** 0.5-2 L NS over 1-2 hr then, D5 ½ NS at 125 cc/hr. NG tube at low intermittent suction (if obstructed).
9. **Special Medications:**
Regimen 1:
   -Gentamicin or tobramycin 100-120 mg IV (1.5-2 mg/kg), then 80 mg IV q8h (5 mg/kg/d) or 7 mg/kg in 50 mL of D5W over 60 min IV q24h **AND EITHER**
   Cefoxitin (Mefoxin) 2 gm IV q6-8h **OR**
   Clindamycin (Cleocin) 600-900 mg IV q8h.
Regimen 2:
   -Metronidazole (Flagyl) 500 mg q8h **AND**
   Ciprofloxacin (Cipro) 250-500 mg PO bid or 200-300 mg IV q12h.
Outpatient Regimen:
   -Metronidazole (Flagyl) 500 mg PO q6h **AND EITHER**
   Ciprofloxacin (Cipro) 500 mg PO bid **OR**
   Trimethoprim/SMX (Bactrim) 1 DS tab PO bid.
10. **Symptomatic Medications:**
    -Meperidine (Demerol) 50-100 mg IM or IV q3-4h prn pain.
    -Zolpidem (Ambien) 5-10 mg qhs prn insomnia.
11. **Extras:** Acute abdomen series, CXR PA and LAT, ECG, CT scan of abdomen, ultrasound, surgery and GI consults.
12. **Labs:** CBC with differential, SMA 7&12, amylase, lipase, blood cultures x 2, drug levels peak and trough 3rd dose. UA, C&S.

Lower Urinary Tract Infection

1. **Admit to:**
2. **Diagnosis:** UTI.
3. **Condition:**
4. **Vital signs:** tid. Call physician if BP <90/60; >160/90; R >30, <10; P >120, <50; T >38.5°C
5. **Activity:** Up ad lib
6. **Nursing:**
7. **Diet:** Regular
8. **IV Fluids:**
9. **Special Medications:**
Lower Urinary Tract Infection (treat for 3-7 days):
   -Trimethoprim-sulfamethoxazole (Septra) 1 double strength tab (160/800 mg) PO bid.
   -Norfloxacin (Noroxin) 400 mg PO bid.
   -Ciprofloxacin (Cipro) 250 mg PO bid.
   -Ofloxacin (Floxin) 200 mg PO bid.
   -Lomefloxacin (Maxaquin) 400 mg PO qd.
   -Enoxacin (Penetrex) 200-400 mg PO q12h; 1h before or 2h after meals.
   -Cefpodoxime (Vantin) 100 mg PO bid.
   -Cephalexin (Keflex) 500 mg PO q6h.
   -Cefixime (Suprax) 200 mg PO q12h or 400 mg PO qd.
   -Cefazolin (Ancef) 1-2 gm IV q8h.
Complicated or Catheter-Associated Urinary Tract Infection:
   -Ceftizoxime (Cefizox) 1 gm IV q8h.

-Gentamicin 2 mg/kg, then 1.5/kg q8h or 7 mg/kg in 50 mL of D5W over 60 min IV q24h.
-Ticarcillin/clavulanate (Timentin) 3.1 gm IV q4-6h
-Ciprofloxacin (Cipro) 500 mg PO bid.
-Ofloxacin (Floxin) 400 mg PO bid.

Prophylaxis (≥3 episodes/yr):
-Trimethoprim/SMX single strength tab PO qhs.

Candida Cystitis
-Fluconazole (Diflucan) 100 mg PO or IV x 1 dose, then 50 mg PO or IV qd for 5 days **OR**
-Amphotericin B continuous bladder irrigation, 50 mg/1000 mL sterile water via 3-way Foley catheter at 1 L/d for 5 days.

10. Symptomatic Medications:
-Phenazopyridine (Pyridium) 100 mg PO tid.

11. Extras: Renal ultrasound.

12. Labs: CBC, SMA 7. UA with micro, urine Gram stain, C&S.

Pyelonephritis

1. **Admit to:**
2. **Diagnosis:** Pyelonephritis
3. **Condition:**
4. **Vital signs:** tid. Call physician if BP <90/60; >160/90; R >30, <10; P >120, <50; T >38.5°C
5. **Activity:**
6. **Nursing:** Inputs and outputs.
7. **Diet:** Regular
8. **IV Fluids:** D5 ½ NS at 125 cc/h.
9. **Special Medications:**
   -Trimethoprim-sulfamethoxazole (Septra) 160/800 mg (10 mL in 100 mL D5W IV over 2 hours) q12h or 1 double strength tab PO bid.
   -Ciprofloxacin (Cipro) 500 mg PO bid or 400 mg IV q12h.
   -Norfloxacin (Noroxin) 400 mg PO bid
   -Ofloxacin (Floxin) 400 mg PO or IV bid.
   -Levofloxacin (Levaquin) 500 mg PO/IV q24h.
   -In more severely ill patients, treatment with an IV third-generation cephalosporin, or ticarcillin/clavulanic acid, or piperacillin/tazobactam or imipenem is recommended with an aminoglycoside.
   -Ceftizoxime (Cefizox) 1 gm IV q8h.
   -Ceftazidime (Fortaz) 1 gm IV q8h.
   -Ticarcillin/clavulanate (Timentin) 3.1 gm IV q6h.
   -Piperacillin/tazobactam (Zosyn) 3.375 gm IV/PB q6h.
   -Imipenem/cilastatin (Primaxin) 0.5-1.0 gm IV q6-8h.
   -Gentamicin or tobramycin, 2 mg/kg IV, then 1.5/kg q8h or 7 mg/kg in 50 mL of D5W over 60 min IV q24h.
10. **Symptomatic Medications:**
    -Phenazopyridine (Pyridium) 100 mg PO tid.
    -Meperidine (Demerol) 50-100 mg IM q4-6h prn pain.
11. **Extras:** Renal ultrasound, intravenous pyelogram, KUB.
12. **Labs:** CBC with differential, SMA 7. UA with micro, urine Gram stain, C&S; blood C&S x 2. Drug levels peak and trough third dose third dose.

Osteomyelitis

1. **Admit to:**
2. **Diagnosis:** Osteomyelitis
3. **Condition:**
4. **Vital signs:** qid. Call physician if BP <90/60; T >38.5°C
5. **Activity:** Bed rest with bathroom privileges.

6. **Nursing:** Keep involved extremity elevated. Range of motion exercises of upper and lower extremities tid.
7. **Diet:** Regular, high fiber.
8. **IV Fluids:** Heparin lock with flush q shift.
9. **Special Medications:**
Adult Empiric Therapy:
   -Nafcillin or oxacillin 2 gm IV q4h **OR**
   -Cefazolin (Ancef) 1-2 gm IV q8h **OR**
   -Vancomycin 1 gm IV q12h (1 gm in 250 cc D5W over 1h).
   -**Add** 3rd generation cephalosporin if gram negative bacilli on Gram stain. Treat for 4-6 weeks.
Post Operative or Post Trauma:
   -Vancomycin 1 gm IV q12h **AND** ceftazidime (Fortaz) 1-2 gm IV q8h.
   -Imipenem/cilastatin (Primaxin)**(single-drug treatment)** 0.5-1.0 gm IV q6-8h.
   -Ticarcillin/clavulanate (Timentin)**(single-drug treatment)** 3.1 gm IV q4-6h.
   -Ciprofloxacin (Cipro) 500-750 mg PO bid or 400 mg IV q12h **AND** Rifampin 600 mg PO qd.
Osteomyelitis with Decubitus Ulcer:
   -Cefoxitin (Mefoxin), 2 gm IV q6-8h.
   -Ciprofloxacin (Cipro) and metronidazole 500 mg IV q8h.
   -Imipenem/cilastatin (Primaxin), see dosage above.
   -Nafcillin, gentamicin and clindamycin; see dosage above.
10. **Symptomatic Medications:**
   -Meperidine (Demerol) 50-100 mg IM q3-4h prn pain.
   -Docusate sodium (Colace) 100 mg PO qhs.
   -Heparin 5000 U SQ bid.
11. **Extras:** Technetium/gallium bone scans, multiple X-ray views, CT/MRI.
12. **Labs:** CBC with differential, SMA 7, blood C&S x 3, MIC, MBC, UA with micro, C&S. Needle biopsy of bone for C&S; trough antibiotic levels.

Active Pulmonary Tuberculosis

1. **Admit to:**
2. **Diagnosis:** Active Pulmonary Tuberculosis
3. **Condition:**
4. **Vital signs:** q shift
5. **Activity:** Up ad lib in room.
6. **Nursing:** Respiratory isolation.
7. **Diet:** Regular
8. **Special Medications:**
   -Isoniazid 300 mg PO qd (5 mg/kg/d, max 300 mg/d) **AND** Rifampin 600 mg PO qd (10 mg/kg/d, 600 mg/d max) **AND** Pyrazinamide 500 mg PO bid-tid (15-30 mg/kg/d, max 2.5 gm) **AND** Ethambutol 400 mg PO bid-tid (15-25 mg/kg/d, 2.5 gm/d max).
   -Empiric treatment consists of a 4-drug combination of isoniazid (INH), rifampin, pyrazinamide (PZA), and either ethambutol or streptomycin. A modified regimen is recommended for patients known to have INH-resistant TB. Patients are treated for 8 weeks with the four-drug regimen, followed by 18 weeks of INH and rifampin.
   -Pyridoxine 50 mg PO qd with INH.
Prophylaxis
   -Isoniazid 300 mg PO qd (5 mg/kg/d) x 6-9 months.
9. **Extras:** CXR PA, LAT, ECG.
10. **Labs:** CBC with differential, SMA7 and 12, LFTs, HIV serology. First AM sputum for AFB x 3 samples.

Cellulitis

1. **Admit to:**
2. **Diagnosis:** Cellulitis
3. **Condition:**
4. **Vital signs:** tid. Call physician if BP <90/60; T >38.5°C
5. **Activity:** Up ad lib.
6. **Nursing:** Keep affected extremity elevated; warm compresses prn.
7. **Diet:** Regular, encourage fluids.
8. **IV Fluids:** Heparin lock with flush q shift.
9. **Special Medications:**

Empiric Therapy Cellulitis
- -Nafcillin or oxacillin 1-2 gm IV q4-6h **OR**
- -Cefazolin (Ancef) 1-2 gm IV q8h **OR**
- -Vancomycin 1 gm q12h (1 gm in 250 cc D5W over 1h) **OR**
- -Erythromycin 500 IV/PO q6h **OR**
- -Dicloxacillin 500 mg PO qid; may add penicillin VK, 500 mg PO qid, to increase coverage for streptococcus **OR**
- -Cephalexin (Keflex) 500 mg PO qid.

Immunosuppressed, Diabetic Patients, or Ulcerated Lesions:
- -Nafcillin or cefazolin and gentamicin or aztreonam. Add clindamycin or metronidazole if septic.
- -Cefazolin (Ancef) 1-2 gm IV q8h.
- -Cefoxitin (Mefoxin) 1-2 gm IV q6-8h.
- -Gentamicin 2 mg/kg, then 1.5 mg/kg IV q8h or 7 mg/kg in 50 mL of D5W over 60 min IV q24h **OR** aztreonam (Azactam) 1-2 gm IV q6h **PLUS**
- -Metronidazole (Flagyl) 500 mg IV q8h or clindamycin 900 mg IV q8h.
- -Ticarcillin/clavulanate (Timentin) **(single-drug treatment)** 3.1 gm IV q4-6h.
- -Ampicillin/Sulbactam (Unasyn) **(single-drug therapy)** 1.5-3.0 gm IV q6h.
- -Imipenem/cilastatin (Primaxin) **(single-drug therapy)** 0.5-1 mg IV q6-8h.
10. **Symptomatic Medications:**
- -Acetaminophen/codeine (Tylenol #3) 1-2 PO q4-6h prn pain.
11. **Extras:** Technetium/Gallium scans, Doppler study (ankle-brachial indices)..
12. **Labs:** CBC, SMA 7, blood C&S x 2. Leading edge aspirate for Gram stain, C&S; UA, antibiotic levels.

Pelvic Inflammatory Disease

1. **Admit to:**
2. **Diagnosis:** Pelvic Inflammatory Disease
3. **Condition:**
4. **Vital signs:** q8h. Call physician if BP >160/90, <90/60; P >120, <50; R>25, <10; T >38.5°C
5. **Activity:**
6. **Nursing:** Inputs and outputs.
7. **Diet:** Regular
8. **IV Fluids:** D5 ½ NS at 100-125 cc/hr.
9. **Special Medications:**
- -Cefoxitin (Mefoxin) 2 gm IV q6h **OR** cefotetan (Cefotan) 1-2 gm IV q12h; **AND** doxycycline (Vibramycin) 100 mg IV q12h (IV for 4 days and 48h after afebrile, then complete 10-14 days of doxycycline 100 mg PO bid) **OR**
- -Clindamycin 900 mg IV q8h **AND** Gentamicin 2 mg/kg IV, then 1.5 mg/kg IV q8h or 7 mg/kg in 50 mL of D5W over 60 min IV q24h, then complete 10-14 d of Clindamycin 300 mg PO qid or Doxycycline 100 mg PO bid **OR**
- -Ceftriaxone (Rocephin) 250 mg IM x 1 and doxycycline 100 mg PO bid for 14 days **OR**
- -Ofloxacin (Floxin) 400 mg PO bid for 14 days.

AND EITHER
- -Clindamycin 300 mg PO qid for 14 days **OR**
- -Metronidazole (Flagyl) 500 mg PO bid for 14 days.

10. Symptomatic Medications:
   -Acetaminophen (Tylenol) 1-2 tabs PO q4-6h prn pain or temperature >38.5°C.
   -Meperidine (Demerol) 25-100 mg IM q4-6h prn pain.
   -Zolpidem (Ambien) 10 mg PO qhs prn insomnia.
11. Labs: CBC, SMA 7&12, ESR. GC culture, chlamydia direct fluorescent antibody stain. UA with micro, C&S, VDRL, HIV, blood cultures x 2. Pelvic ultrasound.

Gastrointestinal Disorders

Peptic Ulcer Disease

1. **Admit to:**
2. **Diagnosis:** Peptic ulcer disease.
3. **Condition:**
4. **Vital Signs:** q4h. Call physician if BP >160/90, <90/60; P >120, <50; T >38.5°C
5. **Activity:** Up ad lib
6. **Nursing:** Guaiac stools.
7. **Diet:** NPO 48h, then regular, no caffeine.
8. **IV Fluids:** D5 ½ NS with 20 mEq KCL at 125 cc/h. NG tube at low intermittent suction (if obstructed).
9. **Special Medications:**
    -Ranitidine (Zantac) 50 mg IV bolus, then continuous infusion at 12.5 mg/h (300 mg in 250 mL D5W at 11 mL/h over 24h) or 50 mg IV q8h **OR**
    -Cimetidine (Tagamet) 300 mg IV bolus, then continuous infusion at 50 mg/h (1200 mg in 250 mL D5W over 24h) or 300 mg IV q6-8h **OR**
    -Famotidine (Pepcid) 20 mg IV q12h **OR**
    -Nizatidine (Axid) 300 mg PO qhs **OR**
    -Omeprazole (Prilosec) 20 mg PO bid (30 minutes prior to meals) **OR**
    -Lansoprazole (Prevacid) 15-30 mg PO qd prior to breakfast [15, 30 mg caps].

Eradication of H. pylori

A. Bismuth, Metronidazole, Tetracycline, Ranitidine
1. 14 day therapy.
2. Bismuth (Pepto bismol) 2 tablets PO qid.
3. Metronidazole (Flagyl) 250 mg PO qid (tid if cannot tolerate the qid dosing).
4. Tetracycline 500 mg PO qid.
5. Ranitidine (Zantac) 150 mg PO bid.
6. Efficacy is greater than 90%.

B. Amoxicillin, Omeprazole, Clarithromycin (AOC)
1. 10 days of therapy.
2. Amoxicillin 1 gm PO bid.
3. Omeprazole (Prilosec) 20 mg PO bid.
4. Clarithromycin (Biaxin) 500 mg PO bid.

C. Metronidazole, Omeprazole, Clarithromycin (MOC)
1. 10 days of therapy
2. Metronidazole 500 mg PO bid.
3. Omeprazole (Prilosec) 20 mg PO bid.
4. Clarithromycin (Biaxin) 500 mg PO bid.
5. Efficacy is >80%
6. Expensive, usually well tolerated.

D. Omeprazole, Clarithromycin (OC)
1. 14 days of therapy.
2. Omeprazole (Prilosec) 40 mg PO qd for 14 days, then 20 mg qd for an additional 14 days of therapy.
3. Clarithromycin (Biaxin) 500 mg PO tid.

E. Ranitidine-Bismuth-Citrate, Clarithromycin (RBC-C)
1. 28 days of therapy.
2. Ranitidine-bismuth-citrate (Tritec) 400 mg PO bid for 28 days.
3. Clarithromycin 500 mg PO tid for 14 days.
4. Efficacy is 70-80%; expensive

10. **Symptomatic Medications:**
    -Trimethobenzamide (Tigan) 100-250 mg PO or 100-200 mg IM/PR q6h prn nausea **OR**
    -Prochlorperazine (Compazine) 5-10 mg IM/IV/PO q4-6h or 25 mg PR q4-6h

    prn nausea.
11. **Extras:** Upright abdomen, KUB, CXR, ECG, endoscopy. GI consult, surgery consult.
12. **Labs:** CBC, SMA 7&12, amylase, lipase, LDH. UA, Helicobacter pylori serology. Fasting serum gastrin qAM for 3 days. Urea breath test for H pylori.

Gastrointestinal Bleeding

1. **Admit to:**
2. **Diagnosis:** Upper/lower GI bleed
3. **Condition:**
4. **Vital signs:** q30min. Call physician if BP >160/90, <90/60; P >120, <50; R>25, <10; T >38.5°C; urine output <15 mL/hr for 4h.
5. **Activity:** Bed rest
6. **Nursing:** Place nasogastric tube, then lavage with 2 L of room temperature normal saline, then connect to low intermittent suction. Repeat lavage q1h. Record volume and character of lavage. Foley to closed drainage; inputs and outputs.
7. **Diet:** NPO
8. **IV Fluids:** Two 16 gauge IV lines. 1-2 L NS wide open; transfuse 2-6 units PRBC to run as fast as possible, then repeat CBC.
9. **Special Medications:**
    -Oxygen 2 L by NC.
    -Ranitidine (Zantac) 50 mg IV bolus, then continuous infusion at 12.5 mg/h [300 mg in 250 mL D5W over 24h (11 cc/h)], or 50 mg IV q6-8h **OR**
    -Cimetidine (Tagamet) 300 mg IV bolus, then continuous infusion at 50 mg/h (1200 mg in 250 cc D5W over 24h), or 300 mg IV q6-8h **OR**
    -Famotidine (Pepcid) 20 mg IV q12h.
    -Vitamin K (Phytonadione) 10 mg IV/SQ qd for 3 days (if INR is elevated).
Esophageal Variceal Bleeds:
    -Somatostatin (Octreotide) 50 mcg IV bolus, followed by 25-50 mcg/h IV infusion (1200 mcg in 250 mL of D5W at 11 mL/h).
    Vasopressin/Nitroglycerine Paste Therapy:
      -Vasopressin (Pitressin) 20 U IV over 20-30 minutes, then 0.2-0.3 U/min [100 U in 250 mL of D5W (0.4 U/mL)] for 30 min, followed by increases of 0.2 U/min until bleeding stops or max of 0.9 U/min. If bleeding stops, taper over 24-48h **AND**
      -Nitroglycerine paste 1 inch q6h **OR** nitroglycerin IV at 10-30 mcg/min continuous infusion (50 mg in 250 mL of D5W).
10. **Extras:** Portable CXR, upright abdomen, ECG. Surgery and GI consults.
Upper GI Bleeds: Esophagogastroduodenoscopy with coagulation or sclerotherapy; Linton-Nachlas tube for tamponade of esophageal varices.
Lower GI Bleeds: Sigmoidoscopy/colonoscopy (after a GoLytely purge 6-8 L over 4-6h), technetium 99m RBC scan, angiography with embolization.
11. **Labs:** Repeat hematocrit q2h; CBC with platelets q12-24h. Repeat INR in 6 hours. SMA 7&12, ALT, AST, alkaline phosphatase, INR/PTT, type and cross for 3-6 U PRBC and 2-4 U FFP.

Cirrhotic Ascites and Edema

1. **Admit to:**
2. **Diagnosis:** Cirrhotic ascites and edema
3. **Condition:**
4. **Vital signs:** Vitals q4-6 hours. Call physician if BP >160/90, <90/60; P >120, <50; T >38.5°C; urine output < 25 cc/hr for 4h.
5. **Activity:** Bed rest with legs elevated.
6. **Nursing:** Inputs and outputs, daily weights, measure abdominal girth qd, guaiac all stools.
7. **Diet:** 2500 calories, 100 gm protein; 500 mg sodium restriction; fluid restric-

tion to 1-1.5 L/d (if hyponatremia, Na <130).
8. **IV Fluids:** Heparin lock with flush q shift.
9. **Special Medications:**
   -Diurese to reduce weight by 0.5-1 kg/d (if edema) or 0.25 kg/d (if no edema).
   -Spironolactone (Aldactone) 25-50 mg PO qid or 200 mg PO qAM, increase by 100 mg/d to max of 400 mg/d.
   -Furosemide (Lasix)(refractory ascites) 40-120 mg PO or IV qd-bid. Add KCL 20-40 mEq PO qAM if renal function is normal **OR**
   -Torsemide (Demadex) 20-40 mg PO/IV qd-bid.
   -Metolazone (Zaroxolyn) 5-10 mg PO qd (max 20 mg/d).
   -Ranitidine (Zantac) 150 mg PO bid.
   -Vitamin K 10 mg SQ qd for 3d.
   -Folic acid 1 mg PO qd.
   -Thiamine 100 mg PO qd.
   -Multivitamin PO qd.

   Paracentesis: Remove up to 5 L of ascites if peripheral edema, tense ascites, or decreased diaphragmatic excursion. If large volume paracentesis without peripheral edema or with renal insuffiencey, give salt-poor albumin, 12.5 gm for each 2 liters of fluid removed (50 mL of 25% solution); infuse 25 mL before paracentesis and 25 mL 6h after.
10. **Symptomatic Medications:**
    -Docusate sodium (Colace) 100 mg PO qhs.
    -Lactulose 30 mL PO bid-qid.
11. **Extras:** KUB, CXR, abdominal ultrasound, liver-spleen scan, GI consult.
12. **Labs:** Ammonia, CBC, SMA 7&12, LFTs, albumin, amylase, lipase, INR/PTT. Urine creatinine, Na, K. HBsAg, anti-HBs, hepatitis C virus antibody, alpha-1-antitrypsin.

Paracentesis Ascitic Fluid
   Tube 1: Protein, albumin, specific gravity, glucose, bilirubin, amylase, lipase, triglyceride, LDH (3-5 mL, red top tube).
   Tube 2: Cell count and differential (3-5 mL, purple top tube).
   Tube 3: C&S, Gram stain, AFB, fungal (5-20 mL); inject 20 mL into blood culture bottles at bedside.
   Tube 4: Cytology (>20 mL).
   Syringe: pH (2 mL).

Viral Hepatitis

1. **Admit to:**
2. **Diagnosis:** Hepatitis
3. **Condition:**
4. **Vital signs:** qid. Call physician if BP <90/60; T >38.5°C
5. **Activity:**
6. **Nursing:** Stool isolation.
7. **Diet:** Clear liquid (if nausea), low fat (if diarrhea).
8. **Special Medications:**
   -Ranitidine (Zantac) 150 mg PO bid.
   -Vitamin K 10 mg SQ qd for 3d.
   -Multivitamin PO qd.
9. **Symptomatic Medications:**
   -Meperidine (Demerol) 50-100 mg IM q4-6h prn pain.
   -Trimethobenzamide (Tigan) 250 mg PO q6-8h prn pruritus or nausea q6-8h prn.
   -Hydroxyzine (Vistaril) 25 mg IM/PO q4-6h prn pruritus or nausea.
   -Diphenhydramine (Benadryl) 25-50 mg PO/IV q4-6h prn pruritus.
10. **Extras:** Ultrasound, GI consult.
11. **Labs:** CBC, SMA 7&12, GGT, LDH, amylase, lipase, INR/PTT, IgM anti-HAV, IgM anti-HBc, HBsAg, anti-HCV; alpha-1-antitrypsin, ANA, ferritin, ceruloplasmin, urine copper.

Cholecystitis and Cholangitis

1. **Admit to:**
2. **Diagnosis:** Bacterial cholangitis
3. **Condition:**
4. **Vital signs:** q4h. Call physician if BP systolic >160, <90; diastolic. >90, <60; P >120, <50; R>25, <10; T >38.5°C
5. **Activity:** Bed rest
6. **Nursing:** Inputs and outputs
7. **Diet:** NPO
8. **IV Fluids:** 0.5-1 L LR over 1h, then D5 ½ NS with 20 mEq KCL/L at 125 cc/h. NG tube at low constant suction. Foley to closed drainage.
9. **Special Medications:**
   - Ticarcillin or piperacillin 3 gm IV q4-6h, and either metronidazole (Flagyl) 500 mg q8h or cefoxitin (Mefoxin) 1-2 gm IV q6h.
   - Ampicillin 1-2 gm IV q4-6h and gentamicin 100 mg (1.5-2 mg/kg), then 80 mg IV q8h (3-5 mg/kg/d) and metronidazole 500 mg IV q8h.
   - Ticarcillin/clavulanate (Timentin) 3.1 g IV q4-6h (single agent).
   - Imipenem/cilastatin (Primaxin) 1.0 gm IV q6h (single agent).
   - Piperacillin/tazobactam (Zosyn) 3.375 IV q6h.
   - Ampicillin/sulbactam (Unasyn) 1.5-3.0 gm IV q6h.
10. **Symptomatic Medications:**
    - Meperidine (Demerol) 50-100 mg IV/IM q4-6h prn pain.
    - Hydroxyzine (Vistaril) 25-50 mg IV/IM q4-6h prn with meperidine.
    - Omeprazole (Prilosec) 20 mg PO bid.
    - Heparin 5000 U SQ q12h.
11. **Extras:** CXR, ECG, RUQ Ultrasound, HIDA scan, acute abdomen series. GI consult, surgical consult.
12. **Labs:** CBC, SMA 7&12, GGT, amylase, lipase, blood C&S x 2. UA, INR/PTT.

Acute Pancreatitis

1. **Admit to:**
2. **Diagnosis:** Acute pancreatitis
3. **Condition:**
4. **Vital signs:** q1-4h, call physician if BP >160/90, <90/60; P >120, <50; R>25, <10; T >38.5°C; urine output < 25 cc/hr for more than 4 hours.
5. **Activity:** Bed rest with bedside commode.
6. **Nursing:** Inputs and outputs, fingerstick glucose qid, guaiac stools. Foley to closed drainage.
7. **Diet:** NPO
8. **IV Fluids:** 1-4 L NS over 1-3h, then D5 ½ NS with 20 mEq KCL/L at 125 cc/hr. NG tube at low constant suction (if obstruction).
9. **Special Medications:**
   - Ranitidine (Zantac) 12.5 mg/h (300 mg in 250 mL D5W at 11 mL/h) IV or 50 mg IV q6-8h **OR**

     Cimetidine (Tagamet) 100 mg/h IV or 300 mg IV q8h **OR**

     Famotidine (Pepcid) 20 mg IV q12h.
   - Ticarcillin/clavulanate (Timentin) 3.1 gm IV or ampicillin/sulbactam (Unasyn) 3.0 gm IV q6h or imipenem (Primaxin) 0.5-1.0 gm IV q6h.
   - Antibiotics are indicated for infected pancreatic pseudocysts or for abscess only. Uncomplicated pancreatitis does not require antibiotics.
   - Heparin 5000 U SQ q12h.
   - Total parenteral nutrition should be provided until the amylase and lipase are normal and symptoms have resolved.
10. **Symptomatic Medications:**
    - Meperidine 50-100 mg IM/IV q3-4h prn pain.
11. **Extras:** Upright abdomen, portable CXR, ECG, ultrasound, CT with contrast. Surgery and GI consults.
12. **Labs:** CBC, platelets, SMA 7&12, calcium, triglycerides, amylase, lipase,

LDH, AST, ALT; blood C&S x 2, hepatitis B surface antigen, INR/PTT, type and hold 4-6 U PRBC and 2-4 U FFP. Pancreatic isoamylase, UA.

Acute Diarrhea

1. **Admit to:**
2. **Diagnosis:** Acute Diarrhea
3. **Condition:**
4. **Vital signs:** q6h; call physician if BP >160/90, <80/60; P >120; R>25; T >38.5°C
5. **Activity:** Up ad lib
6. **Nursing:** Daily weights, inputs and outputs.
7. **Diet:** NPO except ice chips for 24h, then low residual elemental diet; no milk products.
8. **IV Fluids:** 1-2 L NS over 1-2 hours; then D5 ½ NS with 40 mEq KCL/L at 125 cc/h.
9. **Special Medications:**
Febrile or gross blood in stool or neutrophils on microscopic exam or prior travel:
    -Ciprofloxacin (Cipro) 500 mg PO bid **OR**
    -Norfloxacin (Noroxin) 400 mg PO bid **OR**
    -Ofloxacin (Floxin) 300 mg bid **OR**
    -Trimethoprim/SMX (Bactrim DS) (160/800 mg) one DS tab PO bid.
11. **Extras:** Upright abdomen. GI consult.
12. **Labs:** SMA7 and 12, CBC with differential, UA, blood culture x 2.
Stool studies: Wright's stain for fecal leukocytes, ova and parasites x 3, clostridium difficile toxin, culture for enteric pathogens, E coli 0157:H7 culture.

Specific Therapy of Acute Diarrhea

Shigella:
    -Trimethoprim/SMX, (Bactrim) one DS tab PO bid for 5 days **OR**
    -Ciprofloxacin (Cipro) 500 mg PO bid for 5 days **OR**
    -Azithromycin (Zithromax) 500 mg PO x 1, then 250 mg PO qd x 4.
Salmonella (bacteremia):
    -Ofloxacin (Floxin) 400 mg IV/PO q12h for 14 days **OR**
    -Ciprofloxacin (Cipro) 400 mg IV q12h or 750 mg PO q12h for 14 days **OR**
    -Trimethoprim/SMX (Bactrim) one DS tab PO bid for 14 days **OR**
    -Ceftriaxone (Rocephin) 2 gm IV q12h for 14 days.
Campylobacter jejuni:
    -Erythromycin 250 mg PO qid for 5-10 days **OR**
    -Azithromycin (Zithromax) 500 mg PO x 1, then 250 mg PO qd x 4 **OR**
    -Ciprofloxacin (Cipro) 500 mg PO bid for 5 days.
Enterotoxic/Enteroinvasive E coli (Travelers Diarrhea):
    -Ciprofloxacin (Cipro) 500 mg PO bid for 5-7 days **OR**
    -Trimethoprim/SMX (Bactrim), one DS tab PO bid for 5-7 days.
Antibiotic-Associated and Pseudomembranous Colitis (Clostridium difficile):
    -Metronidazole (Flagyl) 250 mg PO or IV qid for 10-14 days **OR**
    -Vancomycin 125 mg PO qid for 10 days (500 PO qid for 10-14 days, if recurrent).
Yersinia Enterocolitica (sepsis):
    -Trimethoprim/SMX (Bactrim), one DS tab PO bid for 5-7 days **OR**
    -Ciprofloxacin (Cipro) 500 mg PO bid for 5-7 days **OR**
    -Ofloxacin (Floxin) 400 mg PO bid **OR**
    -Ceftriaxone (Rocephin) 1 gm IV q12h.

Entamoeba Histolytica (Amebiasis):
Mild to Moderate Intestinal Disease:
-Metronidazole (Flagyl) 750 mg PO tid for 10 days **OR**
-Tinidazole 2 gm per day PO for 3 days **Followed By:**
-Iodoquinol 650 mg PO tid for 20 days **OR**
-Paromomycin 25-30 mg/kg/d PO tid for 7 days.
Severe Intestinal Disease:
-Metronidazole (Flagyl)750 mg PO tid for 10 days **OR**
-Tinidazole 600 mg PO bid for 5 days **Followed By:**
-Iodoquinol 650 mg PO tid for 20 days **OR**
-Paromomycin 25-30 mg/kg/d PO tid for 7 days.
Giardia Lamblia:
-Quinacrine 100 mg PO tid for 5d **OR**
-Metronidazole 250 mg PO tid for 7 days.
Cryptosporidium:
-Paromomycin 500 mg PO qid for 7-10 days [250 mg].

Crohn's Disease

1. **Admit to:**
2. **Diagnosis:** Crohn's disease.
3. **Condition:**
4. **Vital signs:** q8h. Call physician if BP >160/90, <90/60; P >120, <50; R>25, <10; T >38.5°C
5. **Activity:** Up ad lib in room.
6. **Nursing:** Inputs and outputs. NG at low intermittent suction (if obstruction).
7. **Diet:** NPO except for ice chips and medications for 48h, then low residue or elemental diet, no milk products.
8. **IV Fluids:** 1-2 L NS over 1-3h, then D5 ½ NS with 40 mEq KCL/L at 125 cc/hr.
9. **Special Medications:**
-Mesalamine (Asacol) 400-800 mg PO tid or mesalamine (Pentasa) 1000 mg (four 250 mg tabs) PO qid **OR**
-Sulfasalazine (Azulfidine) 0.5-1 gm PO bid; increase over 10 days to 0.5-1 gm PO qid **OR**
-Olsalazine (Dipentum) 500 mg PO bid.
-Infliximab (Remicade) 5 mg/kg IV over 2 hours; MR at 2 and 6 weeks
-Prednisone 40-60 mg/d PO in divided doses **OR**
-Hydrocortisone 50-100 mg IV q6h **OR**
-Methylprednisolone (Solu-Medrol) 10-20 mg IV q6h.
-Metronidazole (Flagyl) 250-500 mg PO q6h.
-Vitamin B_{12}, 100 mcg IM for 5d then 100-200 mcg IM q month.
-Multivitamin PO qAM or 1 ampule IV qAM.
-Folic acid 1 mg PO qd.
10. **Extras:** Abdominal x-ray series, CXR. GI consult.
11. **Labs:** CBC, SMA 7&12, Mg, ionized calcium, blood C&S x 2; stool Wright's stain, stool culture, C difficile antigen assay, stool ova and parasites x 3.

Ulcerative Colitis

1. **Admit to:**
2. **Diagnosis:** Ulcerative colitis
3. **Condition:**
4. **Vital signs:** q4-6h. Call physician if BP >160/90, <90/60; P >120, <50; R>25, <10; T >38.5°C
5. **Activity:** Up ad lib in room.
6. **Nursing:** Inputs and outputs.
7. **Diet:** NPO except for ice chips for 48h, then low residue or elemental diet, no milk products.

8. **IV Fluids:** 1-2 L NS over 1-2h, then D5 ½ NS with 40 mEq KCL/L at 125 cc/hr.
9. **Special Medications:**
    -Mesalamine (Asacol) 400-800 mg PO tid **OR**
    -5-aminosalicylate (Mesalamine) 400-800 mg PO tid or 1 gm PO qid or enema 4 gm/60 mL PR qhs **OR**
    -Sulfasalazine (Azulfidine) 0.5-1 gm PO bid, increase over 10 days as tolerated to 0.5-1.0 gm PO qid **OR**
    -Olsalazine (Dipentum) 500 mg PO bid **OR**
    -Hydrocortisone retention enema, 100 mg in 120 mL saline bid.
    -Methylprednisolone (Solu-Medrol) 10-20 mg IV q6h **OR**
    -Hydrocortisone 100 mg IV q6h **OR**
    -Prednisone 40-60 mg/d PO in divided doses.
    -B12, 100 mcg IM for 5d then 100-200 mcg IM q month.
    -Multivitamin PO qAM or 1 ampule IV qAM.
    -Folate 1 mg PO qd.
10. **Symptomatic Medications:**
    -Loperamide (Imodium) 2-4 mg PO tid-qid prn, max 16 mg/d **OR**
    -Kaopectate 60-90 mL PO qid prn.
11. **Extras:** Upright abdomen. CXR, colonoscopy, GI consult.
12. **Labs:** CBC, SMA 7&12, Mg, ionized calcium, liver panel, blood C&S x 2; stool Wright's stain, stool for ova and parasites x 3, culture for enteric pathogens; Clostridium difficile antigen assay, UA.

Parenteral Nutrition

General Considerations: Daily weights, inputs and outputs. Finger stick glucose q6h.
Central Parenteral Nutrition:
    -Infuse 40-50 mL/h of amino acid-dextrose solution in the first 24h; increase daily by 40 mL/hr increments until providing 1.3-2 x basal energy requirement and 1.2-1.7 gm protein/kg/d (see formula page 97).
Standard solution:

Amino acid sln (Aminosyn) 7-10%	500 mL
Dextrose 40-70%	500 mL
Sodium	35 mEq
Potassium	36 mEq
Chloride	35 mEq
Calcium	4.5 mEq
Phosphate	9 mmol
Magnesium	8.0 mEq
Acetate	82-104 mEq
Multi-trace element formula	1 mL/d
(Zn, copper, manganese, chromium)	
Regular insulin (if indicated)	10-60 U/L
Multivitamin(12)(2 amp)	10 mL/d
Vitamin K (in solution, SQ, IM)	10 mg/week
Vitamin B12	1000 mcg/week
Selenium (after 20 days of continuous TPN)	80 mcg/d

Intralipid 20%, 500 mL/d IVPB; infuse in parallel with standard solution at 1 mL/min for 15 min; if no adverse reactions, increase to 100 mL/hr once daily or 20 mg/hr continuously. Obtain serum triglyceride 6h after end of infusion (maintain <250 mg/dL).
Cyclic Total Parenteral Nutrition:
    -12h night schedule; taper continuous infusion in morning by reducing rate to half of original rate for 1 hour. Further reduce rate by half for an additional hour, then discontinue. Finger stick glucose q4-6h; restart TPN in afternoon. Taper at beginning and end of cycle. Final rate of 185 mL/hr for 9-10 h and 2 hours of taper at each end for total of 2000 mL.

Peripheral Parenteral Supplementation:
-3% amino acid sln (ProCalamine) up to 3 L/d at 125 cc/h **OR**
-Combine 500 mL amino acid solution 7% or 10% (Aminosyn) and 500 mL
   20% dextrose and electrolyte additive. Infuse at up to 100 cc/hr in
   parallel with:
-Intralipid 10% or 20% at 1 mL/min for 15 min (test dose); if no adverse
   reactions, infuse 500 mL/d at 21 mL/h over 24h, or up to 100 mL/h over
   5 hours daily.
-Draw triglyceride level 6h after end of Intralipid infusion.

7. Special Medications:
-Cimetidine (Tagamet) 300 mg IV q6-8h or 1200 mg/day in TPN **OR**
-Ranitidine (Zantac) 50 mg IV q8h or 150 mg/day in TPN.

8. Extras: Nutrition consult.

9. Labs:
Daily labs: SMA7, osmolality, CBC, cholesterol, triglyceride, urine glucose
   and specific gravity.
Twice weekly Labs: Calcium, phosphate, SMA-12, magnesium
Weekly Labs: Serum albumin and protein, pre-albumin, ferritin, INR/PTT,
   zinc, copper, B12, folate, 24h urine nitrogen and creatinine.

Enteral Nutrition

General Considerations: Daily weights, inputs and outputs, nasoduodenal
   feeding tube. Head-of-bed at 30° while enteral feeding and 2 hours after
   completion.
Enteral Bolus Feeding: Give 50-100 mL of enteral solution (Pulmocare, Jevity,
   Vivonex, Osmolite, Vital HN) q3h. Increase amount in 50 mL steps to max
   of 250-300 mL q3-4h; 30 kcal of nonprotein calories/kg/d and 1.5 gm
   protein/kg/d. Before each feeding measure residual volume, and delay
   feeding by 1h if >100 mL. Flush tube with 100 cc of water after each bolus.
Continuous enteral infusion: Initial enteral solution (Pulmocare, Jevity,
   Vivonex, Osmolite) 30 mL/hr. Measure residual volume q1h for 12h then tid;
   hold feeding for 1h if >100 mL. Increase rate by 25-50 mL/hr at 24 hr intervals as tolerated until final rate of 50-100 mL/hr. Three tablespoonfuls of
   protein powder (Promix) may be added to each 500 cc of solution. Flush tube
   with 100 cc water q8h.

Special Medications:
-Metoclopramide (Reglan) 10-20 mg PO or in J-tube q6h **OR**
-Cisapride (Propulsid) 10-20 mg via nasogastric tube qid (concurrent use
   with macrolide antibiotics or azole antifungals may result in prolongation
   of QT interval) **OR**
-Erythromycin 125 mg IV or via nasogastric tube q8h.
-Cimetidine (Tagamet) 400 mg PO bid **OR**
-Ranitidine (Zantac)150 mg PO bid.

Symptomatic Medications:
-Loperamide (Imodium) 2-4 mg PO/J-tube q6h prn, max 16 mg/d **OR**
-Diphenoxylate/atropine (Lomotil) 1-2 tabs or 5-10 mL (2.5 mg/5 mL) PO/J-
   tube q4-6h prn, max 12 tabs/d **OR**
-Kaopectate 30 cc PO or in J-tube q8h.

Extras: CXR, plain abdominal x-ray for tube placement, nutrition consult.

Labs:
Daily labs: SMA7, osmolality, CBC, cholesterol, triglyceride. SMA-12
Weekly Labs when indicated: Protein, Mg, INR/PTT, 24h urine nitrogen
   and creatinine. Pre-albumin, retinol-binding protein.

Hepatic Encephalopathy

1. **Admit to:**
2. **Diagnosis:** Hepatic encephalopathy
3. **Condition:**
4. **Vital signs:** q1-4h, neurochecks q4h. Call physician if BP >160/90,<90/60; P >120,<50; R>25,<10; T >38.5°C
5. **Allergies:** Avoid sedatives, NSAIDS or hepatotoxic drugs.
6. **Activity:** Bed rest.
7. **Nursing:** Keep head-of-bed at 40 degrees, guaiac stools; turn patient q2h while awake, chart stools. Seizure precautions, egg crate mattress, soft restraints prn. Record inputs and outputs.
8. **Diet:** Low protein nasogastric enteral feedings (Hepatic-Aid II) at 30 mL/hr. Increase rate by 25-50 mL/hr at 24 hr intervals as tolerated until final rate of 50-100 mL/hr as tolerated. No dietary protein for 8 hours.
9. **IV Fluids:** D5W at TKO, Foley to closed drainage.
10. **Special Medications:**
    -Sorbitol 500 mL in 200 mL of water PO now.
    -Lactulose 30-45 mL PO q1h for 3 doses, then 15-45 mL PO bid-qid, titrate to produce 3 soft stools/d **OR**
    -Lactulose enema 300 mL in 700 mL of tap water; instill 200-250 mL per rectal tube bid-qid. **AND**
    -Neomycin 1 gm PO q4-6h (4-12 g/d) **OR**
    -Metronidazole (Flagyl) 250 mg PO q6h.
    -Ranitidine (Zantac) 50 mg IV q8h or 150 mg PO bid **OR**
    -Famotidine (Pepcid) 20 mg IV/PO q12h.
    -Flumazenil (Romazicon) 0.2 mg (2 mL) IV over 30 seconds q1min until a total dose of 3 mg; if a partial response occurs, continue 0.5 mg doses until a total of 5 mg. Flumazenil may help reverse hepatic encephalopathy, even in the absence of benzodiazepine use. Excessive doses of flumazenil may precipitate seizures.
    -Multivitamin PO qAM or 1 ampule IV qAM.
    -Folic acid 1 mg PO/IV qd.
    -Thiamine 100 mg PO/IV qd.
    -Vitamin K 10 mg SQ qd for 3 days if elevated INR.
11. **Extras:** CXR, ECG; GI and dietetics consults.
12. **Labs:** Ammonia, CBC, platelets, SMA 7&12, AST, ALT, GGT, LDH, alkaline phosphatase, protein, albumin, bilirubin, INR/PTT, ABG, blood C&S x 2, hepatitis B surface antibody. UA.

Alcohol Withdrawal

1. **Admit to:**
2. **Diagnosis:** Alcohol withdrawals/delirium tremens.
3. **Condition:**
4. **Vital signs:** q4-6h. Call physician if BP >160/90, <90/60; P >130, <50; R>25, <10; T >38.5°C; or increase in agitation.
5. **Activity:**
6. **Nursing:** Seizure precautions. Soft restraints prn.
7. **Diet:** Regular, push fluids.
8. **IV Fluids:** Heparin lock or D5 ½ NS at 100-125 cc/h.
9. **Special Medications:**
Withdrawal syndrome:
    -Chlordiazepoxide (Librium) 50-100 mg PO/IV q6h for 3 days.
Delirium tremens:
    -Chlordiazepoxide (Librium) 100 mg slow IV push or PO, repeat q4-6h prn agitation or tremor for 24h; max 500 mg/d. Then give 50-100 mg PO q6h prn agitation or tremor **OR**
    -Diazepam (Valium) 5 mg slow IV push, repeat q6h until calm, then 5-10 mg PO q4-6h.

Seizures:
- Thiamine 100 mg IV push **AND**
- Dextrose water 50%, 50 mg IV push.
- Lorazepam (Ativan) 0.1 mg/kg IV at 2 mg/min; may repeat x 1 if seizures continue.

Wernicke-Korsakoff Syndrome:
- Thiamine 100 mg IV stat, then 100 mg IV qd.

10. Symptomatic Medications:
- Multivitamin 1 amp IV, then 1 tab PO qd.
- Folate 1 mg PO qd.
- Thiamine 100 mg PO qd.
- Acetaminophen (Tylenol) 1-2 PO q4-6h prn headache.

11. Extras: CXR, ECG. Alcohol rehabilitation and social work consult.

12. Labs: CBC, SMA 7&12, Mg, amylase, lipase, liver panel, urine drug screen. UA, INR/PTT.

Toxicology

Poisoning and Drug Overdose

Decontamination:
-**Gastric Lavage:** Place patient left side down, place nasogastric tube, and check position by injecting air and auscultating. Lavage with normal saline until clear fluid, then leave activated charcoal or other antidote. Gastric lavage is contraindicated for corrosives.
-**Cathartics:**
-Magnesium citrate 6% sln 150-300 mL PO
-Magnesium sulfate 10% solution 150-300 mL PO.
-**Activated Charcoal:** 50 gm PO (first dose should be given using product containing sorbitol). Repeat q2-6h for large ingestions.
-**Hemodialysis:** Indicated for isopropanol, methanol, ethylene glycol, severe salicylate intoxication (>100 mg/dL), lithium, or theophylline (if neurotoxicity, seizures, or coma).

Antidotes:
Narcotic Overdose:
-Naloxone (Narcan) 0.4 mg IV/ET/IM/SC, may repeat q2min.
Methanol Ingestion:
-Ethanol (10% in D5W) 7.5 mL/kg load, then 1.4 mL/kg/hr IV infusion until methanol level <20 mg/dL. Maintain ethanol level of 100-150 mg/100 mL.
Ethylene Glycol Ingestion:
-Fomepizole (Antizol) 15 mg/kg IV over 30 min, then 10 mg/kg IV q12h x 4 doses, then 15 mg/kg IV q12h until ethylene glycol level is less than 20 mg/dL **AND**
-Pyridoxine 100 mg IV q6h for 2 days and thiamine 100 mg IV q6h for 2 days
Carbon Monoxide Intoxication:
-Hyperbaric oxygen therapy or 100% oxygen by mask if hyperbaric oxygen not available.
Tricyclic Antidepressants Overdose:
-Gastric lavage
-Magnesium citrate 300 mg PO/NG x1
-Activated charcoal premixed with sorbitol 50 gm NG q4-6h until level is less than the toxic range.
Benzodiazepine Overdose:
-Flumazenil (Romazicon) 0.2 mg (2 mL) IV over 30 seconds q1min until a total dose of 3 mg; if a partial response occurs, repeat 0.5 mg doses until a total of 5 mg. If sedation persists, repeat the above regimen or start a continuous IV infusion of 0.1-0.5 mg/h. Excessive doses may cause seizures.
Labs: Drug screen (serum, gastric, urine); blood levels, SMA 7, fingerstick glucose, CBC, LFTs, ECG.

Acetaminophen Overdose

1. **Admit to:** Medical intensive care unit.
2. **Diagnosis:** Acetaminophen overdose
3. **Condition:**
4. **Vital signs:** q1h with neurochecks. Call physician if BP >160/90, <90/60; P >130, <50 <50; R>25, <10; urine output <20 cc/h for 3 hours.
5. **Activity:** Bed rest with bedside commode.
6. **Nursing:** Inputs and outputs, aspiration and seizure precautions. Place large bore (Ewald) NG tube, then lavage with 2 L of NS.
7. **Diet:** NPO

8. **IV Fluids:**
9. **Special Medications:**
   -Activated Charcoal 30-100 gm doses, remove via NG suction prior to acetylcysteine.
   -Acetylcysteine (Mucomyst, NAC) 5% solution loading dose 140 mg/kg via NG tube, then 70 mg/kg via NG tube q4h x 17 doses **OR** acetylcysteine 150 mg/kg IV in 200 mL D5W over 15 min, followed by 50 mg/kg in 500 mL D5W, infused over 4h, followed by 100 mg/kg in 1000 mL of D5W over next 16h. Complete all NAC doses even if acetaminophen levels fall below toxic range.
   -Phytonadione 5 mg IV/IM/SQ (if INR increased).
   -Fresh frozen plasma 2-4 U (if INR is unresponsive to phytonadione).
   -Trimethobenzamide (Tigan) 100-200 mg IM/PR q6h prn nausea
10. **Extras:** ECG. Nephrology consult for hemodialysis or charcoal hemoperfusion.
11. **Labs:** CBC, SMA 7&12, LFTs, INR/PTT, acetaminophen level now and in 4h. UA.

Theophylline Overdose

1. **Admit to:** Medical intensive care unit.
2. **Diagnosis:** Theophylline overdose
3. **Condition:**
4. **Vital signs:** Neurochecks q2h. Call physician if BP >160/90, <90/60; P >130; <50; R >25, <10.
5. **Activity:** Bed rest
6. **Nursing:** ECG monitoring until level <20 mcg/mL, aspiration and seizure precautions. Insert single lumen NG tube and lavage with normal saline if recent ingestion.
7. **Diet:** NPO
8. **IV Fluids:** D5 ½ NS at 125 cc/h
9. **Special Medications:**
   -Activated charcoal 50 gm PO q4-6h, with sorbitol cathartic, until theophylline level <20 mcg/mL. Maintain head-of-bed at 30-45 degrees to prevent aspiration of charcoal.
   -Charcoal hemoperfusion is indicated if the serum level is >60 mcg/mL or if signs of neurotoxicity, seizure, coma are present.
   -**Seizure:** Lorazepam 0.1 mg/kg IV at 2 mg/min; may repeat x 1 if seizures continue.
10. **Extras:** ECG.
11. **Labs:** CBC, SMA 7&12, theophylline level now and in q6-8h; INR/PTT, liver panel. UA.

Tricyclic Antidepressant Overdose

1. **Admit to:** Medical intensive care unit.
2. **Diagnosis:** TCA Overdose
3. **Condition:**
4. **Vital Signs:** Neurochecks q1h.
5. **Activity:** Bedrest.
6. **Nursing:** Continuous suicide observation. ECG monitoring, measure QRS width hourly, inputs and outputs, aspiration and seizure precautions. Place single-lumen nasogastric tube and lavage with 2 liters of normal saline if recent ingestion.
7. **Diet:** NPO
8. **IV Fluids:** NS at 100-150 cc/hr.
9. **Special Medications:**
   -Activated charcoal premixed with sorbitol 50 gm via NG tube q4-6h until the TCA level decreases to therapeutic range. Maintain head-of-bed at 30-45

degree angle to prevent charcoal aspiration.
 -Magnesium citrate 300 mL via nasogastric tube x 1 dose.
10. Cardiac Toxicity:
  -If mechanical ventilation is necessary, hyperventilate to maintain pH 7.50-7.55.
  -Administer sodium bicarbonate 50-100 mEq (1-2 amps or 1-2 mEq/kg) IV over 5-10 min, followed by infusion of sodium bicarbonate (2 amps in D5W 1 L) at 100-150 cc/h. Adjust rate to maintain pH 7.50-7.55.
11. Extras: ECG.
12. Labs: Urine toxicology screen, serum TCA levels, liver panel, CBC, SMA-7 and 12, UA.

Neurologic Disorders

Ischemic Stroke

1. **Admit to:**
2. **Diagnosis:** Ischemic stroke
3. **Condition:**
4. **Vital signs:** Vital signs and neurochecks q30minutes for 6 hours, then q60 minutes for 12 hours. Call physician if BP >185/105, <110/60; P >120, <50; R>24, <10; T >38.5°C; or change in neurologic status.
5. **Activity:** Bedrest.
6. **Nursing:** Head-of-bed at 30 degrees, turn q2h when awake, range of motion exercises qid. Foley catheter, eggcrate mattress. Guaiac stools, inputs and outputs's. Oxygen at 2 L per minute by nasal cannula.
   Bleeding precautions: check puncture sites for bleeding or hematomas. Apply digital pressure or pressure dressing to active compressible bleeding sites.
7. **Diet:** NPO except medications for 24 hours, then dysphagia ground diet with thickened liquids.
8. **IV Fluids:** 0.45% normal saline at 100 cc/h.
9. **Special Medications:**

Ischemic Stroke < 3 hours:
   -Tissue plasminogen activator (t-PA, Alteplase) is indicated if the patient presents within 3 hours of onset of symptoms and the stroke is non-hemorrhagic; 0.9 mg/kg (max 90 mg) over 60 min, with 10% of the total dose given as an initial bolus over 1 minute.

Completed Ischemic Stroke >3 hours:
   -Aspirin enteric coated 325 mg PO qd **OR**
   -Clopidogrel (Plavix) 75 mg PO qd **OR**
   -Ticlopidine (Ticlid) 250 mg PO bid.

10. **Symptomatic Medications:**
    -Ranitidine (Zantac) 50 mg IV q8h or 150 mg PO bid
    -Omeprazole (Prilosec) 20 mg PO bid or qhs.
    -Docusate sodium (Colace) 100 mg PO qhs
    -Bisacodyl (Dulcolax) 10-15 mg PO qhs or 10 mg PR prn.
    -Acetaminophen (Tylenol) 650 mg PO/PR q4-6h prn temp >38°C or headache.
11. **Extras:** CXR, ECG, CT without contrast or MRI with gadolinium contrast; carotid duplex scan; echocardiogram, 24-hour Holter monitor; swallowing studies. Physical therapy consult for range of motion exercises; neurology, rehabilitation medicine consults.
12. **Labs:** CBC, glucose, SMA 7&12, fasting lipid profile, VDRL, ESR; drug levels, INR/PTT, UA. Lupus anticoagulant, anticardiolipin antibody.

Transient Ischemic Attack

1. **Admit to:**
2. **Diagnosis:** Transient ischemic attack
3. **Condition:**
4. **Vital signs:** q1h with neurochecks. Call physician if BP >160/90, <90/60; P >120, <50; R>25, <10; T >38.5°C; or change in neurologic status.
5. **Activity:** Up as tolerated.
6. **Nursing:** Guaiac stools.
7. **Diet:** Dysphagia ground with thickened liquids or regular diet.
8. **IV Fluids:** Heparin lock with flush q shift.
9. **Special Medications:**
   -Aspirin 325 mg PO qd **OR**
   -Clopidogrel (Plavix) 75 mg PO qd **OR**
   -Ticlopidine (Ticlid) 250 mg PO bid **OR**
   -Heparin (only if recurrent TIAs or cardiogenic or vertebrobasilar source for emboli) 700-800 U/h (12 U/kg/h) IV infusion without a bolus (25,000 U in 500 mL D5W); adjust q6-12h until PTT 1.2-1.5 x control.
   -Warfarin (Coumadin) 5.0-7.5 mg PO qd for 3d, then 2-4 mg PO qd. Titrate to INR of 2.0-2.5.
10. **Symptomatic Medications:**
    -Ranitidine (Zantac) 150 mg PO bid.
    -Docusate sodium (Colace) 100 mg PO qhs.
    -Milk of magnesia 30 mL PO qd prn constipation.
11. **Extras:** CXR, ECG, CT without contrast; carotid duplex scan, echocardiogram, 24-hour Holter monitor. Physical therapy, neurology consults.
12. **Labs:** CBC, glucose, SMA 7&12, fasting lipid profile, VDRL, drug levels, INR/PTT, UA.

Subarachnoid Hemorrhage

Treatment:
   -Stat neurosurgery consult.
   -Head of bed at 20 degrees, turn patient q2h, range of motion exercises qid, Foley catheter, eggcrate mattress. Guaiac stools.
   -Keep room dark and quiet; strict bedrest. Neurologic checks q1h for 12 hours, then q2h for 12 hours, then q4h. Call physician if abrupt change in neurologic status.
   -Restrict total fluids to 1000 mL/day; diet as tolerated.
   -Nimodipine (Nimotop) 60 mg PO or via NG tube q4h for 21d, must start within 96 hours.
   -Phenytoin (seizures) load 15 mg/kg IV in NS (infuse at max 50 mg/min), then 300 mg PO/IV qAM (4-6 mg/kg/d).
Hypertension:
   -Nitroprusside sodium, 0.1-0.5 mcg/kg/min (50 mg in 250 mL NS), titrate to control blood pressure.
Extras: CXR, ECG, CT without contrast; MRI angiogram; cerebral angiogram. Neurology, neurosurgery consults.
Labs: CBC, SMA 7&12, VDRL, UA.

Seizure and Status Epilepticus

1. **Admit to:**
2. **Diagnosis:** Seizure
3. **Condition:**
4. **Vital signs:** q1h with neurochecks. Call physician if BP >160/90, <90/60; P >120, <50; R>25, <10; T >38.5°C; or any change in neurological status.
5. **Activity:** Bed rest
6. **Nursing:** Finger stick glucose. Seizure precautions with bed rails up; padded tongue blade at bedside. EEG monitoring.
7. **Diet:** NPO for 24h, then regular diet if alert.
8. **IV Fluids:** D5 ½ NS at 100 cc/hr; change to heparin lock when taking PO.
9. **Special Medications:**

Status Epilepticus:
1. Maintain airway.
2. Position the patient laterally with the head down. The head and extremities should be cushioned to prevent injury.
3. During the tonic portion of the seizure, the teeth are tightly clenched. During the clonic phase that follows, however, a bite block or other soft object should be inserted into the mouth to prevent injury to the tongue.
4. 100% O_2 by mask, obtain brief history, and a fingerstick glucose.
5. Secure IV access and draw blood for serum glucose analysis. Give thiamine 100 mg IV push to prevent Wernicke's encephalopathy, then dextrose 50% 50 mL IV push.
6. **Initial Control:**

   Lorazepam (Ativan) 6-8 mg (0.1 mg/kg; not to exceed 2 mg/min) IV at 1-2 mg/min. May repeat 6-8 mg q5-10min (max 80 mg/24h) **OR**

   Diazepam (Valium), 5-10 mg slow IV at 1-2 mg/min. Repeat 5-10 mg q5-10 min prn (max 100 mg/24h).

   Phenytoin (Dilantin) 15-20 mg/kg load in NS at 50 mg/min. Repeat 100-150 mg IV q30min, max 1.5 gm; monitor BP.

   Fosphenytoin (Cerebyx) 20 mg/kg IV/IM (at 150 mg/min), then 4-6 mg/kg/day in 2 or 3 doses (150 mg IV/IM q8h). Fosphenytoin is metabolized to phenytoin; fosphenytoin may be given IM.

   If Seizures Persist, Administer Phenobarbital 20 mg/kg IV at 50 mg/min, repeat 2 mg/kg q15min; additional phenobarbital may be given, up to max of 30-60 mg/kg.

7. **If Seizures Persist, Intubate the Patient and Consider:**
   - Midazolam (Versed) 0.2 mg/kg IV push, then 0.045 mg/kg/hr; titrate up to 0.6 mg/kg/hr **OR**
   -Propofol (Diprivan) 2 mg/kg IV push, then 2 mg/kg/hr; titrate up to 10 mg/kg/hr **OR**
   -Phenobarbital as above.
   -Induction of coma with pentobarbital 10-15 mg/kg IV over 1-2h, then 1-1.5 mg/kg/h continuous infusion. Initiate continuous EEG monitoring.
8. **Consider Intubation and General Anesthesia**

Maintenance Therapy for Epilepsy:

Primary Generalized Seizures -- First-Line Therapy:
   -Carbamazepine (Tegretol) 200-400 mg PO tid [100, 200 mg]. Monitor CBC.
   -Phenytoin (Dilantin) loading dose of 400 mg PO followed by 300 mg PO q4h for 2 doses (total of 1 g), then 300 mg PO qd or 100 mg tid or 200 mg bid [30, 50, 100 mg].
   -Divalproex (Depakote) 250-500 mg PO tid-qid with meals [125, 250, 500 mg].
   -Valproic acid (Depakene) 250-500 mg PO tid-qid with meals [250 mg].

Primary Generalized Seizures -- Second Line Therapy:
   -Phenobarbital 30-120 mg PO bid [8, 16, 32, 65, 100 mg].
   -Primidone (Mysoline) 250-500 mg PO tid [50, 250 mg]; metabolized to phenobarbital.
   -Felbamate (Felbatol) 1200-2400 mg PO qd in 3-4 divided doses, max 3600 mg/d [400, 600 mg; 600 mg/5 mL susp]; adjunct therapy; aplastic anemia, hepatotoxicity.

-Gabapentin (Neurontin), 300-400 mg PO bid-tid; max 1800 mg/day [100, 300, 400 mg]; adjunct therapy.
-Lamotrigine (Lamictal) 50 mg PO qd, then increase to 50-250 mg PO bid [25, 100, 150, 200 mg]; adjunct therapy .

Partial Seizure:

-Carbamazepine (Tegretol) 200-400 mg PO tid [100, 200 mg].
-Divalproex (Depakote) 250-500 mg PO tid with meals [125, 250, 500 mg].
-Valproic acid (Depakene) 250-500 mg PO tid-qid with meals [250 mg].
-Phenytoin (Dilantin) 300 mg PO qd or 200 mg PO bid [30, 50, 100].
-Phenobarbital 30-120 mg PO tid or qd [8, 16, 32, 65, 100 mg].
-Primidone (Mysoline) 250-500 mg PO tid [50, 250 mg]; metabolized to phenobarbital.
-Felbamate (Felbatol) 1200-2400 mg PO qd in 3-4 divided doses, max 3600 mg/d [400,600 mg; 600 mg/5 mL susp]; adjunct therapy; aplastic anemia, hepatotoxicity.
-Gabapentin (Neurontin), 300-400 mg PO bid-tid; max 1800 mg/day [100, 300, 400 mg]; adjunct therapy.
-Lamotrigine (Lamictal) 50 mg PO qd, then increase to 50-250 mg PO bid [25, 100, 150, 200 mg]; adjunct therapy.
-Topiramate (Topamax) 25 mg PO bid; titrate to max 200 mg PO bid [tab 25, 100, 200 mg]; adjunctive therapy.

Absence Seizure:

-Divalproex (Depakote) 250-500 mg PO tid-qid [125, 250, 500 mg].
-Clonazepam (Klonopin) 0.5-5 mg PO bid-qid [0.5, 1, 2 mg].
-Lamotrigine (Lamictal) 50 mg PO qd, then increase to 50-250 mg PO bid [25, 100, 150, 200 mg]; adjunct therapy.

10. Extras: MRI with and without gadolinium or CT with contrast; EEG (with photic stimulation, hyperventilation, sleep deprivation, awake and asleep tracings); portable CXR, ECG.

11. Labs: CBC, SMA 7, glucose, Mg, calcium, phosphate, liver panel, VDRL, anticonvulsant levels. UA, drug screen.

Endocrinologic Disorders

Diabetic Ketoacidosis

1. **Admit to:**
2. **Diagnosis:** Diabetic ketoacidosis
3. **Condition:**
4. **Vital signs:** q1h, postural BP and pulse. Call physician if BP >160/90, <90/60; P >140, <50; R >30, <10; T >38.5°C; or urine output < 20 mL/hr for more than 2 hours.
5. **Activity:** Bed rest with bedside commode.
6. **Nursing:** Inputs and outputs. Foley to closed drainage. Record labs on flow sheet.
7. **Diet:** NPO for 12 hours, then clear liquids as tolerated.
8. **IV Fluids:**
1-2 L NS over 1-3h (≥16 gauge), infuse at 400-1000 mL/h until hemodynamically stable, then change to 0.45% saline at 125-150 cc/hr; keep urine output >30-60 mL/h.
Add KCL when serum potassium is <5.0 mEq/L.
    Concentration.......20-40 mEq KCL/L
May use K phosphate, 20-40 mEq/L, in place of KCL if low phosphate.
Change to 5% dextrose in 0.45% saline with 20-40 mEq KCL/liter when blood glucose 250-300.
9. **Special Medications:**
   -Oxygen at 2 L/min by NC.
   -Insulin Regular (Humulin) 7-10 units (0.1 U/kg) IV bolus, then 7-10 U/h IV infusion (0.1 U/kg/h); 50 U in 250 mL of 0.9% saline; flush IV tubing with 20 mL of insulin sln before starting infusion. Adjust insulin infusion to decrease serum glucose by 100 mg/dL or less per hour. When bicarbonate level is >16 mEq/L and anion gap <16 mEq/L, decrease insulin infusion rate by half
   -When the glucose level reaches 250 mg/dL, 5% dextrose should be added to the replacement fluids with KCL 20-40 mEq/L.
   -Use 10% glucose at 50-100 mL/h if anion gap persists and serum glucose has decreased to less than 100 mg/dL while on insulin infusion.
   -Change to subcutaneous insulin when anion gap cleared; discontinue insulin infusion 1-2h after subcutaneous dose.
10. **Extras:** Portable CXR, ECG.
11. **Labs:** Fingerstick glucose q1-2h. SMA 7 q4-6h. SMA 12, pH, bicarbonate, phosphate, amylase, lipase, hemoglobin A1c; CBC. UA, serum pregnancy test.

Nonketotic Hyperosmolar Syndrome

1. **Admit to:**
2. **Diagnosis:** Nonketotic hyperosmolar syndrome
3. **Condition:**
4. **Vital signs:** q1h. Call physician if BP >160/90, <90/60; P >140, <50; R>25, <10; T >38.5° C; or urine output <20 cc/hr for more than 4 hours.
5. **Activity:** Bed rest with bedside commode.
6. **Nursing:** Input and output measurement. Foley to closed drainage. Record labs on flow sheet.
7. **Diet:** NPO.
8. **IV Fluids:**
   -1-2 L NS over 1h (≥16 gauge IV catheter), then give 0.45% saline at 125 cc/hr. Maintain urine output ≥50 mL/hr.
   -Add 20-40 mEq/L KCL when urine output adequate.
9. **Special Medications:**
   -Insulin regular 2-3 U/h IV infusion (50 U in 250 mL of 0.9% saline).

-Ranitidine (Zantac) 50 mg IV q8h or 150 mg PO bid.
-Heparin 5000 U SQ q12h.
10. **Extras:** Portable CXR, ECG.
11. **Labs:** Fingerstick glucose q1-2h x 6h, then q6h. SMA 7, osmolality. SMA 12, phosphate, ketones, hemoglobin A1C, CBC. UA.

Thyroid Storm and Hyperthyroidism

1. **Admit to:**
2. **Diagnosis:** Thyroid Storm
3. **Condition:**
4. **Vital signs:** q1-4h. Call physician if BP >160/90, <90/60; P >130, <50; R>25, <10; T >38.5°C
5. **Activity:** Bed rest
6. **Nursing:** Cooling blanket prn temp >39°C, inputs and outputs. Oxygen 2 L/min by nasal canula.
7. **Diet:** Regular
8. **IV Fluids:** D5 ½ NS at 125 mL/h.
9. **Special Medications:**
Thyroid Storm and Hyperthyroidism:
-Propylthiouracil (PTU) 1000 mg PO, then 50-250 mg PO q4-8h, up to 1200 mg/d; usual maintenance dose 50 mg PO tid **OR**
-Methimazole (Tapazole) 30-60 mg PO, then maintenance of 15 mg PO qd-bid **AND**
-Iodide solution (Lugol's solution), 3-6 drops tid; one hour after propylthiouracil **AND**
-Dexamethasone (Solu-Medrol) 2 mg IV q6h **AND**
-Propranolol 40-160 mg PO q6h or 5-10 mg/h, max 2-5 mg IV q4h or propranolol-LA (Inderal-LA), 80-120 mg PO qd [60, 80, 120, 160 mg].
-Acetaminophen (Tylenol) 1-2 tabs PO q4-6h prn temp >38°C.
-Triazolam (Halcion) 0.125-0.5 mg PO qhs prn sleep **OR**
-Lorazepam (Ativan) 1-2 mg IV/IM/PO q4-8h prn anxiety.
10. **Extras:** CXR PA and LAT, ECG, endocrine consult. If visual symptoms, obtain ophthalmology consult.
11. **Labs:** CBC, SMA 7&12; sensitive TSH, free T4. UA.

Myxedema Coma and Hypothyroidism

1. **Admit to:**
2. **Diagnosis:** Myxedema Coma
3. **Condition:**
4. **Vital signs:** q1h. Call physician if BP systolic >160/90, <90/60; P >130, <50; R>25, <10; T >38.5°C
5. **Activity:** Bed rest
6. **Nursing:** Triple blankets prn temp <36°C, inputs and outputs, aspiration precautions.
7. **Diet:** NPO
8. **IV Fluids:** IV D5 NS TKO.
9. **Special Medications:**
Myxedema Coma and Hypothyroidism:
-Volume replacement with NS 1-2 L rapid IV, then 125 mL/h.
-Levothyroxine (Synthroid, Levoxine) 300-500 mcg IV, then 100 mcg PO or IV qd.
-Hydrocortisone 100 mg IV loading dose, then 50-100 mg IV q8h.
Hypothyroidism in Medically Stable Patient:
-Levothyroxine (Synthroid, T4) 50-75 mcg PO qd, increase by 25 mcg PO qd at 2-4 week intervals, to 75-150 mcg qd until TSH normalized.
11. **Extras:** ECG, endocrine consult.
12. **Labs:** CBC, SMA 7&12; sensitive TSH, free T4. UA, RA factor, ANA.

Nephrologic Disorders

Renal Failure

1. **Admit to:**
2. **Diagnosis:** Renal Failure
3. **Condition:**
4. **Vital signs:** q8h. Call physician if QRS complex >0.14 sec; urine output <20 cc/hr; BP >160/90, <90/60; P >120, <50; R>25, <10; T >38.5°C
5. **Allergies:** Avoid magnesium containing antacids, salt substitutes, NSAIDS, and other nephrotoxins. Discontinue phosphate or potassium supplements unless depleted.
6. **Activity:** Bed rest.
7. **Nursing:** Daily weights, inputs and outputs, chart urine output. If no urine output for 4h, inputs and outputs catheterize. Guaiac stools.
8. **Diet:** Renal diet of high biologic value protein of 0.6-0.8 g/kg, sodium 2 g, potassium 1 mEq/kg, and at least 35 kcal/kg of nonprotein calories. In oliguric patients, daily fluid intake should be restricted to less than 1 L after volume has been normalized.
9. **IV Fluids:** D5W at TKO.
10. **Special Medications:**
    -Consider fluid challenge (to rule out pre-renal azotemia if not fluid over-loaded) with 500-1000 mL NS IV over 30 min. In acute renal failure, inputs and outputs catheterize and check postvoid residual to rule out obstruction.
    -Furosemide (Lasix) 80-320 mg IV bolus over 10-60 min, double the dose if no response after 2 hours to total max 1000 mg/24h, or furosemide 1000 mg in 250 mL D5W at 20-40 mg/hr continuous IV infusion **OR**
    -Torsemide (Demadex) 20-40 mg IV bolus over 5-10 min, double the dose up to max 200 mg/day.
    -Bumetanide (Bumex) 1-2 mg IV bolus over 1-20 min; double the dose if no response in 1-2 h to total max 10 mg/day.
    -Metolazone (Zaroxolyn) 5-10 mg PO (max 20 mg/24h) 30 min before a loop diuretic.
    -Dopamine (Intropin) 1-3 mcg/kg per minute IV.
    -Hyperkalemia is treated with sodium polystyrene sulfonate (Kayexalate), 15-30 g PO/NG/PR q4-6h.
    -Hyperphosphatemia is controlled with calcium acetate (Phoslo), 2-3 tabs with meals.
    -Metabolic acidosis is treated with sodium bicarbonate to maintain the serum pH >7.2 and the bicarbonate level >20 mEq/L. 1-2 amps (50-100 mEq) IV push, followed by infusion of 2-3 amps in 1000 mL of D5W at 150 mL/hr.
    -Adjust all medications to creatinine clearance, and remove potassium phosphate and magnesium from IV. Avoid NSAIDs and nephrotoxic drugs.
11. **Extras:** CXR, ECG, renal ultrasound, nephrology and dietetics consults.
12. **Labs:** CBC, platelets, SMA 7&12, creatinine, BUN, potassium, magnesium, phosphate, calcium, uric acid, osmolality, ESR, INR/PTT, ANA.
Urine specific gravity, UA with micro, urine C&S; 1st AM spot urine electrolytes, creatinine, pH, osmolality; Wright's stain, urine electrophoresis. 24h urine protein, creatinine, sodium.

Nephrolithiasis

1. **Admit to:**
2. **Diagnosis:** Nephrolithiasis
3. **Condition:**
4. **Vital signs:** q6h. Call physician if urine output <30 cc/hr; BP >160/90, <90/60; T >38.5°C
5. **Activity:** Up ad lib.

6. **Nursing:** Strain urine, measure inputs and outputs. Place Foley if no urine for 4 hours.
7. **Diet:** Regular, push oral fluids.
8. **IV Fluids:** IV D5 ½ NS at 100-125 cc/hr (maintain urine output of 80 mL/h).
9. **Special Medications:**
   -Cefazolin (Ancef) 1-2 gm IV q8h
   -Meperidine (Demerol) 75-100 mg and hydroxyzine 25 mg IM/IV q2-4h prn pain **OR**
   -Butorphanol (Stadol) 0.5-2 mg IV q3-4h.
   -Hydrocodone/acetaminophen (Vicodin), 1-2 tab q4-6h PO prn pain **OR**
   -Hydromorphone (Dilaudid) 1-2 tabs q4-6h PO prn pain **OR**
   -Acetaminophen with codeine (Tylenol 3) 1-2 tabs PO q3-4h prn pain.
   -Ketorolac (Toradol) 10 mg PO q4-6h prn pain, or 30-60 mg IV/IM then 15-30 mg IV/IM q6h (max 5 days).
   -Zolpidem (Ambien) 10 mg PO qhs prn insomnia.
Note: If stone <5 mm without sepsis then discharge home with analgesics and increase PO fluids. If stone >10 mm and/or fever or increased WBC or signs of ureteral dilation, admission for urology evaluation is indicated.
11. **Extras:** Intravenous pyelogram, KUB, CXR, ECG.
12. **Labs:** CBC, SMA 6 and 12, calcium, uric acid, phosphorous, UA with micro, urine C&S, urine pH, INR/PTT. Urine cystine (nitroprusside test), send stones for X-ray crystallography. 24 hour urine collection for uric acid, calcium, creatinine.

Hypercalcemia

1. **Admit to:**
2. **Diagnosis:** Hypercalcemia
3. **Condition:**
4. **Vital signs:** q4h. Call physician if BP >160/90, <90/60; P >120, <50; R>25, <10; T >38.5°C; or tetany or any abnormal mental status.
5. **Activity:** Encourage ambulation; up in chair at other times.
6. **Nursing:** Seizure precautions, weigh patient bid, measure inputs and outputs.
7. **Diet:** Restrict dietary calcium to 400 mg/d, push PO fluids.
8. **Special Medications:**
   -1-2 L of 0.9% saline over 1-4 hours until no longer hypotensive, then saline diuresis with 0.9% saline infused at 125 cc/h **AND**
   -Furosemide (Lasix) 20-80 mg IV q4-12h. Maintain urine output of 200 mL/h; monitor serum sodium, potassium, magnesium
   -Calcitonin (Calcimar) 4-8 IV kg IM q12h or SQ q6-12h.
   -Etidronate (Didronel) 7.5 mg/kg/day in 250 mL of normal saline IV infusion over 2 hours for 3 days.
   -Pamidronate (Aredia) 60 mg in 1 liter of NS infused over 4 hours or 90 mg in 1 liter of NS infused over 24 hours x one dose.
9. **Extras:** CXR, ECG, mammogram.
10. **Labs:** Total and ionized calcium, SMA 7&12, phosphate, Mg, alkaline phosphatase, prostate specific antigen. 24h urine calcium, phosphate, parathyroid hormone.

Hypocalcemia

1. **Admit to:**
2. **Diagnosis:** Hypocalcemia
3. **Condition:**
4. **Vital signs:** q4h. Call physician if BP >160/90, <90/60; P >120, <50; R>25, <10; T >38.5°C; or any abnormal mental status.
5. **Activity:** Up ad lib
6. **Nursing:** I and O.
7. **Diet:** No added salt diet.
8. **Special Medications:**

Symptomatic Hypocalcemia:
   -Calcium chloride, 10% (270 mg calcium/10 mL vial) give 5-10 mL slowly over 10 min or dilute in 50-100 mL of D5W and infuse over 20 min, repeat q20-30 min if symptomatic, or hourly if asymptomatic. Correct hyperphosphatemia before hypocalcemia **OR**
   -Calcium gluconate, 20 mL of 10% solution IV (2 vials)(90 mg elemental calcium/10 mL vial) infused over 10-15 min, followed by infusion of 60 mL of calcium gluconate in 500 cc of D5W (1 mg/mL) at 0.5-2.0 mg/kg/h.

Chronic Hypocalcemia:
   -Calcium carbonate with vitamin D (Oscal-D) 1-2 tab PO tid **OR**
   -Calcium carbonate (Oscal) 1-2 tab PO tid **OR**
   -Calcium citrate (Citracal) 1 tab PO q8h or Extra strength Tums 1-2 PO with meals.
   -Vitamin D2 (Ergocalciferol) 1 tab PO qd.
   -Calcitriol (Rocaltrol) 0.25 mcg PO qd, titrate up to 0.5-2.0 mcg qid.
   -Docusate sodium (Colace) 1 tab PO bid.
9. **Extras:** CXR, ECG.
10. **Labs:** SMA 7&12, phosphate, Mg. 24h urine calcium, potassium, phosphate, magnesium.

Hyperkalemia

1. **Admit to:**
2. **Diagnosis:** Hyperkalemia
3. **Condition:**
4. **Vital signs:** q4h. Call physician if QRS complex >0.14 sec or BP >160/90, <90/60; P >120, <50; R>25, <10; T >38.5°C.
5. **Activity:** Bed rest; up in chair as tolerated.
6. **Nursing:** Inputs and outputs. Chart QRS complex width q1h.
7. **Diet:** Regular, no salt substitutes.
8. **IV Fluids:** D5NS at 125 cc/h
9. **Special Medications:**
   -Consider discontinuing ACE inhibitors, angiotensin II receptor blockers, beta-blockers, potassium sparing diuretics.
   -Calcium gluconate (10% sln) 10-30 mL IV over 2-5 min; second dose may be given in 5 min. Contraindicated if digoxin toxicity is suspected. Keep 10 mL vial of calcium gluconate at bedside for emergent use.
   -Sodium bicarbonate 1 amp (50 mEq) IV over 5 min (give after calcium in separate IV).
   -Regular insulin 10 units IV push with 1 ampule of 50% glucose IV push.
   -Kayexalate 30-45 gm premixed in sorbitol solution PO/NG/PR now and in q3-4h prn, up to 5 times per day.
   -Furosemide 40-80 mg IV, repeat prn.
   -Consider emergent dialysis if cardiac complications or renal failure.
10. **Extras:** ECG.
11. **Labs:** CBC, platelets, SMA7, magnesium, calcium, SMA-12. UA, specific gravity, Urine sodium, pH, 24h urine potassium, creatinine.

Hypokalemia

1. **Admit to:**
2. **Diagnosis:** Hypokalemia
3. **Condition:**
4. **Vital signs:** Vitals, urine output q4h. Call physician if BP >160/90, <90/60; P>120, <50; R>25, <10; T >38.5°C.
5. **Activity:** Bed rest; up in chair as tolerated.
6. **Nursing:** Inputs and outputs
7. **Diet:** Regular
8. **Special Medications:**
Acute Therapy:
    -KCL 20-40 mEq in 100 cc saline infused IVPB over 2 hours; or add 40-80 mEq to 1 liter of IV fluid and infuse over 4-8 hours.
    -KCL 40 mEq PO tid (in addition to IV); max total dose 100-200 mEq/d (3 mEq/kg/d).
Chronic Therapy:
    -KCL elixir 1-3 tablespoon qd-tid PO after meals (20 mEq/Tbsp of 10% sln) **OR**
    -Micro-K 10 mEq tabs 2-3 tabs PO tid after meals (40-100 mEq/d) **OR**
    -K-Dur 20 mEq tabs 1 PO bid-tid.
Hypokalemia with metabolic acidosis:
    -Potassium citrate 15-30 mL in juice PO qid after meals (1 mEq/mL).
    -Potassium gluconate 15 mL in juice PO qid after meals (20 mEq/15 mL).
9. **Extras:** ECG, dietetics consult.
10. **Labs:** CBC, magnesium, SMA 7&12. UA, urine Na, pH, 24h urine for K, creatinine.

Hypermagnesemia

1. **Admit to:**
2. **Diagnosis:** Hypermagnesemia
3. **Condition:**
4. **Vital signs:** q6h. Call physician if QRS >0.14 sec.
5. **Activity:** Up ad lib
6. **Nursing:** Inputs and outputs, daily weights.
7. **Diet:** Regular
8. **Special Medications:**
    -Saline diuresis 0.9% saline infused at 100-200 cc/h to replace urine loss **AND**
    -Calcium chloride, 1-3 gm added to saline infusate (10% sln; 1 gm per 10 mL amp) to run at 1 gm/hr **AND**
    -Furosemide (Lasix) 20-40 mg IV q4-6h as needed.
    -Magnesium >9.0 requires stat hemodialysis because of risk of respiratory failure.
9. **Extras:** ECG
10. **Labs:** Magnesium, calcium, SMA 7&12, creatinine. 24 hour urine magnesium, creatinine.

Hypomagnesemia

1. **Admit to:**
2. **Diagnosis:** Hypomagnesemia
3. **Condition:**
4. **Vital signs:** q6h
5. **Activity:** Up ad lib
6. **Diet:** Regular
7. **Special Medications:**

-Magnesium sulfate 4-6 gm in 500 mL D5W IV at 1 gm/hr. Hold if no patellar reflex. (Estimation of Mg deficit = 0.2 x kg weight x desired increase in Mg concentration; give deficit over 2-3d) **OR**

-Magnesium sulfate (severe hypomagnesemia <1.0) 1-2 gm (2-4 mL of 50% sln) IV over 15 min, **OR**

-Magnesium chloride (Slow-Mag) 65-130 mg (1-2 tabs) PO tid-qid (64 mg or 5.3 mEq/tab) **OR**

-Milk of magnesia 5 mL PO qd-qid.

8. **Extras:** ECG
9. **Labs:** Magnesium, calcium, SMA 7&12. Urine Mg, electrolytes, 24h urine magnesium, creatinine.

Hypernatremia

1. **Admit to:**
2. **Diagnosis:** Hypernatremia
3. **Condition:**
4. **Vital signs:** q2h. Call physician if BP >160/90, <70/50; P >140, <50; R>25, <10; T >38.5°C.
5. **Activity:** Bed rest; up in chair as tolerated.
6. **Nursing:** Inputs and outputs, daily weights.
7. **Diet:** No added salt.
8. **Special Medications:**

Hypernatremia with Hypovolemia:

If volume depleted, give 1-2 L NS IV over 1-3 hours until not orthostatic, then give D5W IV or PO to replace half of body water deficit over first 24hours (attempt to correct sodium at 1 mEq/L/h), then remaining deficit over next 1-2 days.

Body water deficit (L) = $\frac{0.6(\text{weight kg})([\text{Na serum}]-140)}{140}$

Hypernatremia with ECF Volume Excess:

-Furosemide 40-80 mg IV or PO qd-bid.
-Salt poor albumin (25%) 50-100 mL bid-tid x 48-72 h.

Hypernatremia with Diabetes Insipidus:

-D5W to correct body water deficit (see above).
-Pitressin 5-10 U IM/IV q6h or desmopressin (DDAVP) 4 mcg IV/SQ q12h; keep urine specific gravity >1.010.

9. **Extras:** CXR, ECG.
10. **Labs:** SMA 7&12, serum osmolality, liver panel, ADH, plasma renin activity. UA, urine specific gravity. Urine osmolality, Na, 24h urine K, creatinine.

Hyponatremia

1. **Admit to:**
2. **Diagnosis:** Hyponatremia
3. **Condition:**
4. **Vital signs:** q4h. Call physician if BP >160/90, <70/50; P >140, <50; R>25, <10; T >38.5°C.
5. **Activity:** Up in chair as tolerated.
6. **Nursing:** Inputs and outputs, daily weights.
7. **Diet:** Regular diet.
8. **Special Medications:**

Hyponatremia with Hypervolemia and Edema (low osmolality <280, UNa <10 mmol/L: nephrosis, heart failure, cirrhosis):

-Water restrict to 0.5-1.0 L/d.
-Furosemide 40-80 mg IV or PO qd-bid.

Hyponatremia with Normal Volume Status (low osmolality <280, UNa <10 mmol: water intoxication; UNa >20: SIADH, diuretic-induced):

-Water restrict to 0.5-1.5 L/d.

Hyponatremia with Hypovolemia (low osmolality <280) UNa <10 mmol/L: vomiting, diarrhea, third space/respiratory/skin loss; UNa >20 mmol/L: diuretics, renal injury, RTA, adrenal insufficiency, partial obstruction, salt wasting:

If volume depleted, give 0.5-2 L of 0.9% saline over 1-2 hours until no longer hypotensive, then 0.9% saline at 125 cc/h or 100-500 cc 3% hypertonic saline over 4h.

Severe Symptomatic Hyponatremia:

If volume depleted, give 1-2 L of 0.9% saline (154 mEq/L) over 1-2 hours until no longer orthostatic.

Determine volume of 3% hypertonic saline (513 mEq/L) to be infused:

$$\text{Na (mEq) deficit} = 0.6 \times (\text{wt kg}) \times (\text{desired [Na]} - \text{actual [Na]})$$

$$\frac{\text{Volume of sln (L)}}{\text{Number of hrs}} = \frac{\text{Sodium to be infused (mEq)}}{(\text{mEq/L in sln}) \times \text{Number of hrs}}$$

-Correct half of sodium deficit intravenously over 24 hours until serum sodium is 120 mEq/L; increase sodium by 12-20 mEq/L over 24 hours (1 mEq/L/h).
-Alternative Method: 3% saline 100-300 cc over 4-6h, repeated as needed.
9. **Extras:** CXR, ECG, head/chest CT scan.
10. **Labs:** SMA 7&12, osmolality, triglyceride, liver panel. UA, urine specific gravity. Urine osmolality, Na.

Hyperphosphatemia

1. **Admit to:**
2. **Diagnosis:** Hyperphosphatemia
3. **Condition:**
4. **Vital signs:** qid
5. **Activity:** Up ad lib
6. **Nursing:** Inputs and outputs
7. **Diet:** Low phosphorus diet with 0.7-1 gm/d
8. **Special Medications:**
Moderate Hyperphosphatemia:
-Restrict dietary phosphate to 0.7-1.0 gm/d.
-Calcium acetate (Phoslo) 1-3 tabs PO tid with meals, **OR**
-Aluminum hydroxide (Amphojel) 5-10 mL or 1-2 tablets PO before meals tid.
Severe Hyperphosphatemia:
-Volume expansion with 0.9% saline 1-2 L over 1-2h.
-Acetazolamide (Diamox) 500 mg PO or IV q6h.
-Consider dialysis.
9. **Extras:** CXR PA and LAT, ECG.
10. **Labs:** Phosphate, SMA 7&12, magnesium, calcium. UA, parathyroid hormone.

Hypophosphatemia

1. **Admit to:**
2. **Diagnosis:** Hypophosphatemia
3. **Condition:**
4. **Vital signs:** qid
5. **Activity:** Up ad lib
6. **Nursing:** Inputs and outputs.
7. **Diet:** Regular diet.
8. **Special Medications:**
Mild to Moderate Hypophosphatemia (1.0-2.2 mg/dL):
-Sodium or potassium phosphate 0.25 mMoles/kg in 150-250 mL of NS or D5W at 10 mMoles/h.
-Neutral phosphate (Nutra-Phos), 2 tab PO bid (250 mg elemental phospho-

rus/tab) **OR**
-Phospho-Soda 5 mL (129 mg phosphorus) PO bid-tid.
Severe Hypophosphatemia (<1.0 mg/dL):
  -Na or K phosphate 0.5 mMoles/kg in 250 mL D5W or NS, IV infusion at 10 mMoles/hr **OR**
  -Add potassium phosphate to IV solution in place of maintenance KCL; max IV dose 7.5 mg phosphorus/kg/6h.
9. Extras: CXR PA and LAT, ECG.
10. Labs: Phosphate, SMA 7&12, Mg, calcium, UA.

Rheumatologic Disorders

Systemic Lupus Erythematosus

1. **Admit to:**
2. **Diagnosis:** Systemic Lupus Erythematosus
3. **Condition:**
4. **Vital signs:** tid
5. **Allergies:**
6. **Activity:** Up as tolerated with bathroom privileges
7. **Nursing:**
8. **Diet:** No added salt, low psoralen diet.
9. **Special Medications:**
   -Ibuprofen (Motrin) 400 mg PO qid (max 2.4 g/d) **OR**
   -Indomethacin (Indocin) 25-50 mg tid-qid.
   -Hydroxychloroquine (Plaquenil) 200-600 mg/d PO
   -Prednisone 60-100 mg PO qd, may increase to 200-300 mg/d. Maintenance 10-20 mg PO qd or 20-40 mg PO qOD **OR**
   -Methylprednisolone (pulse therapy) 500 mg IV over 30 min q12h for 3-5d, then prednisone 50 mg PO qd.
   -Betamethasone dipropionate (Diprolene) 0.05% ointment applied bid.
10. **Extras:** CXR PA, LAT, ECG. Rheumatology consult.
11. **Labs:** CBC, platelets, SMA 7&12, INR/PTT, ESR, complement CH-50, C3, C4, C-reactive protein, LE prep, Coombs test, VDRL, rheumatoid factor, ANA, DNA binding, lupus anticoagulant, anticardiolipin, antinuclear cytoplasmic antibody. UA.

Acute Gout Attack

1. **Admit to:**
2. **Diagnosis:** Acute gout attack
3. **Condition:**
4. **Vital signs:** tid
5. **Activity:** Bed rest with bedside commode
6. **Nursing:** Keep foot elevated; support sheets over foot; guaiac stools.
7. **Diet:** Low purine diet.
8. **Special Medications:**
   -Ibuprofen (Motrin) 800 mg, then 400-800 mg PO q4-6h **OR**
   -Diclofenac (Voltaren) 25-75 mg tid-qid with food **OR**
   -Indomethacin (Indocin) 25-50 mg PO q6h for 2d, then 50 mg tid for 2 days, then 25 mg PO tid **OR**
   -Ketorolac (Toradol) 30-60 mg IV/IM, then 15-30 mg IV/IM q6h or 10 mg PO tid-qid **OR**
   -Naproxen sodium (Anaprox, Anaprox-DS) 550 mg PO bid **OR**
   -Methylprednisolone (SoluMedrol) 125 mg IV x 1 dose **THEN**
   -Prednisone 60 mg PO qd for 5 days, followed by tapering.
   -Colchicine 2 tablets (0.5 mg or 0.6 mg), followed by 1 tablet q1h until relief, max dose of 9.6 mg/24h. Maintenance colchicine: 0.5-0.6 mg PO qd-bid.
   Hypouricemic Therapy:
   -Probenecid (Benemid), 250 mg bid. Increase the dosage to 500 mg bid after 1 week, then increase by 500-mg increments every 4 weeks until the uric acid level is below 6.5 mg/dL. Max dose 2 g/d. Contraindicated during acute attack.
   -Allopurinol (Zyloprim) 300 mg PO qd, may increase by 100-300 mg q2weeks. Usually initiated after the acute attack.
9. **Symptomatic Medications:**
   -Ranitidine (Zantac) 150 mg PO bid.
   -Meperidine (Demerol) 50-100 mg IM/IV q4-6h prn pain **OR**
   -Hydrocodone/acetaminophen (Vicodin), 1-2 tab q4-6h PO prn pain

10. **Labs:** CBC, SMA 7, uric acid. UA with micro. Synovial fluid for light and polarizing micrography for crystals; C&S, Gram stain, glucose, protein, cell count. X-ray views of joint. 24 hour urine for uric acid.

PEDIATRICS

General Pediatrics

Pediatric History and Physical Examination

History

Identifying Data: Patient's name; age, sex. List the patient's significant medical problems. Name and relationship to child of informant (patient, mother).
Chief Compliant: Reason given by patient/informant for seeking medical care and the duration of the symptom(s).
History of Present Illness (HPI): Describe the course of the patient's illness, including when it began, character of the symptom(s); aggravating or alleviating factors; pertinent positives and negatives. Past diagnostic testing.
Past Medical History (PMH): Past diseases, surgeries, hospitalizations; medical problems; history of asthma.
Birth History: Gestational age at birth, preterm, obstetrical problems.
Developmental History: Motor skills, language development, self-care skills.
Medications: Include prescription and OTC drugs, vitamins, herbal products, natural remedies, nutritional supplements.
Feedings: Diet, volume of formula per day.
Immunizations: Up-to-date?
Drug Allergies: Penicillin, codeine?
Food Allergies:
Family History: Medical problems in family, including the patient's disorder. Asthma, cancer, tuberculosis, allergies.
Social History: Family situation, alcohol, smoking, drugs. Level of education.
Review of Systems (ROS):
  General: Weight loss, fever, chills, fatigue, night sweats.
  Skin: Rashes, skin discolorations.
  Head: Headaches, dizziness, seizures.
  Eyes: Visual changes.
  Ears: Tinnitus, vertigo, hearing loss.
  Nose: Nose bleeds, discharge.
  Mouth and Throat: Dental disease, hoarseness, throat pain.
  Respiratory: Cough, shortness of breath, sputum (color and consistency).
  Cardiovascular: Dyspnea on exertion, edema, valvular disease.
  Gastrointestinal: Abdominal pain, vomiting, diarrhea, constipation.
  Genitourinary: Dysuria, frequency, hematuria.
  Gynecological: Last menstrual period (frequency, duration), age of menarche; dysmenorrhea, contraception, vaginal bleeding, breast masses.
  Endocrine: Polyuria, polydipsia.
  Musculoskeletal: Joint pain or swelling, arthritis, myalgias.
  Skin and Lymphatics: Easy bruising, lymphadenopathy.
  Neuropsychiatric: Weakness, seizures.
  Pain: quality (sharp/stabbing, aching, pressure), location, duration

Physical Examination

General appearance: Note whether the patient looks "ill," well, or malnourished.
Physical Measurements: weight, height, head circumference (plot on growth charts).
Vital Signs: Temperature, heart rate, respiratory rate, blood pressure.
Skin: Rashes, scars, moles, skin turgor, capillary refill (in seconds).
Lymph Nodes: Cervical, axillary, inguinal nodes: size, tenderness.
Head: Bruising, masses, fontanels.
Eyes: Pupils: equal, round, and reactive to light and accommodation (PERRLA); extra ocular movements intact (EOMI). Funduscopy (papilledema, hemorrhages, exudates).
Ears: Acuity, tympanic membranes (dull, shiny, intact, infected, bulging).

Mouth and Throat: Mucus membrane color and moisture; oral lesions, dentition, pharynx, tonsils.
Neck: Thyromegaly, lymphadenopathy, masses.
Chest: Equal expansion, rhonchi, crackles, rubs, breath sounds.
Heart: Regular rate and rhythm (RRR), first and second heart sounds (S1, S2); gallops (S3, S4), murmurs (grade 1-6), pulses (graded 0-2+).
Breast: Discharge, masses; axillary masses.
Abdomen: Bowel sounds, bruits, tenderness, masses; hepatomegaly, splenomegaly; guarding, rebound, percussion note (tympanic), suprapubic tenderness.
Genitourinary: Inguinal masses, hernias, scrotum, testicles.
Pelvic Examination: Vaginal mucosa, cervical discharge, uterine size, masses, adnexal masses, ovaries.
Extremities: Joint swelling, range of motion, edema (grade 1-4+); cyanosis, clubbing, edema (CCE); pulses.
Rectal Examination: Sphincter tone, masses, fissures; test for occult blood
Neurological: Mental status and affect; gait, strength (graded 0-5), sensation, deep tendon reflexes (biceps, triceps, patellar, ankle; graded 0-4+).
Labs: Electrolytes (sodium, potassium, bicarbonate, chloride, BUN, creatinine), CBC (hemoglobin, hematocrit, WBC count, platelets, differential); x-rays, ECG, urine analysis (UA), liver function tests (LFTs).
Assessment (Impression): Assign a number to each problem and discuss separately. Discuss differential diagnosis and give reasons that support the working diagnosis; give reasons for excluding other diagnoses.
Plan: Describe therapeutic plan for each numbered problem, including testing, laboratory studies, medications.

Progress Notes

Daily progress notes should summarize developments in a patient's hospital course, problems that remain active, plans to treat those problems, and arrangements for discharge. Progress notes should address every element of the problem list.

Example Progress Note

Date/time:
Identify Discipline and Level of Education: e.g. Pediatric resident PL-3
Subjective: Any problems and symptoms of the patient should be charted. Appetite, pain, or fussiness may be included.
Objective:
General appearance.
Vitals, including highest temperature (T^{max}) over past 24 hours. Feedings, fluid inputs and outputs (I/O), including oral and parenteral intake and urine and stool volume output.
Physical exam, including chest and abdomen, with particular attention to active problems. Emphasize changes from previous physical exams.
Labs: Include new test results and flag abnormal values.
Current Medications: List all medications and dosages.
Assessment and Plan: This section should be organized by problem. A separate assessment and plan should be written for each problem.

Discharge Note

The discharge note should be written in the patient's chart prior to discharge.

Discharge Note

Date/time:
Diagnoses:
Treatment: Briefly describe treatment provided during hospitalization, including surgical procedures and antibiotic therapy.
Studies Performed: Electrocardiograms, CT scans.
Discharge Medications:
Follow-up Arrangements:

Prescription Writing

- Patient's name:
- Date:
- Drug name, dosage form, dose, route, frequency (include concentration for oral liquids or mg strength for oral solids): Amoxicillin 125mg/5mL 5 mL PO tid
- Quantity to dispense: mL for oral liquids, # of oral solids
- Refills: If appropriate
- Signature

Procedure Note

A procedure note should be written in the chart after a procedure is performed (eg, lumbar puncture).

Procedure Note

Date and time:
Procedure:
Indications:
Patient Consent: Document that the indications, risks and alternatives to the procedure were explained to the parents and patient. Note that the parents and the patient were given the opportunity to ask questions and that the parents consented to the procedure in writing.
Lab tests: Relevant labs, such as the CBC
Anesthesia: Local with 2% lidocaine
Description of Procedure: Briefly describe the procedure, including sterile prep, anesthesia method, patient position, devices used, ana-tomic location of procedure, and outcome.
Complications and Estimated Blood Loss (EBL):
Disposition: Describe how the patient tolerated the procedure.
Specimens: Describe any specimens obtained and labs tests which were ordered.

Developmental Milestones

Age	Milestones
1 month	Raises head slightly when prone; alerts to sound; regards face, moves extremities equally.
2-3 months	Smiles, holds head up, coos, reaches for familiar objects, recognizes parent.
4-5 months	Rolls front to back and back to front; sits well when propped; laughs, orients to voice; enjoys looking around; grasps rattle, bears some weight on legs.
6 months	Sits unsupported; passes cube hand to hand; babbles; uses raking grasp; feeds self crackers.
8-9 months	Crawls, cruises; pulls to stand; pincer grasp; plays pat-a-cake; feeds self with bottle; sits without support; explores environment.
12 months	Walking, talking a few words; understands "no"; says "mama/dada" discriminantly; throws objects; imitates actions, marks with crayon, drinks from a cup.
15-18 months	Comes when called; scribbles; walks backward; uses 4-20 words; builds tower of 2 blocks.
24-30 months	Removes shoes; follows 2 step command; jumps with both feet; holds pencil, knows first and last name; knows pronouns. Parallel play; points to body parts, runs, spoon feeds self, copies parents.
3 years	Dresses and undresses; walks up and down steps; draws a circle; uses 3-4 word sentences; takes turns; shares. Group play.
4 years	Hops, skips, catches ball; memorizes songs; plays cooperatively; knows colors; copies a circle; uses plurals.
5 years	Jumps over objects; prints first name; knows address and mother's name; follows game rules; draws three part man; hops on one foot.

Immunizations

Immunization Schedule for Infants and Children		
Age	**Immunizations**	**Comments**
Birth - 2 mo	HBV	If mother is HbsAg positive or unknown status, the first dose of HBV should be given within 12 hours of birth along with hepatitis B immune globulin 0.5 mL.
1-4 mo	HBV	The second HBV dose should be given at least one month after the first dose. For infants of HbsAg positive or unknown status mothers, the second dose should be given at 1-2 months of age.
2 mo	DTaP, Hib, IPV, PCV	DTP and Hib are available combined as Tetramune. The pneumococcal vaccine recommendation is new for 2001.
4 mo	DTaP, Hib, IPV, PCV	
6 mo	DTaP, (Hib), PCV	Dose 3 of Hib is not indicated if the product for doses 1 and 2 was PedvaxHIB.
6-18 mo	HBV, IPV	The third HBV dose should be administered at least 4 months after the first dose and at least 2 months after the second dose. For infants of HbsAg positive or unknown status mothers, the third dose should be given at 6 months of age.
12-15 mo 12-18 mo	Hib, PCV, MMR VAR	Tuberculin testing may be done at the same visit if indicated. Varicella vaccine is recommended in children who do not have a reliable history of having had the clinical disease.
15-18 mo	DTaP	The 4th dose of DTaP should be given 6-12 mo after the third dose of DTaP and may be given as early as 12 mo, provided that the interval between doses 3 and 4 is at least 6 mo.
4-6 yr	DTaP, IPV, MMR	DTaP and IPV should be given at or before school entry. DTaP should not be given after the 7th birthday
11-12 yr	MMR	Omit if MMR dose was given at age 4-6 years.
14-16 yr	Td	Repeat every 10 yrs throughout life

Age	Immunizations	Comments
HBV = Hepatitis B virus vaccine; DTaP = diphtheria and tetanus toxoids and acellular pertussis vaccine; Hib = Haemophilus influenzae type b conjugate vaccine; IPV = inactivated polio vaccine; MMR = live measles, mumps, and rubella viruses vaccine; PCV = pneumococcal conjugate vaccine (Prevnar); Td = adult tetanus toxoid (full dose) and diphtheria toxoid (reduced dose), for children >7 yr and adults; VAR = varicella virus vaccine		

Recommended Schedule for Children Younger than 7 Years Not Immunized in the First Year of Life

Age	Immunizations	Comments
First visit	DTaP, (Hib), HBV, MMR, IPV, (PCV), VAR	If indicated, tuberculin testing may be done at the same visit. If child is ≥5 years, Hib is not indicated. PCV recommended for all children < 2 yrs or 24-59 months of age and at high risk for invasive pneumococcal disease (e.g. sickle cell anemia, HIV, immunocompromised). Varicella vaccine if child has not had varicella disease.
Interval after 1st visit 1 month 2 months ≥8 months	DTaP, HBV DTaP, Hib, IPV, (PCV) DTaP, HBV, IPV	Second dose of Hib is indicated only if first dose was received when <15 months. Second dose of PCV 6-8 weeks after first dose (if criteria met above).
4-6 years (at or before school entry)	DTaP, IPV, MMR	DTaP is not necessary if the fourth dose was given after the fourth birthday. IPV is not necessary if the third dose was given after the fourth birthday.
11-12 yr	MMR	MMR should be given at entry to middle school or junior high school if it wasn't given at age 4-6 years.
10 yr later	Td	Repeat every 10 yrs
HBV = Hepatitis B virus vaccine; DTaP = diphtheria and tetanus toxoids and acellular pertussis vaccine; Hib = Haemophilus influenzae type b conjugate vaccine; IPV = inactivated polio vaccine; MMR = live measles, mumps, and rubella viruses vaccine; PCV = pneumococcal conjugate vaccine (Prevnar); Td = adult tetanus toxoid (full dose) and diphtheria toxoid (reduced dose), for children >7 yr and adults; VAR = varicella virus vaccine		

Recommended Schedule for Children >7 Years Who Were Not Immunized Previously		
Age	**Immunizations**	**Comments**
First visit	HBV, IPV, MMR, Td, VAR	Varicella vaccine if child has not had varicella disease.
Interval after First visit 2 months 8-14 months	HBV, IPV, Td, VAR, MMR HBV, Td, IPV	If child is ≥ 13 years old, a second varicella vaccine dose is needed 4-8 weeks after the first dose.
11-12 yrs old	MMR	Omit if MMR dose was given at age 4-6 years.
10 yr later	Td	Repeat every 10 years
HBV = Hepatitis B virus vaccine; DTaP = diphtheria and tetanus toxoids and acellular pertussis vaccine; Hib = Haemophilus influenzae type b conjugate vaccine; IPV = inactivated polio vaccine; MMR = live measles, mumps, and rubella viruses vaccine; PCV = pneumococcal conjugate vaccine (Prevnar); Td = adult tetanus toxoid (full dose) and diphtheria toxoid (reduced dose), for children >7 yr and adults; VAR = varicella virus vaccine		

Haemophilus Immunization

H influenzae type b Vaccination in Children Immunized Beginning at 2 to 6 Months of Age		
Vaccine Product	**Total Number of Doses**	**Regimens**
PedvaxHIB (PRP-OMP)	3	2 doses two months apart plus booster at 12-15 months which must be at least two months after previous dose. Any vaccine may be used for the booster.
HibTITER (HbOC), ActHIB (PRP-T), OmniHIB (PRP-T)	4	3 doses two months apart plus booster at 12-15 months which must be at least two months after previous dose. Any vaccine may be used for the booster.

H influenzae type b Vaccination When the Initial Vaccination was Delayed Until 7 Months of Age or Older			
Age at Initiation	**Vaccine Product**	**Total Doses**	**Regimens**
7-11 mo	any vaccine (PedvaxHIB or HibTITER or ActHIB or OmniHIB)	3	2 doses at 2-month intervals plus booster at 12-18 months (at least 2 months after previous dose)

Age at Initiation	Vaccine Product	Total Doses	Regimens
12-14 mo	any vaccine	2	2 doses 2 months apart
15-59 mo	any vaccine	1	Single dose of any product
≥5 years	Any vaccine	1	Only recommended for children with chronic illness known to be associated with an increased risk for H flu disease.

Varicella Immunization

Indications for Varicella Immunization:
- A. Age 12 to 18 months: One dose of varicella vaccine is recommended for universal immunization for all healthy children who lack a reliable history of varicella.
- B. Age 19 months to the 13th birthday: Vaccination of susceptible children is recommended and may be given any time during childhood but before the 13th birthday because of the potential increased severity of natural varicella after this age. Susceptible is defined by either lack of proof of either varicella vaccination or a reliable history of varicella. One dose is recommended.
- C. Healthy adolescents and young adults: Healthy adolescents past their 13th birthday who have not been immunized previously and have no history of varicella infection should be immunized against varicella by administration of two doses of vaccine 4 to 8 weeks apart. Longer intervals between doses do not necessitate a third dose, but may leave the individual unprotected during the intervening months.
- D. All susceptible children aged 1 year to 18 years old who are in direct contact with people at high risk for varicella related complications (eg, immunocompromised individuals) and who have not had a documented case of varicella.

Influenza Immunization

Indications for Influenza Vaccination
- A. Targeted high-risk children and adolescents (eg, chronic pulmonary disease including asthma, sickle cell anemia, HIV infection).
- B. Other high-risk children and adolescents (eg, diabetes mellitus, chronic renal disease, chronic metabolic disease).
- C. Close contacts of high risk patients.
- D. Foreign travel if exposure is likely.

Vaccine Administration. Administer in the Fall, usually October 1 - November 15, before the start of the influenza season.

Influenza Immunization Administration			
Age	Vaccine Type	Dosage (mL)	Number of Doses
6-35 months	Split virus only	0.25	1-2*
3-8 yrs	Split virus only	0.5	1-2*
9-12 yrs	Split virus only	0.5	1
> 12 yrs	Whole or split virus	0.5	1

*Two doses administered at least one month apart are recommended for children who are receiving influenza vaccine for the first time.

Pediatric Symptomatic Care

Antipyretics

Analgesics/Antipyretics:
-Acetaminophen (Tylenol) 10-20 mg/kg/dose PO/PR q4-6h, max 5 doses/day or 80 mg/kg/day or 4 gm/day (whichever is smaller) **OR**
-Acetaminophen dose by age (if weight appropriate for age):

AGE:	mg/dose PO/PR q4-6h prn:
0-3 mo	40 mg/dose
4-11 mo	80 mg/dose
1-2 yr	120 mg/dose
2-3 yr	160 mg/dose
4-5 yr	240 mg/dose
6-8 yr	320 mg/dose
9-10 yr	400 mg/dose
11-12 yr	480 mg/dose
>12 yr	325-650 mg/dose

-Preparations: caplets: 160, 500 mg; caplet, ER: 650 mg; drops: 80 mg/0.8 mL; elixir: 80 mg/2.5 mL, 80 mg/5 mL, 120 mg/5 mL, 160 mg/5 mL, 325 mg/5 mL, 500 mg/15 mL; suppositories: 80, 120, 325, 650 mg; tabs: 325, 500 mg; tabs, chewable: 80, 120, 160 mg.
-Ibuprofen (Motrin, Advil, Nuprin, Medipren, Children's Motrin)
    Analgesic: 4-10 mg/kg/dose PO q6-8h prn
    Antipyretic: 5-10 mg/kg/dose PO q6-8h.
-Preparations: cap: 200 mg; caplet: 100 mg; oral drops: 40 mg/mL; susp: 100 mg/5 mL; tabs: 100, 200, 300, 400, 600, 800 mg; tabs, chewable: 50, 100 mg.
May cause GI distress, bleeding.

Antitussives, Decongestants, Expectorants, and Antihistamines

Antihistamines:
    -Brompheniramine (Dimetane) [elixir: 2 mg/5 mL; tab: 4, 8, 12 mg; tab, SR: 8, 12 mg]
      < 6 yr: 0.5 mg/kg/day PO q6h prn (max 8 mg/day)
      6-11 yr: 2-4 mg PO q6-8h
      ≥12 yr: 4-8 mg PO q4-6h or 8 mg SR PO q8-12h or 12 mg SR PO q12h (max 24 mg/day).
    -Chlorpheniramine (Chlor-Trimeton) [cap, SR: 8, 12 mg; syrup 2mg/5mL; tabs: 4, 8, 12 mg; tab, chew: 2 mg; tab, SR: 8, 12 mg]
      2-5 yr: 1 mg PO q4-6h prn
      6-11 yr: 2 mg PO q4-6h prn
      ≥ 12 yr: 4 mg PO q4-6h prn or 8-12 mg SR PO q8-12h
Antitussives (Pure) - Dextromethorphan:
    -Benylin DM Cough Syrup [syrup: 10 mg/5mL]
    -Benylin Pediatric [syrup: 37.5mg/5mL]
    -Robitussin Pediatric [syrup: 7.5 mg/5mL]
    -Vick's Formula 44 Pediatric Formula [syrup: 3 mg/5mL]
      2-5 yr: 2.5-5 mg PO q4h prn or 7.5 mg PO q6-8h prn
      6-11 yr 5-10 mg PO q4h prn or 15 mg PO q6-8h prn
      ≥12 yr: 10-20 mg PO q4h prn or 30 mg PO q6-8h prn.
Expectorants:
    -Guaifenesin (Robitussin) [syrup: 100 mg/5 mL]
      <2 yr: 12 mg/kg/day PO q4-6h prn
      2-5 yr: 50-100 mg PO q4h prn (max 600 mg/day)

6-11 yr: 100-200 mg PO q4h prn (max 1.2 gm/day)

≥12 yr: 100-400 mg PO q4h prn (max 2.4 gm/day)

May irritate gastric mucosa; take with large quantities of fluids.

Decongestants:

-Pseudoephedrine (Sudafed, Novafed): [cap: 60 mg; cap, SR: 120, 240 mg; drops: 7.5 mg/0.8 mL; syrup: 15 mg/5 mL, 30 mg/5 mL; tabs: 30, 60 mg].
<2 yr: 4 mg/kg/day PO q6h.
2-5 yr: 15 mg po q6h
6-11 yr: 30 mg po q6h
>12 yr: 30-60 mg/dose PO q6h or sustained release 120 mg PO q12h or sustained release 240 mg PO q24h.

-Phenylephrine (Neo-synephrine) [nasal drops: 1/4, 1/2, 1%; nasal spray: 1/4, 1/2, 1%].
Children: Use 1/4 % spray or drops, 1-2 drops/spray in each nostril q3-4h.
Adults: Use 1/4-1/2% drops/spray, 1-2 drops/sprays in each nostril q3-4h
Discontinue use after 3 days to avoid rebound congestion.

Combination Products:

-Actifed [per cap or tab or 10 mL syrup: Triprolidine 2.5 mg, Pseudoephedrine 60 mg].
4 mth-2 yr: 1.25 mL PO q6-8h
2-4 yr: 2.5 mL PO q6-8h
4-6 yr: 3.75 mL PO q6-8h
6-11y: 5 mL or ½ tab PO q6-8h

≥12 yr: 10 mL or 1 cap/tab PO q6-8h **OR**
4 mg pseudoephedrine/kg/day PO tid-qid

-Actifed with Codeine cough syrup [syrup/5 mL: Codeine 10 mg, Triprolidine 1.25 mg, Pseudoephedrine 30 mg].
4 mth-2 yr: 1.25 mL PO q6-8h
2-4 yr: 2.5 mL PO q6-8h
4-6 yr: 3.75 mL PO q6-8h
6-11y: 5 mL PO q6-8h

≥12 yr: 10 mL PO q6-8h **OR**
4 mg pseudoephedrine/kg/day PO tid-qid.

-Dimetane Decongestant [cap/cplt or 10 mL: Brompheniramine 4 mg, Phenylephrine 5 mg].
6-11 yr: 5 mL or ½ cap/caplet PO q4-6h prn

≥ 12 yr: 10 mL or 1 cap/caplet PO q4-6h prn

-Dimetane DX [syrup per 5 mL: Brompheniramine 2 mg, Dextromethorphan 10 mg, Pseudoephedrine 30 mg].
2-5 yrs: 2.5 mL PO q4-6h prn
6-11 yrs: 5 mL PO q4-6h prn

≥ 12 yrs: 10 mL PO q4-6h prn

-PediaCare Cough-Cold Chewable Tablets: [tab, chew: Pseudoephedrine 15 mg, Chlorpheniramine 1 mg, Dextromethorphan 5 mg].
3-5 yr: 1 tab PO q4-6h prn (max 4 tabs/day)
6-11 yr: 2 tabs PO q4-6h (max 8 tabs/day)

≥12 yr: 4 tabs PO q4-6h (max 16 tabs/day)

-PediaCare Cough-Cold Liquid [liquid per 5 mL: Pseudoephedrine 15 mg, Chlorpheniramine 1 mg, Dextromethorphan 5 mg].
3-5 yr: 5 mL PO q6-8h prn
6-11 yr: 10 mL PO q6-8h prn

≥12 yr: 20 mL PO q6-8h prn

-PediaCare Night Rest Cough-Cold Liquid [liquid per 5 mL: Pseudoephedrine 15 mg, Chlorpheniramine 1 mg, Dextromethorphan 7.5 mg].
3-5 yr: 5 mL PO q6-8h prn
6-11 yr: 10 mL PO q6-8h prn

≥12 yr: 20 mL PO q6-8h prn

-Phenergan VC [syrup per 5 mL: Phenylephrine 5 mg, Promethazine 6.25 mg].

2-5 yr: 1.25 mL PO q4-6h prn
6-11 yr: 2.5 mL PO q4-6h prn

≥12 yr: 5 mL PO q4-6h prn
-Phenergan VC with Codeine [per 5 mL: Promethazine 6.25 mg, Codeine 10 mg, Phenylephrine 5 mg].
2-5 yr: 1.25 mL PO q4-6h prn
6-11 yr: 2.5 mL PO q4-6h prn

≥12 yr: 5 mL PO q4-6h prn
Adults: 5-10 mL q4-6h prn (max 120 mg codeine per day)
-Phenergan with Codeine [syrup per 5 mL: Promethazine 6.25 mg, Codeine 10 mg].
2-5 yr: 1.25 mL PO q4-6h prn
6-11 yr: 2.5 mL PO q4-6h prn

≥12 yr: 5 mL PO q4-6h prn
Adults: 5-10 mL q4-6h prn (max 120 mg codeine per day)
-Phenergan with Dextromethorphan [syrup per 5 mL: Promethazine 6.25 mg, Dextromethorphan 15 mg].
2-5 yr: 1.25 mL PO q4-6h prn
6-11 yr: 2.5 mL PO q4-6h prn

≥12 yr: 5 mL PO q4-6h prn
-Robitussin AC [syrup per 5 mL: Guaifenesin 100 mg, Codeine 10 mg].
6 mos-2 yr: 1.25-2.5 mL PO q4h prn
2-5 yrs: 2.5 mL PO q4h prn
6-11 yrs: 5 mL PO q4h prn

≥12 yrs: 10 mL PO q4-6h prn.
-Robitussin-DAC [syrup per 5 mL: Codeine 10mg, Guaifenesin 100 mg, Pseudoephedrine 30 mg].
2-5 yrs: 1-1.5 mg/kg/day of codeine PO q4-6h prn (max 30 mg/day)
6-11 yrs: 5 mL PO q4-6h prn

≥12 yrs: 10 mL PO q4-6h prn
-Robitussin DM [syrup per 5 mL: Guaifenesin 100 mg, Dextromethorphan 10 mg].
2-5 yr: 2.5 mL PO q4h prn, max 10 mL/day
6-11 yr: 5 mL PO q4h prn, max 20 mL/day

≥12 yr: 10 mL PO q4h prn, max 40 mL/day
-Robitussin Pediatric Cough and Cold [syrup per 5 mL: Dextromethorphan 7.5mg, Pseudoephedrine 15 mg].
2-5 yr: 5 mL PO q4-6h prn
6-11 yr: 10 mL PO q4-6h prn

≥12 yr: 15 mL po q4-6h prn
Maximum four doses daily.
-Rondec drops [drops per 1 mL: Carbinoxamine maleate 2 mg, Pseudoephedrine 25 mg].
4-5 mg pseudoephedrine/kg/day PO q6h prn **OR**
1-3 m: 1/4 dropperful (1/4 mL) PO q6h prn
3-6 m: 1/2 dropperful (1/2 mL) PO q6h prn
6-9 m: 3/4 dropperful (0.75 mL) PO q6h prn
9-18 m: 1 dropperful (1 mL) PO q6h prn
-Rondec syrup [syrup per 5 mL: Pseudoephedrine 60 mg, Carbinoxamine maleate 4 mg].
4-5 mg pseudoephedrine/kg/day PO q6h prn.
-Rondec DM drops [drops per mL: Carbinoxamine maleate 2 mg, Pseudoephedrine 25 mg, Dextromethorphan 4 mg].
4-5 mg pseudoephedrine/kg/day PO q6h prn **OR**
1-3 m: 1/4 dropperful (1/4 mL) PO q6h prn
3-6 m: 1/2 dropperful (1/2 mL) PO q6h prn
6-9 m: 3/4 dropperful (0.75 mL) PO q6h prn
9-18 m: 1 dropperful (1 mL) PO q6h prn.

-Rondec DM syrup [syrup per 5 mL: Carbinoxamine maleate 4 mg, Pseudoephedrine 60 mg, Dextromethorphan 15 mg].
4-5 mg pseudoephedrine/kg/day PO q6h prn.

-Ryna Liquid [liquid per 5 mL: Chlorpheniramine 2 mg; Pseudoephedrine 30 mg].
6-11 yrs: 5 mL PO q6h prn

≥12 yr: 10 mL PO q6h prn

-Ryna-C [liquid per 5 mL: Chlorpheniramine 2mg, Codeine 10 mg, Pseudoephedrine 30 mg].
4-5 mg/kg/day of pseudoephedrine component PO q6h prn

-Ryna-CS [liquid per 5 mL: Codeine 10 mg, Guaifenesin 100 mg, Pseudoephedrine 30 mg].
4-5 mg pseudoephedrine/kg/day PO q6h prn

-Rynatan Pediatric [susp per 5 mL: Chlorpheniramine 2 mg, Phenylephrine 5 mg, Pyrilamine 12.5 mg].
2-5 yr: 2.5-5 mL PO bid prn
6-11 yr: 5-10 mL PO bid prn

≥12 yr: 10-15 mL PO bid prn

-Tylenol Cold Multi-Symptom Plus Cough Liquid, Children's [liquid per 5 mL: Acetaminophen 160 mg, Chlorpheniramine 1 mg, Pseudoephedrine 15 mg].
2-5 yr: 5 mL PO q4h prn
6-11 yr: 10 mL PO q4h prn

≥12 yr: 20 mL po q4h prn
Maximum four doses daily.

-Tylenol Cold Plus Cough Chewable Tablet, Children's [tab, chew: Acetaminophen 80 mg, Chlorpheniramine 0.5 mg, Dextromethorphan 2.5 mg, Pseudoephedrine 7.5 mg].
2-5 yr: 2 tabs PO q4h prn
6-11 yr: 4 tabs PO q4h prn

≥12 yr: 4 tabs PO q4h prn
Maximum four doses daily.

-Vick's Children's NyQuil Night-time Cough/Cold [liquid per 5 mL: Chlorpheniramine 0.67 mg; Dextromethorphan 5 mg, Pseudoephedrine 10 mg].
6-11 yr: 15 mL PO q6-8h prn

≥12 yr: 30 mL PO q6-8h prn

-Vicks Pediatric Formula 44D [liquid per 5 mL: Dextromethorphan 5 mg, Pseudoephedrine 10 mg].
2-5 yr: 3.75 mL PO q6h prn
6-11 yr: 7.5 mL po q6h prn

≥12 yr: 15 mL PO q6h prn

-Vicks Pediatric Formula 44E [syrup per 5 mL: Dextromethorphan 3.3 mg, Guaifenesin 33.3 mg].
2-5 yr: 5 mL PO q4h prn
6-11 yr: 10 mL PO q4h prn

≥12 yr: 15 mL po q4h prn

-Vick's Pediatric Formula 44M Multi-Symptom Cough and Cold Liquid [liquid per 5 mL: Chlorpheniramine 0.67 mg, Dextromethorphan 5 mg, Pseudoephedrine 10 mg].
2-5 yr: 7.5 mL PO q6h prn
6-11 yr: 15 mL PO q6h prn

≥12 yr: 30 mL PO q6h prn

Analgesia and Sedation

Analgesics/Anesthetic Agents:
  -Acetaminophen (Tylenol) 10-15 mg/kg PO/PR q4-6h prn (see page 97 for detailed list of available products)
  -Acetaminophen/Codeine [per 5 mL: Acetaminophen 120 mg, Codeine 12 mg; tabs: Tylenol #2: 15 mg codeine/300 mg acetaminophen; #3: 30 mg codeine/300 mg acetaminophen; #4: 60 mg codeine/300 mg acetaminophen]
  0.5-1.0 mg codeine/kg/dose PO q4h prn.
  -Acetaminophen/Hydrocodone [elixir per 5 mL: hydrocodone 2.5 mg, acetaminophen 167 mg]
  Tab:
  Lortab 2.5/500: Hydrocodone 2.5 mg, acetaminophen 500 mg
  Lortab 5/500 and Vicodin: Hydrocodone 5 mg, acetaminophen 500 mg
  Lortab 7.5/500: Hydrocodone 7.5 mg, acetaminophen 500 mg
  Vicodin ES: Hydrocodone 7.5 mg, acetaminophen 750 mg
  Lortab 10/500: Hydrocodone 10 mg, acetaminophen 500 mg
  Lortab 10/650: Hydrocodone 10 mg, acetaminophen 650 mg
  Children: 0.6 mg hydrocodone/kg/day PO q6-8h prn
    <2 yr: do not exceed 1.25 mg/dose
    2-12 yr: do not exceed 5 mg/dose
    >12 yr: do not exceed 10 mg/dose
  -ELAMax [lidocaine 4% cream (liposomal): 5, 30 gm]
  Apply 10-60 minutes prior to procedure. Occlusive dressing is optional. Available OTC.
  -EMLA cream (eutectic mixture of local anesthetics) [cream: 2.5% lidocaine and 2.5% prilocaine: 5, 30 gm; transdermal disc]. Apply and cover with occlusive dressing at least 1 hour (max 4 hours) prior to procedure.
  -Fentanyl 1-2 mcg/kg IV q1-2h prn or 1-3 mcg/kg/hr continuous IV infusion.
  -Hydromorphone (Dilaudid) 0.015 mg/kg IV/IM/SC q3-4h or
  0.0075 mg/kg/hr continuous IV infusion titrated as necessary for pain relief or 0.03-0.08 mg/kg PO q6h prn.
  -Ketamine 4 mg/kg IM or 0.5-1 mg/kg IV. Onset for IV administration is 30 seconds, duration is 5-15 minutes.
  -Lidocaine, buffered: Add sodium bicarbonate 1 mEq/mL 1 part to 9 parts lidocaine 1% for local infiltration (eg, 2 mL lidocaine 1% and 0.22 mL sodium bicarbonate 1 mEq/mL) to raise the pH of the lidocaine to neutral and decrease the "sting" of subcutaneous lidocaine.
  -Meperidine (Demerol) 1 mg/kg IV/IM q2-3h prn pain.
  -Morphine 0.05-0.1 mg/kg IV q2-4h prn or 0.02-0.06 mg/kg/hr continuous IV infusion or 0.1-0.15 mg/kg IM/SC q3-4h or 0.2-0.5 mg/kg PO q4-6h.

Sedation:
Fentanyl and Midazolam Sedation:
  -Fentanyl 1 mcg/kg IV slowly, may repeat to total of 3 mcg/kg **AND**
  -Midazolam (Versed) 0.05-0.1 mg/kg slow IV [inj: 1 mg/mL, 5 mg/mL].
  Have reversal agents available: naloxone 0.1 mg/kg (usual max 2 mg) IM/IV for fentanyl reversal and flumazenil 0.01 mg/kg (usual max 5 mg) IM/IV for midazolam reversal.
Benzodiazepines:
  -Diazepam (Valium) 0.2-0.5 mg/kg/dose PO/PR or 0.05-0.2 mg/kg/dose IM/IV, max 10 mg.
  -Lorazepam (Ativan) 0.05-0.1 mg/kg/dose IM/IV/PO, max 4 mg.
  -Midazolam (Versed) 0.08-0.2 mg/kg/dose IM/IV over 10-20 min, max 5 mg; or 0.2-0.4 mg/kg/dose PO x 1, max 15 mg, 30-45 min prior to procedure; or 0.2 mg/kg intranasal (using 5 mg/mL injectable solution, insert into nares with needleless tuberculin syringe.)
Phenothiazines:
  -Promethazine (Phenergan) 0.5-1 mg/kg/dose IM or slow IV over 20 min, max 50 mg/dose.

-Chlorpromazine (Thorazine) 0.5-1 mg/kg/dose IM or slow IV over 20min, max 50 mg/dose.

Antihistamines:
  -Diphenhydramine (Benadryl) 1 mg/kg/dose IV/IM/PO, max 50 mg.
  -Hydroxyzine (Vistaril) 0.5-1 mg/kg/dose IM/PO, max 50 mg.

Barbiturates:
  -Methohexital (Brevital)
    IM: 5-10 mg/kg
    IV: 1-2 mg/kg
    PR: 25 mg/kg (max 500 mg/dose)
  -Thiopental (Pentothal): Sedation, rectal: 5-10 mg/kg; seizures, IV: 2-3 mg/kg

Other Sedatives:
  -Chloral hydrate 25-100 mg/kg/dose PO/PR (max 1.5 gm/dose), allow 30 min for absorption.

Nonsteroidal Anti-inflammatory Drugs:
  -Ibuprofen (Motrin, Advil, Nuprin, Medipren, Children's Motrin)
    Anti-inflammatory: 30-50 mg/kg/day PO q6h, max 2400 mg/day.
    [cap: 200 mg; caplet: 100 mg; oral drops: 40 mg/mL; susp: 100 mg/5 mL; tabs: 100, 200, 300, 400, 600, 800 mg; tabs, chewable: 50, 100 mg].
  -Ketorolac (Toradol)
    Single dose: 0.4-1 mg/kg IV/IM (max 30 mg/dose IV, 60 mg/dose IM)
    Multiple doses: 0.4-0.5 mg/kg IV/IM q6h prn (max 30 mg/dose)
    [inj: 15 mg/mL, 30 mg/mL].
    Do not use for more than three days because of risk of GI bleed.
  -Naproxen (Naprosyn)
    Analgesia: 5-7 mg/kg/dose PO q8-12h
    Inflammatory disease: 10-15 mg/kg/day PO q12h, max 1000 mg/day
    [susp: 125 mg/5mL; tab: 250, 375, 500 mg; tab, DR: 375, 500 mg].
  -Naproxen sodium (Aleve, Anaprox, Naprelan)
    Analgesia: 5-7 mg/kg/dose PO q8-12h
    Inflammatory disease: 10-15 mg/kg/day PO q12h, max 1000 mg/day
    [tab: 220, 275, 550 mg; tab, ER: 375, 500, 750 mg]. Naproxen sodium 220 mg = 200 mg base.

Antiemetics

  -Chlorpromazine (Thorazine)
    0.25-1 mg/kg/dose slow IV over 20 min/IM/PO q4-8h prn, max 50 mg/dose
    [inj: 25 mg/mL,,; oral concentrate 30 mg/mL; supp: 25,100 mg; syrup: 10 mg/5 mL; tabs: 10, 25, 50, 100, 200 mg].
  -Diphenhydramine (Benadryl)
    1 mg/kg/dose IM/IV/PO q6h prn, max 50 mg/dose
    [caps: 25, 50 mg; inj: 10 mg/mL, 50 mg/mL; liquid: 12.5 mg/5 mL; tabs: 25, 50 mg].
  -Dimenhydrinate (Dramamine)

    ≥12 yrs: 5 mg/kg/day IM/IV/PO q6h prn, max 300 mg/day
    Not recommended in <12y due to high incidence of extrapyramidal side effects.
    [cap: 50 mg; inj: 50 mg/mL; liquid 12.5 mg/4 mL; tab: 50 mg; tab, chew: 50mg].
  -Prochlorperazine (Compazine)

    ≥12 yrs: 0.1-0.15 mg/kg/dose IM, max 10 mg/dose or 5-10 mg PO q6-8h, max 40 mg/day OR 5-25 mg PR q12h, max 50 mg/day
    Not recommended in <12y due to high incidence of extrapyramidal side effects
    [caps, SR: 10, 15, 30 mg; inj: 5 mg/mL; supp: 2.5, 5, 25 mg; syrup: 5 mg/5 mL; tabs: 5, 10, 25 mg].
  -Promethazine (Phenergan)
    0.25-1 mg/kg/dose PO/IM/IV over 20 min or PR q4-6h prn, max 50 mg/dose

[inj: 25,50 mg/mL; supp: 12.5, 25, 50 mg; syrup 6.25 mg/5 mL, 25 mg/5 mL; tabs: 12.5, 25, 50 mg].

-Trimethobenzamide (Tigan)

15 mg/kg/day IM/PO/PR q6-8h, max 100 mg/dose if <13.6 kg or 200 mg/dose if 13.6-41kg.

[caps: 100, 250 mg; inj: 100 mg/mL; supp: 100, 200 mg].

Post-Operative Nausea and Vomiting:

-Ondansetron (Zofran) 0.1 mg/kg IV x 1, max 4 mg.

-Droperidol (Inapsine) 0.01-0.05 mg/kg IV/IM q4-6h prn, max 5 mg [inj: 2.5 mg/mL].

Chemotherapy-Induced Nausea:

-Dexamethasone

10 mg/m^2/dose (max 20 mg) IV x 1, then 5 mg/m^2/dose (max 10 mg) IV q6h prn

[inj: 4 mg/mL, 10 mg/mL]

-Dronabinol (Marinol)

5 mg/m^2/dose PO 1-3 hrs prior to chemotherapy, then q4h prn afterwards. May titrate up in 2.5 mg/m^2/dose increments to max of 15 mg/m^2/dose.

[cap: 2.5, 5, 10 mg]

-Granisetron (Kytril)

10-20 mcg/kg IV given just prior to chemotherapy (single dose) [inj: 1 mg/mL]

Adults (oral) 1 mg PO bid or 2 mg PO qd [tab: 1 mg]

-Metoclopramide (Reglan)

0.5-1 mg/kg/dose IV q6h prn.

Pretreatment with diphenhydramine 1 mg/kg IV is recommended to decrease the risk of extrapyramidal reactions.

[inj: 5 mg/mL]

-Ondansetron (Zofran)

0.15 mg/kg/dose IV 30 minutes before chemotherapy and repeated 4 hr and 8 hr later (total of 3 doses) OR

0.3 mg/kg/dose IV x 1 30 minutes before chemotherapy OR

0.45 mg/kg/day as a continuous IV infusion OR

Oral:

<0.3 m^2: 1 mg PO three times daily

0.3-0.6 m^2: 2 mg PO three times daily

0.6-1 m^2: 3 mg PO three times daily

>1 m^2: 4 mg PO three times daily OR

4-11 yr: 4 mg PO three times daily

>11 yr: 8 mg PO three times daily

[inj: 2 mg/mL; oral soln: 4mg/5 mL; tab: 4, 8, 24 mg; tab, orally disintegrating: 4, 8 mg]

Cardiology

Pediatric Advanced Life Support

I. **Cardiopulmonary assessment**
   A. **Airway (A) assessment**. The airway should be assessed and cleared.
   B. **Breathing (B) assessment**. A respiratory rate of less than 10 or greater than 60 is a sign of impending respiratory failure.
   C. **Circulation (C) assessment**. In infants, chest compressions should be initiated if the heart rate is less than 80 beats/minute (bpm). In children, chest compressions should be initiated if the heart rate is less than 60 bpm.

II. **Respiratory failure**
   A. An open airway should be established. Bag-valve-mask ventilation should be initiated if the respiratory rate is less than 10. Intubation is performed if prolonged ventilation is required. Matching the endotracheal tube to the size of the nares or fifth finger provides an estimate of tube size.

Intubation			
Age	**ETT**	**Laryngoscope Blade**	**NG Tube Size**
Premature	2.0-2.5	0	8
Newborn >2 kg	3.0-3.5	1	10
Infant	3.5-4.0	1	10
12 mo	4.0-4.5	1.5	12
36 mo	4.5-5.0	2	12-14
6 yr	5.0-5.5	2	14-16
10 yr	6.0-6.5	2	16-18
Adolescent	.0-7.5	3	18-20
Adult	7.5-8.0	3	20

Uncuffed ET tube in children <8 yrs.
Straight laryngoscope blade if <6-10 yrs; curved blade if older.

   B. Vascular access should be obtained. Gastric decompression with a nasogastric or oral gastric tube is necessary.

III. **Shock**
   A. If the child is in shock, oxygen administration and monitoring are followed by initiation of vascular access. Crystalloid (normal saline or lactated Ringer's) solutions are used for rapid fluid boluses of 20 mL/kg over less than 20 minutes until the shock is resolved.
   B. Shock secondary to traumatic blood loss may require blood replacement if perfusion parameters have not normalized after a total of 40 to 60 mL/kg of crystalloid has been administered.

IV. **Cardiopulmonary failure**
   A. Oxygen is delivered at a concentration of 100%.
   B. Intubation and foreign body removal are completed. If signs of shock persist, crystalloid replacement is initiated with boluses of 20 mL/kg over less than 20 minutes. Inotropic agents are added if indicated.

Inotropic Agents Used in Resuscitation of Children		
Agent	**Intravenous dosage**	**Indications**
Epinephrine	0.1 to 1.0 µg/kg/minute (continuous infusion)	Symptomatic bradycardia, shock (cardiogenic, septic, anaphylactic), hypotension
Dopamine	2 to 5 µg/kg/minute (continuous infusion) 10 to 20 µg/kg/minute (continuous infusion)	Low dose: improve renal and splanchnic blood flow High dose: useful in the treatment of hypotension and shock in the presence of adequate intravascular volume
Dobutamine	2 to 20 µg/kg/minute (continuous infusion)	Normotensive cardiogenic shock

V. Dysrhythmias

A. Bradycardia

1. Bradycardia is the most common dysrhythmia in children. Initial management is ventilation and oxygenation. Chest compressions should be initiated if the heart rate is <60 bpm in a child or <80 bpm in an infant.
2. If bradycardia persists, epinephrine is administered. Intravenous or intraosseous epinephrine is given in a dose of 0.1 mL/kg of the 1:10,000 concentration (0.01 mg/kg). Endotracheal tube epinephrine is given as a dose of 0.1 mL/kg of the 1:1,000 concentration (0.1 mg/kg) diluted to a final volume of 3-5 mL in normal saline. This dose may be repeated every three to five minutes.
3. Atropine may be tried if multiple doses of epinephrine are unsuccessful. Atropine is given in a dose of 0.2 mL/kg IV/IO/ET of the 1:10,000 concentration (0.02 mg/kg). The minimum dose is 0.1 mg; the maximum single dose is 0.5 mg for a child and 1 mg for an adolescent. Endotracheal tube administration of atropine should be further diluted to a final volume of 3-5 mL in normal saline.
4. Pacing may be attempted if drug therapy has failed.

B. Asystole

1. Epinephrine is the drug of choice for asystole. The initial dose of intravenous or intraosseous epinephrine is given in a dose of 0.1 mL/kg of the 1:10,000 concentration of epinephrine (0.01 mg/kg). Endotracheal tube administration of epinephrine is given as a dose of 0.1 mL/kg of the 1:1,000 concentration of epinephrine (0.1 mg/kg), further diluted to a final volume of 3-5 mL in normal saline.
2. Subsequent doses of epinephrine are administered every three to five minutes at 0.1 mL/kg IV/IO/ET of the 1:1,000 concentration (0.1 mg/kg).

C. Supraventricular tachycardia

1. Supraventricular tachycardia presents with a heart rate >220 beats/minute in infants and >180 beats/minute in children. Supraventricular tachycardia is the most common dysrhythmia in the first year of life.
2. **Stable children with no signs of respiratory compromise or shock and a normal blood pressure**
   a. Initiate 100% oxygen and cardiac monitoring, and obtain pediatric cardiology consultation.

      b. Administer adenosine 0.1 mg/kg (max 6 mg) by rapid intravenous push. The dose of adenosine may be doubled to 0.2 mg/kg (max 12 mg) and repeated if supraventricular tachycardia is not converted.

      c. **Verapamil (Calan)** may be used; however, it is contraindicated under one year; in congestive heart failure or myocardial depression; in children receiving beta- adrenergic blockers; and in the presence of a possible bypass tract (ie, Wolff-Parkinson-White syndrome). Dose is 0.1-0.3 mg/kg/dose (max 5 mg) IV; may repeat dose in 30 minutes prn (max 10 mg).

   3. **Supraventricular tachycardia in unstable child with signs of shock**: Administer synchronized cardioversion at 0.5 joules (J)/kg. If supraventricular tachycardia persists, cardioversion is repeated at double the dose: 1.0 J/kg.

D. Ventricular tachycardia with palpable pulse

   1. A palpable pulse with heart rate ≥ 120 bpm with a wide QRS (>0.08 seconds) is present. Initiate cardiac monitoring, administer oxygen and ventilate.

   2. If vascular access is available, administer a lidocaine bolus of 1 mg/kg; if successful, begin lidocaine infusion at 20-50 µg/kg/minute.

   3. If ventricular tachycardia persists, perform synchronized cardioversion using 0.5 J/kg.

   4. If ventricular tachycardia persists, repeat synchronized cardioversion using 1.0 J/kg.

   5. If ventricular tachycardia persists, administer a lidocaine bolus of 1.0 mg/kg, and begin lidocaine infusion at 20-50 µg/kg/min.

   6. Repeat synchronized cardioversion as indicated.

E. Ventricular fibrillation and pulseless ventricular tachycardia

   1. Apply cardiac monitor, administer oxygen, and ventilate.

   2. Perform defibrillation using 2 J/kg. Do not delay defibrillation.

   3. If ventricular fibrillation persists, perform defibrillation using 4 J/kg.

   4. If ventricular fibrillation persists, perform defibrillation using 4 J/kg.

   5. If ventricular fibrillation persists, perform intubation, continue CPR, and obtain vascular access. Administer epinephrine, 0.1 mL/kg of 1:10,000 IV or IO (0.01 mg/kg); or 0.1 mL/kg of 1:1000 ET (0.1 mg/kg).

   6. If ventricular fibrillation persists, perform defibrillation using 4 J/kg.

   7. If ventricular fibrillation persists, administer lidocaine 1 mg/kg IV or IO, or 2 mg/kg ET.

   8. If ventricular fibrillation persists, perform defibrillation using 4 J/kg.

   9. If ventricular fibrillation persists, continue epinephrine, 0.1 mg/kg IV/IO/ET, 0.1 mL/kg of 1:1,000; administer every 3 to 5 minutes.

  10. If ventricular fibrillation persists, alternate defibrillation (4 J/kg) with lidocaine and epinephrine. Consider bretylium 5 mg/kg IV first dose, 10 mg/kg IV second dose.

F. Pulseless electrical activity is uncommon in children. It usually occurs secondary to hypoxemia, hypovolemia, hypothermia, hypoglycemia, hyperkalemia, cardiac tamponade, tension pneumothorax, severe acidosis or drug overdose. Successful resuscitation depends on treatment of the underlying etiology.

   1. The initial dose of IV or IO epinephrine is given in a dose of 0.1 mL/kg of the 1:10,000 concentration (0.01 mg/kg). Endotracheal epinephrine is given as a dose of 0.1 mL/kg of the 1:1,000 concentration (0.1 mg/kg) diluted to a final volume of 3-5 mL in normal saline.

   2. Subsequent doses are administered every three to five minutes as 0.1 mL/kg of the 1:1,000 concentration IV/IO/ET (0.1 mg/kg).

VI. **Serum glucose concentration** should be determined in all children undergoing resuscitation. Glucose replacement is provided with 25% dextrose in water, 2 to 4 mL/kg (0.5 to 1 g/kg) IV over 20 to 30 minutes for hypoglycemia. In neonates, 10% dextrose in water, 5 to 10 mL/kg (0.5 to 1 g/kg), is recommended.

Congestive Heart Failure

1. Admit to:
2. Diagnosis: Congestive Heart Failure
3. Condition:
4. Vital signs: Call MD if:
5. Activity:
6. Nursing: Daily weights, inputs and outputs
7. Diet: Low salt diet
8. IV Fluids:
9. Special Medications:
   -Oxygen 2-4 L/min by NC.
   -Furosemide (Lasix) 1 mg/kg/dose IV/IM/PO q6-12h prn, max 80 mg PO, 40 mg IV; may increase to 2 mg/kg/dose IV/IM/PO
      [inj: 10 mg/mL; oral liquid: 10 mg/mL, 40 mg/5 mL; tabs: 20, 40, 80 mg] **OR**
   -Bumetanide (Bumex) 0.015-0.1 mg/kg PO/IV/IM q12-24h, max 10 mg/day [inj: 0.25 mg/mL; tabs: 0.5, 1, 2 mg].

Digoxin:
   -Obtain a baseline ECG, serum electrolytes (potassium), and serum creatinine before administration.
   Initial digitalization is given over 24 hours in three divided doses: ½ total digitalizing dose (TDD) at time 0 hours, 1/4 TDD at 8-12 hours, and 1/4 TDD 8-12 hours later.
   Maintenance therapy is then started.

Total Digitalizing Dose

	PO	IV
Premature infant	20-30 mcg/kg	10-30 mcg/kg
Full term newborn (0-2 weeks)	30 mcg/kg	20-25 mcg/kg
2 wks-2 yr	40-50 mcg/kg	30-40 mcg/kg
2-10 yr 30-40 mcg/kg	25-30 mcg/kg	
>10 yr 0.75-1.5 mg	10 mcg/kg (max 1 mg)	

Maintenance digoxin dose

	PO	IV
Preterm neonate	4-10 mcg/kg/day	4-9 mcg/kg/day
Term neonate (0-2 wks)	6-10 mcg/kg/day	6-8 mcg/kg/day
2 weeks - 2 yr	10-12 mcg/kg/day	8-10 mcg/kg/day
2-10 yr 8-10 mcg/kg/day	6-8 mcg/kg/day	
>10 yr 5 mcg/kg/day	2-3 mcg/kg/day	
Adult 0.125-0.5 mg/day	0.1-0.4 mg/day	

   Divide bid if <10 yrs or qd if ≥ 10 yrs.
   [caps: 50, 100, 200 mcg; elixir: 50 mcg/mL; inj: 100 mcg/mL, 250 mcg/mL; tabs: 0.125, 0.25, 0.5 mg].

Other Agents:
   -Dopamine (Intropin) 2-20 mcg/kg/min continuous IV infusion, titrate cardiac output and BP.
   -Dobutamine (Dobutrex) 2-20 mcg/kg/min continuous IV infusion, max of 40 mcg/kg/min.
   -Nitroglycerin 0.5 mcg/kg/min continuous IV infusion, may increase by 1 mcg/kg q20min; usual max 5 mcg/kg/min.
   -Captopril (Capoten)
      Neonates: 0.05-0.1 mg/kg/dose PO q6-8h
      Infants: 0.15-0.3 mg/kg/dose PO q8h.
      Children: 0.5 mg/kg/dose PO q6-12h. Titrate as needed up to max of 6 mg/kg/day
      [tabs: 12.5, 25, 50,100 mg]. Tablets can be crushed and made into extemporaneous suspension.
   -KCl 1-4 mEq/kg/day PO q6-24h.
10. Extras and X-rays: CXR PA and LAT, ECG, echocardiogram.
11. Labs: ABG, SMA 7, Mg, Ca, CBC, iron studies, digoxin level, UA.

Atrial Fibrillation

1. **Admit to:**
2. **Diagnosis:** Atrial fibrillation
3. **Condition:**
4. **Vital signs:** Call MD if:
5. **Activity:**
6. **Nursing:**
7. **Diet:**
8. **IV Fluids:**
9. **Special Medications:**

Cardioversion (if unstable or refractory to drug treatment):

1. If unstable, **synchronized cardioversion** using 0.5 J/kg immediately. In stable patient with atrial fibrillation, consider starting quinidine or procainamide 24-48h prior to cardioversion.

   -Quinidine gluconate 2-10 mg/kg/dose IV q3-6h
   -Procainamide: loading dose: 3-6 mg/kg IV over 5 min (max 100 mg), may repeat every 5-10 minutes to max of 15 mg/kg (max 500 mg). Maintenance: 20-80 mcg/kg/min continuous IV infusion (max 2 gm/24 hrs)
2. Midazolam (Versed) 0.1 mg/kg (max 5 mg) IV over 2 min, repeat prn until amnesic.
3. Synchronized cardioversion using 0.5 J/kg. Increase stepwise by 0.5 J/kg if initial dosage fails to convert the patient. Consider esophageal overdrive pacing.

Digoxin Rate Control:

   Initial digitalization is given over 24 hours in three divided doses: 1/2 total digitalizing dose (TDD) at time 0 hours, 1/4 TDD at 8-12 hours, and 1/4 TDD 8-12 hours later. Maintenance therapy is then started.

Total Digitalizing Dose

	PO	IV
Premature infant	20-30 mcg/kg	10-30 mcg/kg
Full term newborn (0-2 weeks)	30 mcg/kg	20-25 mcg/kg
2 wks-2 yr	40-50 mcg/kg	30-40 mcg/kg
2-10 yr 30-40 mcg/kg	25-30 mcg/kg	
>10 yr 0.75-1.5 mg	10 mcg/kg (max 1 mg)	

Maintenance Digoxin Dose

	PO	IV
Preterm neonate	4-10 mcg/kg/day	4-9 mcg/kg/day
Term neonate (0-2 wks)	6-10 mcg/kg/day	6-8 mcg/kg/day
2 weeks - 2 yr	10-12 mcg/kg/day	8-10 mcg/kg/day
2-10 yr 8-10 mcg/kg/day	6-8 mcg/kg/day	
>10 yr 5 mcg/kg/day	2-3 mcg/kg/day	

   Divide bid if <10 yrs or qd if ≥10 yrs.
   [caps: 50, 100, 200 mcg; elixir: 50 mcg/mL; inj: 100 mcg/mL, 250 mcg/mL; tabs: 0.125, 0.25, 0.5 mg].

Other Rate Control Agents:

   -Propranolol 0.01-0.1 mg/kg slow IV push over 10 minutes, repeat q6-8h prn (max 1 mg/dose) or 0.5-4 mg/kg/day PO q6-8h (max 60 mg/day)
   [inj: 1 mg/mL; oral solutions: 4 mg/mL, 8 mg/mL; oral concentrate: 80 mg/mL; tabs: 10, 20, 40, 60, 80, 90 mg].

Pharmacologic Conversion (after rate control):

   -Procainamide (Pronestyl): Loading dose of 2-6 mg/kg/dose IV over 5 min, then 20-80 mcg/kg/min IV infusion (max 100 mg/dose or 2 gm/24h). Oral maintenance: 15-50 mg/kg/day PO q3-6h (max 4 gm/day).
   [caps: 250, 375, 500 mg; inj: 100 mg/mL, 500 mg/mL; tabs: 250, 375, 500 mg; tabs, SR: 250, 500, 750, 1000 mg].

10. **Extras and X-rays:** Portable CXR, ECG, echocardiogram.
11. **Labs:** CBC, SMA 7, Mg, Ca, UA, ABG. Serum drug levels.

Hypertensive Emergencies

1. **Admit to:**
2. **Diagnosis:** Hypertensive Emergency
3. **Condition:**
4. **Vital signs:** Call MD if systolic BP >150 mmHg, diastolic bp >90 mmHg, MAP > 120 mmHg.
5. **Activity:**
6. **Nursing:** BP q1h, ECG, daily weights, inputs and outputs.
7. **Diet:**
8. **IV Fluids:**
9. **Special Medications:**
   -Nitroprusside (Nipride) 0.5-10 mcg/kg/min continuous IV infusion. Titrate to desired blood pressure. Cyanide and thiocyanate toxicity may develop with prolonged use or in renal impairment.
   -Labetalol (Trandate) 0.2 mg/kg (max 20 mg) IV over 2 min or 0.4-1 mg/kg/hr continuous infusion.
   -Enalaprilat (Vasotec IV) 5-10 mcg/kg/dose IV q8-24h prn.
   -Nifedipine (Adalat, Procardia): 0.25-0.5 mg/kg/dose PO (max 10 mg/dose) q4h prn [trade name capsules: 10 mg/0.34 mL, 20 mg/0.45 mL; may puncture capsule with tuberculin syringe and draw up partial oral dosages].
10. **Extras and X-rays:** CXR, ECG, renal Doppler and ultrasound. Hypertensive intravenous pyelography.
11. **Labs:** CBC, SMA 7, BUN, creatinine, UA with micro. Urine specific gravity, thyroid panel, 24h urine for metanephrines; ANA, complement, ASO titer; toxicology screen.

Pulmonology

Asthma

1. **Admit to:**
2. **Diagnosis:** Exacerbation of asthma
3. **Condition:**
4. **Vital signs:** Call MD if:
5. **Activity:**
6. **Nursing:** Pulse oximeter, measure peak flow rate in older patients.
7. **Diet:**
8. **IV Fluids:** D5 1/4 NS or D5 ½ NS at maintenance rate.
9. **Special Medications:**
   -Oxygen humidified prn, 1-6 L/min by NC or 25-80% by mask, keep sat >92%.

Aerosolized and Nebulized Beta 2 Agonists:
   -Albuterol (Ventolin) (using 0.5% = 5 mg/mL soln) nebulized 0.2-0.5 mL in
    2 mL NS q1-4h and prn; may also be given by continuous aerosol.
    [soln for inhalation: 0.83 mg/3 mL unit dose; 5 mg/mL 20 mL multidose
    bulk bottle]
   -Albuterol (Ventolin, Proventil) 2 puffs q1-6h prn with spacer and mask.
    [capsule for inhalation (Rotacaps) using Rotahaler inhalation device: 200
    mcg; MDI: 90 mcg/puff, 200 puffs/17 gm]
   -Levalbuterol (Xopenex)
    2-11 yrs: 0.16-1.25 mg nebulized

    ≥12 yrs: 0.63-1.25mg nebulized q6-8h
    [soln for inhalation: 0.63 mg/3 mL, 1.25 mg/3 mL]. Levalbuterol 0.63 mg is
    comparable to albuterol 2.5 mg.
   -Salmeterol (Serevent) > 4 yrs: 2 puffs bid. Not indicated for acute treatment.
    [Serevent Diskus: 50 mcg/puff; MDI: 21 mcg/puff, 60 puffs/6.5gm or 120
    puffs/13 gm]

   -Formoterol (Foradil): ≥5 yrs: 12 mcg capsule aerosolized using dry powder
    inhaler bid. [capsule for aerosolization: 12 mcg]
   -Metaproterenol (Alupent, Metaprel)
    > 12 yrs: 2-3 puffs q3-4h prn, max 12 puffs/24 hrs. [MDI: 0.65 mg/puff]
   -Racemic epinephrine (2.25% sln) 0.05 mL/kg/dose (max 0.5 mL) in 2-3 mL
    saline nebulized q1-6h.

Intravenous Beta-2 Agonist:
   -Terbutaline (Brethaire, Brethine, Bricanyl)
    Loading dose: 2-10 mcg/kg IV
    Maintenance continuous IV infusion: 0.08-6 mcg/kg/min
    Monitor heart rate and blood pressure closely.
    [inj: 1 mg/mL]

Corticosteroid (systemic) Pulse Therapy:
   -Prednisolone 1-2 mg/kg/day PO q12-24h x 3-5 days
    [syrup: 5 mg/5 mL; Orapred 20.2 mg/5mL; Prelone 15 mg/5 mL] **OR**
   -Prednisone 1-2 mg/kg/day PO q12-24h x 3-5 days
    [oral solution: 1 mg/mL, 5 mg/mL; tabs: 1, 2, 5, 10, 20, 50 mg] **OR**
   -Methylprednisolone (Solu-Medrol) 2 mg/kg/dose IV/IM q6h x 4 doses, then
    1 mg/kg/dose IV/IM q6h x 3-5 days.

Aminophylline and theophylline:
   -Therapeutic range 10-20 mcg/mL. Concomitant drugs (e.g. erythromycin or
    carbamazepine) may increase serum theophylline levels by decreasing
    drug metabolism.
   -Aminophylline loading dose 5-6 mg/kg **total** body weight IV over 20-30 min
    [1 mg/kg of aminophylline will raise serum level by 2 mcg/mL].
   -Aminophylline maintenance as continuous IV infusion (based on ideal body
    weight)
    1-6 mth: 0.5 mg/kg/hr

6-12 mth: 0.6-0.75 mg/kg/hr
1-10 yr: 1.0 mg/kg/hr
10-16 yr: 0.75-0.9 mg/kg/hr
>16 yr: 0.7 mg/kg/hr **OR**
-Theophylline PO maintenance
80% of total daily maintenance IV aminophylline dose in 2-4 doses/day **OR**
1-6 mth: 9.6 mg/kg/day.
6-12 mth: 11.5-14.4 mg/kg/day.
1-10 yr: 19.2 mg/kg/day.
10-16 yr: 14.4-17.3 mg/kg/day.
>16 yr: 10 mg/kg/day.
-Give theophylline as sustained release theophylline preparation: q8-12h or
liquid immediate release: q6h.
-Slo-Phyllin Gyrocaps, may open caps and sprinkle on food [60, 125, 250 mg
caps] q8-12h
-Slobid Gyrocaps, may open caps and sprinkle on food [50, 75, 100, 125,
200, 300 mg caps] q8-12h
-Theophylline oral liquid: 80 mg/15 mL, 10 mg/mL] q6-8h.
-Theo-Dur [100, 200, 300, 450 mg tabs; scored, may cut in half, but do not
crush] q8-12h.
-Theophylline Products
Cap: 100, 200 mg
Cap, SR: 50, 60, 65, 75, 100, 125, 130, 200, 250, 260, 300 mg
Liquid: 80 mg/15 mL, 10 mg/mL
Tab: 100, 125, 200, 250, 300 mg
Tab, SR: 50, 75, 100, 125, 130, 200, 250, 260, 300, 400, 450, 500 mg
Corticosteroid metered dose inhalers or nebulized solution:
-Beclomethasone (Beclovent, Vanceril) MDI 1-4 puffs bid-qid with spacer and
mask, followed by gargling with water. [42 mcg/puff].
-Beclomethasone (Vanceril Double Strength) MDI 2 puffs bid [84 mcg/puff]
-Budesonide (Pulmicort Turbohaler) MDI 1-2 puffs bid [200 mcg/puff]
-Budesonide (Pulmicort) 0.25-0.5 mg nebulized bid [0.25 mg/2mL, 0.5
mg/2mL]
-Flunisolide (Aerobid) MDI 2-4 puffs bid [250 mcg/puff]
-Fluticasone (Flovent) MDI 1-2 puffs bid [44, 110, 220 mcg/actuation]
-Triamcinolone (Azmacort) MDI 1-4 puffs bid-qid [100 mcg/puff]
Cromolyn/nedocromil:
-Cromolyn sodium (Intal) MDI 2-4 puffs qid [800 mcg/puff] or nebulized 20 mg
bid-qid [10 mg/mL 2 mL unit dose ampules]
-Nedocromil (Tilade) MDI 2 puffs bid-qid [1.75 mg/puff]
Oral beta-2 agonists:
-Albuterol (Proventil)
2-6 years: 0.1-0.2 mg/kg/dose PO q6-8h
6-12 years: 2 mg PO tid-qid
>12 years: 2-4 mg PO tid-qid or 4-8 mg ER tab PO bid
[soln: 2 mg/5 mL; tab: 2, 4 mg; tab, ER: 4, 8 mg]
-Metaproterenol (Alupent, Metaprel)
< 2 yrs: 0.4 mg/kg/dose PO tid-qid
2-6 yrs: 1.3-2.6 mg PO q6-8h
6-9 yrs: 10 mg PO q6-8h
[syrup: 10 mg/5mL; tabs: 10, 20 mg]
Leukotriene receptor antagonists:
-Montelukast (Singulair)
2-5 yr: 4 mg PO qPM
6-14 yr: 5 mg PO qPM
> 14 yr: 10 mg PO qPM
[tab: 10 mg; tab, chew : 4, 5 mg]
-Zafirlukast (Accolate)
7-11 yr: 10 mg PO bid
≥12 yr: 20 mg PO bid
[tabs: 10, 20 mg]

-Zileuton (Zyflo)
≥ 12 yr: 600 mg PO qid (with meals and at bedtime)
[tab: 600 mg]
10. Extras and X-rays: CXR, pulmonary function test, peak flow rates.
11. Labs: CBC, CBG/ABG. Urine antigen screen, UA, theophylline level.

Allergic Rhinitis and Conjunctivitis

Antihistamines:
-Astemizole (Hismanal):
6-12 yr: 5 mg/day PO qd
>12 yr: 10 mg PO qd
[tab: 10 mg].
-Loratadine (Claritin)
>3 yrs and < 30 kg: 5 mg PO qd
>30 kg: 10 mg PO qd.
[syrup: 1mg/mL; tab: 10 mg; tab, rapidly disintegrating: 10 mg]
-Cetirizine (Zyrtec)
12 y: 5-10 mg qd
6-11 y: 5-10 mg qd
[tabs: 5, 10 mg Syrup: 5 mg/5 mL]
-Fexofenadine (Allegra), 12 y: 60 mg bid [60 mg]
-Actifed [per cap or tab or 10 mL syrup: triprolidine 2.5 mg, pseudoephedrine 60 mg]
4 mg pseudoephedrine/kg/day PO tid-qid **OR**
4 m-2 yr: 1.25 mL PO q6-8h
2-4 yr: 2.5 mL PO q6-8h
4-6 yr: 3.75 mL PO q6-8h
6-11y: 5 mL or ½ tab PO q6-8h
>12 yr: 10 mL or 1 cap/tab PO q6-8h.
-Chlorpheniramine maleate (Chlor-Trimeton):
0.35 mg/kg/day PO q4-6h OR
2-5 yr: 1 mg PO q4-6h (max 4 mg/day)
6-11y: 2 mg PO q4-6h (max 12 mg/day)

≥12y: 4 mg PO q4-6h or 8-12 mg SR q8-12h (max 24 mg/day).
[cap, SR: 8,12 mg; soln: 2 mg/5 mL; tab: 4, 8, 12 mg; tab, chew: 2 mg; tab, SR: 8, 12 mg]
-Diphenhydramine (Benadryl)
1 mg/kg/dose PO q6h prn, max 50 mg/dose
[elixir/liquid: 12.5 mg/5 mL; tab, cap: 25, 50 mg].
Intranasal Therapy:
-Azelastine (Astelin)
3-12 yr: 1 spray in each nostril bid
> 12 yr: 2 sprays in each nostril bid
[nasal soln: 1 mg/mL, 17 mL (137 mcg/spray)]
-Beclomethasone (Beconase, Vancenase)
6-11 yrs: 1 spray into each nostril tid

≥12 yrs: 1 spray into each nostril bid-qid
[42 mcg/actuation]
-Beclomethasone aqueous (Beconase AQ)
6-11 yrs: 1-2 sprays into each nostril bid

≥12 yrs: 1-2 sprays into each nostril bid
[42 mcg/actuation]
-Beclomethasone Double Strength (Vancenase AQ)
6-11 yrs: 1-2 puffs into each nostril qd

≥12 yrs: 1-2 sprays into each nostril qd
[84 mcg/actuation]

-Budesonide (Rhinocort)
  6-11 yrs: 2 sprays into each nostril bid or 4 sprays into each nostril qAM

  ≥12 yrs: 2 sprays into each nostril bid or 4 sprays into each nostril qAM
  [32 mcg/actuation]
-Budesonide aqueous(Rhinocort AQ)
  6-11 yrs: 1-2 sprays into each nostril bid

  ≥12 yrs: 1 sprays into each nostril qd, may increase up to 4 sprays into
  each nostril qAM
  [32 mcg/actuation]
-Cromolyn (Nasalcrom)
  1 puff into each nostril q3-4h
  [40 mg/mL 13 mL].
-Flunisolide (Nasalide, Nasarel)
  6-11 yrs: 1 spray into each nostril tid or 2 sprays into each nostril bid

  ≥12 yrs: 2 sprays into each nostril bid-tid
  [25 mcg/actuation].
-Fluticasone (Flonase)
  4-6 yrs: 1-2 sprays into each nostril qd
  6-11 yrs: 1-2 sprays into each nostril qd

  ≥ 12 yrs: 1 spray into each nostril bid or 2 sprays into each nostril qd
  [50 mcg/actuation]
-Mometasone (Nasonex)
  4-6 yrs: 1 spray into each nostril qd
  6-11 yrs: 1 spray into each nostril qd

  ≥12 yrs: 2 sprays into each nostril qd
  [50 mcg/actuation]
-Triamcinolone (Nasacort)
  6-11 yr: 2 sprays into each nostril qd
  >12 yr: 2 sprays into each nostril qd.
  [55 mcg/actuation]
-Triamcinolone aqueous (Nasacort AQ)
  6-11 yr: 2 spray into each nostril qd
  >12 yr: 2 sprays into each nostril qd.
  [55 mcg/actuation]
Allergic Conjunctivitis Therapy:
-Azelastine (Optivar)

  ≥3 yr: instill 1 drop into affected eye(s) bid
  [ophth soln: 0.05% 6 mL]
-Cromolyn ophthalmic (Crolom, Opticrom)
  Instill 2 drops into each affected eye(s) q4-6h
  [ophth soln: 4% 2.5, 10 mL].
Decongestants:
-Pseudoephedrine (Sudafed, Novafed)
  <12 yr: 4 mg/kg/day PO q6h.
  >12 yr and adults: 30-60 mg/dose PO q6-8h or sustained release 120 mg
  PO q12h or sustained release 240 mg PO q24h
  [cap/cplt, SR: 120, 240 mg; drops: 7.5 mg/0.8mL; syrup: 15 mg/5mL, 30
  mg/5mL; tabs: 30, 60 mg]

Anaphylaxis

1. **Admit to:**
2. **Diagnosis:** Anaphylaxis
3. **Condition:**
4. **Vital signs:** Call MD if:
5. **Activity:**
6. **Nursing:** Inputs and outputs, ECG monitoring, pulse oximeter.

7. Diet:
8. IV Fluids: 2 IV lines. Normal saline or LR 10-20 mL/kg rapidly over 1h, then D5 ½ NS at 1-1.5 times maintenance.
9. Special Medications:
-O_2 at 4 L/min by NC or mask.
-Epinephrine, 0.01 mg/kg [0.01 mL/kg of 1 mg/mL = 1:1000] (maximum 0.5 mL) subcutaneously, repeat every 15-20 minutes prn. Usual dose for infants is 0.05-0.1mL, for children 0.1-0.3 mL, and for adolescents 0.3-0.5 mL. If anaphylaxis is caused by an insect sting or intramuscular injection, inject an additional 0.1 mL of epinephrine at the site to slow antigen absorption.
-Epinephrine racemic (if stridor is present), 2.25% nebulized, 0.25-0.5 mL in 2.5 mL NS over 15 min q30 min-4h.
-Albuterol (Ventolin) (0.5%, 5 mg/mL sln) nebulized 0.01-0.03 mL/kg (max 1 mL) in 2 mL NS q1-2h and prn; may be used in addition to epinephrine if necessary.
Corticosteroids:
-For severe symptoms, give hydrocortisone 5 mg/kg IV q8h until stable, then change to oral prednisone. If symptoms are mild, give prednisone: initially 2 mg/kg/day (max 40 mg) PO q12h, then taper the dose over 4-5 days.
Antihistamines:
-Diphenhydramine (Benadryl) 1 mg/kg/dose IV/IM/IO/PO q6h, max 50 mg/dose; antihistamines are not a substitute for epinephrine **OR**
-Hydroxyzine (Vistaril) 0.5-1 mg/kg/dose IM/IV/PO q4-6h, max 50 mg/dose.
10. Extras and X-rays: Portable CXR.
11. Labs: CBC, SMA 7, CBG.

Pleural Effusion

1. Admit to:
2. Diagnosis: Pleural effusion
3. Condition:
4. Vital signs: Call MD if:
5. Activity:
6. Diet:
7. IV Fluids:
8. Extras and X-rays: CXR PA and LAT, lateral decubitus, ultrasound, sputum AFB. Pulmonary consult.
9. Labs: CBC with differential, SMA 7, protein, albumin, ESR, UA.
Pleural fluid:
Tube 1 - LDH, protein, amylase, triglycerides, glucose, specific gravity (10 mL red top).
Tube 2 - Gram stain, culture and sensitivity, AFB, fungal culture and sensitivity (20-60 mL).
Tube 3 - Cell count and differential (5-10 mL, EDTA purple top).
Tube 4 - Cytology (25-50 mL, heparinized).
Syringe - pH (2 mL, heparinized).

Evaluation of Thoracentesis Fluid		
	Transudate	**Exudate**
Specific gravity	<1.016	>1.016
Protein ratio pleural fluid/serum	<0.5	>0.5

	Transudate	Exudate
Protein (gm/100 mL)	<3.0	>3.0
LDH ratio pleural fluid/serum	<0.6	>0.6
WBC	<1,000/mm^3	>1,000/mm^3
Glucose	Equivalent to serum	Less than serum

Infectious Diseases

Suspected Sepsis

1. **Admit to:**
2. **Diagnosis:** Suspected sepsis
3. **Condition:**
4. **Vital signs:** Call MD if:
5. **Activity:**
6. **Nursing:** Inputs and outputs, daily weights, cooling measures prn temp >38°C, consent for lumbar puncture.
7. **Diet:**
8. **IV Fluids:** Correct hypovolemia if present; NS 10-20 mL/kg IV bolus, then IV fluids at 1-1.5 times maintenance.
9. **Special Medications:**
Term newborns <1 month old (Group B strep, E coli, Group D strep, gram negatives, Listeria monocytogenes): Ampicillin and gentamicin or cefotaxime.
   - Ampicillin IV/IM: <7d: 150 mg/kg/day q8h; >7d: 200 mg/kg/day q6h.
   - Cefotaxime (Claforan) IV/IM: <7 days: 100 mg/kg/day q12h; >7 days: 150 mg/kg/day q8h.
   - Gentamicin (Garamycin) IV/IM: 5 mg/kg/day q12h.
   - Also see page 171.
Infant 1-2 months old (H. flu, strep pneumonia, N meningitidis, Group B strep):
   - Ampicillin 100 mg/kg/day IV/IM q6h **AND EITHER**
   - Cefotaxime (Claforan) 100 mg/kg/day IV/IM q6h **OR**
   - Ceftriaxone (Rocephin) 50-75 mg/kg/day IV/IM q12-24h **OR**
   - Gentamicin (Garamycin) 7.5 mg/kg/day IV/IM q8h
Children 2 months to 18 years old (S pneumonia, H flu, N. meningitidis):
   - Cefotaxime (Claforan) 100 mg/kg/day IV/IM q6h, max 12 gm/day **OR**
   - Ceftriaxone (Rocephin) 50-75 mg/kg/day IV/IM q 12-24h, max 4 gm/day.
Immunocompromised Patients (Gram negative bacilli, Pseudomonas, Staph, Strep viridans):
   - Ticarcillin (Ticar) 200-300 mg/kg/day IV/IM q6h, max 24 gm/day
   - Ticarcillin/clavulanate (Timentin) 200-300 mg/kg/day of ticarcillin IV/IM q6-8h, max 24gm/day **OR**
   - Piperacillin (Pipracil) 200-300 mg/kg/day IV/IM q6h, max 24 gm/day **OR**
   - Piperacillin/tazobactam (Zosyn) 240 mg/kg/day of piperacillin IV/IM q6-8h, max 12 gm/day **OR**
   - Ceftazidime (Fortaz) 100-150 mg/kg/day IV/IM q8h, max 12 gm/day **AND**
   - Tobramycin (Nebcin) or Gentamicin (Garamycin) (normal renal function):
     <5 yr (except neonates): 7.5 mg/kg/day IV/IM q8h.
     5-10 yr: 6.0 mg/kg/day IV/IM q8h.
     >10 yr: 5.0 mg/kg/day IV/IM q8h **AND (if gram positive infection strongly suspected)**
   - Vancomycin (Vancocin) (central line infection) 40-60 mg/kg/day IV q6-8h, max 4 gm/day
10. **Symptomatic Medications:**
   - Ibuprofen (Advil) 5-10 mg/kg/dose PO q6h-8h prn temp >38°C **OR**
   - Acetaminophen (Tylenol) 10-15 mg/kg PO/PR q4-6h prn temp >38°C or pain.
11. **Extras and X-rays:** CXR.
12. **Labs:** CBC, SMA 7. Blood culture and sensitivity x 2. UA, urine culture and sensitivity; antibiotic levels. Stool for Wright stain if diarrhea. Nasopharyngeal washings for direct fluorescent antibody (RSV, chlamydia).
   CSF Tube 1 - Gram stain, culture and sensitivity for bacteria, antigen screen (1-2 mL).
   CSF Tube 2 - Glucose, protein (1-2 mL).
   CSF Tube 3 - Cell count and differential (1-2 mL).

Meningitis

1. **Admit to:**
2. **Diagnosis:** Meningitis.
3. **Condition:** Guarded.
4. **Vital signs:** Call MD if:
5. **Activity:**
6. **Nursing:** Strict isolation precautions. Inputs and outputs, daily weights; cooling measures prn temp >38°C; consent for lumbar puncture. Monitor for signs of increased intracranial pressure.
7. **Diet:**
8. **IV Fluids:** Isotonic fluids at maintenance rate.
9. **Special Medications:**
Term Newborns <1 months old (Group B strep, E coli, gram negatives, Listeria):
-Ampicillin, 0-7 d: 150 mg/kg/day IV/IM q8h; >7d: 200 mg/kg/day IV/IM q6h **AND**
-Cefotaxime (Claforan): <7d: 100 mg/kg/day IV/IM q12h; >7 days: 150 mg/kg/day q8h IV/IM.
Infants 1-3 months old (H. flu, strep pneumonia, N. Meningitidis, group B strep, E coli):
-Cefotaxime (Claforan) 200 mg/kg/day IV/IM q6h **OR**
-Ceftriaxone (Rocephin) 100 mg/kg/day IV/IM q12-24h **AND**
-Vancomycin (Vancocin) 40-60 mg/kg/day IV q6h.
-Dexamethasone 0.6 mg/kg/day IV q6h x 4 days. Initiate before or with the first dose of parenteral antibiotic.
Children 3 months to 18 years old (S pneumonia, H flu, N. meningitidis):
-Cefotaxime (Claforan) 200 mg/kg/day IV/IM q6h, max 12 gm/day or ceftriaxone (Rocephin) 100 mg/kg/day IV/IM q12-24h, max 4 gm/day **AND**
-Vancomycin (Vancocin) 60 mg/kg/day IV q6h, max 4gm/day.
-Dexamethasone 0.6 mg/kg/day IV q6h x 4 days. Initiate before or with the first dose of parenteral antibiotic.
10. **Symptomatic Medications:**
-Ibuprofen (Advil) 5-10 mg/kg/dose PO q6-8h prn **OR**
-Acetaminophen (Tylenol) 15 mg/kg PO/PR q4h prn temp >38°C or pain.
11. **Extras and X-rays:** CXR, MRI.
12. **Labs:** CBC, SMA 7. Blood culture and sensitivity x 2. UA, urine culture and sensitivity; urine specific gravity. Antibiotic levels. Urine and blood antigen testing.
Lumbar Puncture:
CSF Tube 1 - Gram stain, culture and sensitivity, bacterial antigen screen (1-2 mL).
CSF Tube 2 - Glucose, protein (1-2 mL).
CSF Tube 3 - Cell count and differential (1-2 mL).

Specific Therapy for Meningitis and Encephalitis

Dexamethasone (0.6 mg/kg/day IV q6h x 4 days) given before the first dose of antibiotics decreases hearing deficits and possibly other neurologic sequelae in Haemophilus influenzae meningitis.
Streptococcus pneumoniae:
Until sensitivities are available, combination therapy with vancomycin and cefotaxime/ceftriaxone is recommended. For children with severe hypersensitivity to beta-lactams, the combination of vancomycin and rifampin is recommended.
-Penicillin G 250,000-400,000 U/kg/day IV/IM q4-6h, max 24 MU/day
-Cefotaxime (Claforan) 200-300 mg/kg/day IV/IM q6h, max 12 gm/day
-Ceftriaxone (Rocephin) 100 mg/kg/day IV/IM q12-24h, max 4 gm/day
-Vancomycin (Vancocin) 60 mg/kg/day IV q6h, max 4 gm/day

-Rifampin 20 mg/kg/day IV q12h, max 600 mg/day
-Meropenem (Merrem) 120 mg/kg/day IV q8h, max 6 gm/day
-Chloramphenicol (Chloromycetin) 75-100 mg/kg/day IV q6h, max 4 gm/day
Neisseria meningitidis:
Penicillin is the drug of choice. Cefotaxime and ceftriaxone are acceptable alternatives.
-Penicillin G 250,000-400,000 U/kg/day IV/IM q4h x 7-10d, max 24 MU/d.
-Cefotaxime (Claforan) 200-300 mg/kg/day IV/IM q6h, max 12 gm/day
-Ceftriaxone (Rocephin) 100 mg/kg/day IV/IM q12-24h, max 4 gm/day
Meningococcal exposure prophylaxis (see H flu prophylaxis below):

-Ceftriaxone (Rocephin) IM x 1 dose; ≤12y: 125 mg; >12y: 250 mg **OR**

-Rifampin, ≤1 mth: 5 mg/kg/dose PO bid x 2 days; >1 mth: 10 mg/kg/dose (max 600 mg/dose) PO q12h x 2 days [caps: 150 mg, 300 mg; extemporaneous suspension] **OR**

-Ciprofloxacin (Cipro) 500 mg PO x 1 for adults (>18 yr).
Haemophilus influenzae
Ampicillin should not be used alone as initial therapy until sensitivities are available as 10-40% of isolates are ampicillin-resistant.
-Cefotaxime (Claforan) 200-300 mg/kg/day IV/IM q6h, max 12 gm/day **OR**
-Ceftriaxone (Rocephin) 100 mg/kg/day IV/IM q12-24h, max 4 gm/day **OR**
-Ampicillin (beta-lactamase negative) 200-400 mg/kg/day IV/IM q4-6h, max 12 gm/day.
H influenzae type B exposure prophylaxis and eradication of nasopharyngeal carriage:
-Rifampin <1 month: 10 mg/kg/day PO q24h x 4 days; >1 month: 20 mg/kg/day PO qd x 4 doses (max 600 mg/dose). [caps: 150, 300 mg; extemporaneous suspension].
Group A or non-enterococcal Group D Streptococcus:
-Penicillin G 250,000 U/kg/day IV/IM q4-6h, max 24 MU/d.
Listeria monocytogenes or Group B Streptococcus:
-Ampicillin 200 mg/kg/day IV/IM q6h, max 12 gm/day **AND**
-Gentamicin (Garamycin) or Tobramycin (Nebcin) (normal renal function):
<5 yr (except neonates): 7.5 mg/kg/day IV/IM q8h.
5-10 yr: 6.0 mg/kg/day IV/IM q8h.
>10 yr: 5.0 mg/kg/day IV/IM q8h
Staphylococcus aureus:
-Nafcillin (Nafcil) or Oxacillin (Bactocill, Prostaphlin)150-200 mg/kg/day IV/IM q4-6h, max 12 gm/day **OR**
-Vancomycin (Vancocin) 40-60 mg/kg/day IV q6h, max 4 gm/day (may require concomitant intrathecal therapy).
Herpes Simplex Encephalitis:
-Acyclovir (Zovirax) 1500 mg/m^2/day or 30 mg/kg/day IV over 1h q8h x 14-21 days

Infective Endocarditis

1. **Admit to:**
2. **Diagnosis:** Infective endocarditis
3. **Condition:**
4. **Vital signs:** Call MD if:
5. **Activity:**
6. **Diet:**
7. **IV Fluids:**
8. **Special Medications:**
Subacute Bacterial Endocarditis Empiric Therapy:
-Penicillin G 250,000 U/kg/day IV/IM q4-6, max 24 MU/day **AND**
-Gentamicin (Garamycin) or Tobramycin (Nebcin) (normal renal function):
<5 yr (except neonates): 7.5 mg/kg/day IV/IM q8h.
5-10 yr: 6.0 mg/kg/day IV/IM q8h.

>10 yr: 5.0 mg/kg/day IV/IM q8h
Acute Bacterial Endocarditis Empiric Therapy (including IV drug user):
  -Gentamicin (Garamycin) or Tobramycin (Nebcin), see above for dose **AND
    EITHER**
  -Nafcillin (Nafcil) or oxacillin (Bactocill, Prostaphlin) 150 mg/kg/day IV/IM q6h,
    max 12 gm/day **OR**
  -Vancomycin (Vancocin) 40-60 mg/kg/day IV q6-8h, max 4 gm/day
Streptococci viridans/bovis:
  -Penicillin G 150,000 u/kg/day IV/IM q4-6h, max 24 MU/day **OR**
  -Vancomycin (Vancocin) 40-60 mg/kg/day IV q6-8h, max 4 gm/day.
Staphylococcus aureus (methicillin sensitive):
  -Nafcillin (Nafcil) or oxacillin (Bactocill, Prostaphlin) 150 mg/kg/day IV/IM q6h,
    max 12 gm/day **AND**
  -Gentamicin (Garamycin) or Tobramycin (Nebcin), see above for dose.
Methicillin-resistant Staphylococcus aureus:
  -Vancomycin (Vancocin) 40-60 mg/kg/day IV q6h, max 4 gm/day.
Staphylococcus epidermidis:
  -Vancomycin (Vancocin) 40-60 mg/kg/day IV q6h max 4 gm/day **AND**
  -Gentamicin (Garamycin) or Tobramycin (Nebcin), see above for dose.
9. **Extras and X-rays:** CXR PA and LAT, echocardiogram, ECG. Cardiology and
    infectious disease consultation.
10. **Labs:** CBC, ESR. Bacterial culture and sensitivity x 3-4 over 24h, MBC.
    Antibiotic levels. UA, urine culture and sensitivity.

Endocarditis Prophylaxis

Prophylactic Regimens for Dental, Oral, Respiratory Tract, or Esophageal Procedures			
Situation	**Drug**	**Regimen**	**Maximum Dose**
Standard general prophylaxis	Amoxicillin	50 mg/kg PO as a single dose 1 hr before procedure	2000 mg
Unable to take oral medication	Ampicillin	50 mg/kg IV/IM within 30 minutes before procedure	2000 mg
Allergic to penicillin	Clindamycin **or**	20 mg/kg PO as a single dose 1 hour before procedure	600 mg
	Cephalexin (Keflex) or cefadroxil (Duricef) **or**	50 mg/kg PO as a single dose 1 hour before procedure	2000 mg
	Azithromycin (Zithromax) or clarithromycin (Biaxin)	15 mg/kg PO as a single dose 1 hour before procedure	500 mg

Situation	Drug	Regimen	Maximum Dose
Allergic to penicillin and unable to take oral medications	Clindamycin or	20 mg/kg IV 30 minutes before procedure	600 mg
	Cefazolin (Ancef)	25 mg/kg IV/IM within 30 minutes before procedure	1000 mg

Prophylactic Regimens for Genitourinary/Gastrointestinal Procedures

Situation	Drug	Regimen	Maximum Dose
High-risk patients	Ampicillin **plus**	50 mg/kg IV/IM	2000 mg
	Gentamicin followed by	1.5 mg/kg IV/IM within 30 minutes before starting procedure	120 mg
	Ampicillin or Amoxicillin	25 mg/kg IV/IM 25 mg/kg PO six hours later	1000 mg 1000 mg
High-risk patients allergic to penicillin	Vancomycin **plus**	20 mg/kg IV over 1-2 hours	1000 mg
	Gentamicin	1.5 mg/kg IV/IM to be completed within 30 minutes before starting procedure	120 mg
Moderate-risk patients	Amoxicillin **or**	50 mg/kg PO one hour before procedure	2000 mg
	Ampicillin	50 mg/kg IV/IM within 30 minutes of starting procedure	2000 mg
Moderate-risk patients allergic to penicillin	Vancomycin	20 mg/kg IV over 1-2 hours, completed within 30 minutes of starting the procedure	1000 mg

Pneumonia

1. **Admit to:**
2. **Diagnosis:** Pneumonia
3. **Condition:**
4. **Vital signs:** Call MD if:
5. **Activity:**
6. **Nursing:** Pulse oximeter, inputs and outputs. Bronchial clearance techniques, vibrating vest.
7. **Diet:**
8. **IV Fluids:**
9. **Special Medications:**
   -Humidified O_2 by NC at 2-4 L/min or 25-100% by mask, adjust to keep saturation >92%

Term Neonates <1 month:
-Ampicillin 100 mg/kg/day IV/IM q6h **AND**
-Cefotaxime (Claforan) <1 wk: 100 mg/kg/day IV/IM q12h; >1 wk: 150 mg/kg/day IV/IM q8h **OR**
-Gentamicin (Garamycin) 5 mg/kg/day IV/IM q12h.

Children 1 month-5 years old:
-Cefuroxime (Zinacef) 100-150 mg/kg/day IV/IM q8h **OR**
-Ampicillin 100 mg/kg/day IV/IM q6h **AND**
-Gentamicin (Garamycin) or Tobramycin (Nebcin):
  7.5 mg/kg/day IV/IM q8h (normal renal function).
-If chlamydia is strongly suspected, add erythromycin 40 mg/kg/day IV q6h.

Oral Therapy:
-Cefuroxime axetil (Ceftin)
  tab: child: 125-250 mg PO bid; adult: 250-500 mg PO bid
  susp: 30 mg/kg/day PO q12h, max 1000 mg/day
  [susp: 125 mg/5 mL; tabs: 125, 250,500 mg] **OR**
-Loracarbef (Lorabid)
  30 mg/kg/day PO q12h, max 800 mg/day
  [cap: 200, 400 mg; susp: 100 mg/5 mL, 200 mg/5mL]
-Cefpodoxime (Vantin)
  10 mg/kg/day PO q12h, max 800 mg/day
  [susp: 50 mg/5 mL, 100 mg/5 mL; tabs: 100, 200 mg]
-Cefprozil (Cefzil)
  30 mg/kg/day PO q12h, max 1000 mg/day
  [susp: 125 mg/5 mL, 250 mg/5 mL; tabs: 250, 500 mg].
-Cefixime (Suprax)
  8 mg/kg/day PO qd-bid, max 400 mg/day
  [susp: 100 mg/5 mL; tabs: 200, 400 mg].
-Clarithromycin (Biaxin)
  15-30 mg/kg/day PO bid, max 1000 mg/day
  [susp: 125 mg/5 mL, 250 mg/5 mL; tabs: 250, 500 mg].
-Azithromycin (Zithromax)

  Children ≥2 yrs: 12 mg/kg/day PO qd x 5 days, max 500 mg/day

  ≥16 yrs: 500 mg PO on day 1, 250 mg PO qd on days 2-5
  [cap: 250 mg; susp: 100 mg/5mL, 200 mg/5mL; tabs: 250, 600 mg]
-Amoxicillin/clavulanate (Augmentin)
  30-40 mg/kg/day of amoxicillin PO q8h , max 500 mg/dose
  [elixir 125 mg/5 mL, 250 mg/5 mL; tabs: 250, 500 mg; tabs, chew: 125, 250 mg;]
-Amoxicillin/clavulanate (Augmentin BID)
  30-40 mg/kg/day PO q12h, max 875 mg (amoxicillin)/dose
  [susp 200 mg/5 mL, 400 mg/5 mL; tab: 875 mg; tabs, chew: 200, 400 mg]

Community Acquired Pneumonia 5-18 years old (viral, Mycoplasma pneumoniae, chlamydia pneumoniae, pneumococcus, legionella):
-Cefuroxime (Zinacef) 100-150 mg/kg/day IV/IM q8h, max 9 gm/day **OR**
-Erythromycin estolate (Ilosone) 30-50 mg/kg/day PO q8-12h, max 2 gm/day

[caps: 125, 250 mg; drops: 100 mg/mL; susp: 125 mg/5 mL, 250 mg/5 mL; tab: 500 mg; tabs, chew: 125,250 mg]
-Erythromycin ethylsuccinate (EryPed, EES)
   30-50 mg/kg/day PO q6-8h, max 2gm/day
   [susp: 200 mg/5 mL, 400 mg/5 mL; tab: 400 mg; tab, chew: 200 mg]
-Erythromycin base (E-mycin, Ery-Tab, Eryc)
   30-50 mg/kg/day PO q6-8h, max 2gm/day
   [cap, DR: 250 mg; tabs: 250, 333, 500 mg]
-Erythromycin lactobionate
   20-40 mg/kg/day IV q6h, max 4 gm/day
   [inj: 500 mg, 1 gm]
-Clarithromycin (Biaxin)
   15-30 mg/kg/day PO bid, max 1000 mg/day
   [susp: 125 mg/5 mL, 250 mg/5 mL; tabs: 250, 500 mg]

Immunosuppressed, Neutropenic Pneumonia (S. pneumoniae, group A strep, H flu, gram neg enterics, Klebsiella, Mycoplasma Pneumonia, Legionella, Chlamydia pneumoniae, S aureus):
-Tobramycin (Nebcin) (normal renal function):
   <5 yr (except neonates): 7.5 mg/kg/day IV/IM q8h.
   5-10 yr: 6.0 mg/kg/day IV/IM q8h.
   >10 yr: 5.0 mg/kg/day IV/IM q8h **OR**
-Ceftazidime (Fortaz)150 mg/kg/day IV/IM q8h, max 12 gm/day **AND**
-Ticarcillin/clavulanate (Timentin) 200-300 mg/kg/day of ticarcillin IV q6-8h, max 24 gm/day **OR**
-Nafcillin (Nafcil) or oxacillin (Bactocill, Prostaphlin) 150 mg/kg/day IV/IM q6h, max 12 gm/day **OR**
-Vancomycin (Vancocin) 40 mg/kg/day IV q6h, max 4 gm/day.

Cystic Fibrosis Exacerbation (Pseudomonas aeruginosa):
-Ticarcillin/clavulanate (Timentin) 200-300 mg/kg/day of ticarcillin IV q6-8h, max 24 gm/day **OR**
-Piperacillin/tazobactam (Zosyn) 300 mg/kg/day of piperacillin IV q6-8h, max 12 gm/day **OR**
-Piperacillin (Pipracil) 200-300 mg/kg/day IV/IM q4-6h, max 24 gm/day **AND**
-Tobramycin (Nebcin):
   <5 yr (except neonates): 7.5 mg/kg/day IV/IM q8h.
   5-10 yr: 6.0 mg/kg/day IV/IM q8h.
   >10 yr: 5.0 mg/kg/day IV/IM q8h **OR**
-Ceftazidime (Fortaz) 150 mg/kg/day IV/IM q8h, max 12 gm/day **OR**
-Aztreonam (Azactam) 150-200 mg/kg/day IV/IM q6-8h, max 8 gm/day **OR**
-Imipenem/Cilastatin (Primaxin) 60-100 mg/kg/day imipenem component IV q6-8h, max 4 gm/day **OR**
-Meropenem (Merrem) 60-120 mg/kg/day IV q8h, max 6gm/day.

10. Symptomatic Medications:
-Acetaminophen (Tylenol) 10-15 mg/kg PO/PR q4h prn temp >38°C or pain.
11. Extras and X-rays: CXR PA and LAT, PPD.
12. Labs: CBC, ABG, blood culture and sensitivity x 2. Sputum gram stain, culture and sensitivity, AFB. Antibiotic levels. Nasopharyngeal washings for direct fluorescent antibody (RSV, adenovirus, parainfluenza, influenza virus, chlamydia) and cultures for respiratory viruses. UA.

Specific Therapy for Pneumonia

Pneumococcal pneumonia:
-Erythromycin estolate (Ilosone)
30-50 mg/kg/day PO q8-12h, max 2 gm/day
[caps: 125, 250 mg; drops: 100 mg/mL; susp: 125 mg/5 mL, 250 mg/5 mL; tab: 500 mg; tabs, chew: 125,250 mg]
-Erythromycin ethylsuccinate (EryPed, EES)
30-50 mg/kg/day PO q6-8h, max 2gm/day
[susp: 200 mg/5 mL, 400 mg/5 mL; tab: 400 mg; tab, chew: 200 mg]
-Erythromycin base (E-Mycin, Ery-Tab, Eryc)
30-50 mg/kg/day PO q6-8h, max 2gm/day
[tab: 250, 333, 500 mg]
-Erythromycin lactobionate
20-40 mg/kg/day IV q6h, max 4 gm/day
[inj: 500 mg, 1 g m] **OR**
-Vancomycin (Vancocin) 40 mg/kg/day IV q6h, max 4 gm/day **OR**
-Cefotaxime (Claforan) 100-150 mg/kg/day IV/IM q6h, max 12 gm/day **OR**
-Penicillin G 150,000 U/kg/day IV/IM q4-6h, max 24 MU/day.

Staphylococcus aureus:
-Oxacillin (Bactocill, Prostaphlin) or Nafcillin (Nafcil) 150-200 mg/kg/day IV/IM q4-6h, max 12 gm/day **OR**
-Vancomycin (Vancocin) 40 mg/kg/day IV q6h, max 4 gm/day

Haemophilus influenzae (<5 yr of age):
-Cefotaxime (Claforan) 100-150 mg/kg/day IV/IM q8h, max 12 gm/day **OR**
-Cefuroxime (Zinacef) 100-150 mg/kg/day IV/IM q8h (beta-lactamase pos), max 9 gm/day **OR**
-Ampicillin 100-200 mg/kg/day IV/IM q6h (beta-lactamase negative), max 12 gm/day

Pseudomonas aeruginosa:
-Tobramycin (Nebcin):
<5 yr (except neonates): 7.5 mg/kg/day IV/IM q8h.
5-10 yr: 6.0 mg/kg/day IV/IM q8h.
>10 yr: 5.0 mg/kg/day IV/IM q8h **AND**
-Piperacillin (Pipracil) or ticarcillin (Ticar) 200-300 mg/kg/day IV/IM q4-6h, max 24 gm/day **OR**
-Ceftazidime (Fortaz) 150 mg/kg/day IV/IM q8h, max 12 gm/day.

Mycoplasma pneumoniae:
-Clarithromycin (Biaxin) 15-30 mg/kg/day PO q12h, max 1 gm/day
[susp: 125 mg/5 mL, 250 mg/5 mL; tabs: 250, 500 mg].
-Erythromycin estolate (Ilosone)
30-50 mg/kg/day PO q8-12h, max 2 gm/day
[caps: 125, 250 mg; drops: 100 mg/mL; susp: 125 mg/5 mL, 250 mg/5 mL; tab: 500 mg; tabs, chew: 125,250 mg]
-Erythromycin ethylsuccinate (EryPed, EES)
30-50 mg/kg/day PO q6-8h, max 2gm/day
[susp: 200 mg/5 mL, 400 mg/5 mL; tab: 400 mg; tab, chew: 200 mg]
-Erythromycin base (E-Mycin, Ery-Tab, Eryc)
30-50 mg/kg/day PO q6-8h, max 2gm/day
[cap, DR: 250 mg; tabs: 250, 333, 500 mg]
-Erythromycin lactobionate (Erythrocin)
20-40 mg/kg/day IV q6h, max 4 gm/day
[inj: 500 mg, 1 gm]
-Tetracycline (Achromycin)
>8 yrs only
25-50 mg/kg/day PO q6h, max 2 gm/day
[caps: 100, 250, 500 mg; susp: 125 mg/5 mL; tabs: 250, 500 mg]

Moraxella catarrhalis:
  -Clarithromycin (Biaxin)
    15 mg/kg/day PO q12h, max 1 gm/day
    [susp: 125 mg/5 mL, 250 mg/5 mL; tabs: 250, 500 mg] **OR**
  -Cefuroxime (Zinacef) 100-150 mg/kg/day IV/IM q8h, max 9 gm/day **OR**
  -Erythromycin estolate (Ilosone)
    30-50 mg/kg/day PO q8-12h, max 2 gm/day
    [caps: 125, 250 mg; drops: 100 mg/mL; susp: 125 mg/5 mL, 250 mg/5 mL;
    tab: 500 mg; tabs, chew: 125,250 mg]
  -Erythromycin ethylsuccinate (EryPed, EES)
    30-50 mg/kg/day PO q6-8h, max 2gm/day
    [susp: 200 mg/5 mL, 400 mg/5 mL; tab: 400 mg; tab, chew: 200 mg]
  -Erythromycin base (E-Mycin, Ery-Tab, Eryc)
    30-50 mg/kg/day PO q6-8h, max 2gm/day
    [cap, DR: 250 mg; tabs: 250, 333, 500 mg]
  -Erythromycin lactobionate (Erythrocin)
    20-40 mg/kg/day IV q6h, max 4 gm/day
    [inj: 500 mg, 1 gm] **OR**
  -Trimethoprim/Sulfamethoxazole (Bactrim, Septra)
    6-12 mg TMP/kg/day PO/IV q12h, max 320 mg TMP/day
    [inj per mL: TMP 16 mg/SMX 80 mg; susp per 5 mL: TMP 40 mg/SMX 200
    mg; tab DS: TMP 160 mg/SMX 800 mg; tab SS: TMP 80mg/SMX 400 mg]
Chlamydia pneumoniae (TWAR), psittaci, trachomatous:
  -Erythromycin estolate (Ilosone)
    30-50 mg/kg/day PO q8-12h, max 2 gm/day
    [caps: 125, 250 mg; drops: 100 mg/mL; susp: 125 mg/5 mL, 250 mg/5 mL;
    tab: 500 mg; tabs, chew: 125,250 mg]
  -Erythromycin ethylsuccinate (EryPed, EES)
    30-50 mg/kg/day PO q6-8h, max 2gm/day
    [susp: 200 mg/5 mL, 400 mg/5 mL; tab: 400 mg; tab, chew: 200 mg]
  -Erythromycin base (E-Mycin, Ery-Tab, Eryc)
    30-50 mg/kg/day PO q6-8h, max 2gm/day
    [cap, DR: 250 mg; tabs: 250, 333, 500 mg]
  -Erythromycin lactobionate (Erythrocin)
    20-40 mg/kg/day IV q6h, max 4 gm/day
    [inj: 500 mg, 1 gm] **OR**
  -Azithromycin (Zithromax)

    children ≥2 yrs: 12 mg/kg/day PO qd x 5 days, max 500 mg/day

    ≥16 yrs: 500 mg PO on day one, then 250 mg PO qd on days 2-5
    [cap: 250 mg; susp: 100 mg/5mL, 200 mg/5mL; tabs: 250, 600 mg]
Influenza Virus:
  -Oseltamivir (Tamiflu)

    ≥1 yr and <15 kg: 30 mg PO bid
    15-23 kg: 45 mg PO bid
    >23 - 40 kg: 60 mg PO bid
    >40 kg: 75 mg PO bid
    >18 yr: 75 mg PO bid
    [cap: 75 mg; susp: 12 mg/mL]
    Approved for treatment of uncomplicated influenza A or B when patient
    has been symptomatic no longer than 48 hrs. **OR**
  -Rimantadine (Flumadine)
    <10 yr: 5 mg/kg/day PO qd, max 150 mg/day
    >10 yr: 100 mg PO bid
    [syrup: 50 mg/5 mL; tab: 100 mg].
    Approved for treatment or prophylaxis of Influenza A. Not effective against
    Influenza B. **OR**
  -Amantadine (Symmetrel)
    1-9 yr: 5 mg/kg/day PO qd-bid, max 150 mg/day
    >9 yr: 5 mg/kg/day PO qd-bid, max 200 mg/day
    [cap: 100 mg; syr: 50 mg/5 mL].

Approved for treatment or prophylaxis of Influenza A. Not effective against Influenza B.

Bronchiolitis

1. **Admit to:**
2. **Diagnosis:** Bronchiolitis
3. **Condition:**
4. **Vital signs:** Call MD if:
5. **Activity:**
6. **Nursing:** Pulse oximeter, peak flow rate. Respiratory isolation.
7. **Diet:**
8. **IV Fluids:**
9. **Special Medications:**
   -Oxygen, humidified 1-4 L/min by NC or 40-60% by mask, keep sat >92%.

Nebulized Beta 2 Agonists:
   -Albuterol (Ventolin, Proventil) (5 mg/mL sln) nebulized 0.2-0.5 mL in 2 mL NS (0.10-0.15 mg/kg) q1-4h prn.

Treatment of Respiratory Syncytial Virus (severe lung disease or underlying cardiopulmonary disease):
   -Ribavirin (Virazole) therapy should be considered in high risk children <2 yrs with bronchopulmonary dysplasia or with history of premature birth less than 35 weeks gestational age. Ribavirin is administered as a 6 gm vial, aerosolized by SPAG nebulizer over 18-20h qd x 3-5 days or 2 gm over 2 hrs q8h x 3-5 days.

Prophylaxis Against Respiratory Syncytial Virus:
   -Recommended use in high risk children <2 yrs with BPD who required medical management within the past six months, or with history of premature birth less than or equal to 28 weeks gestational age who are less than one year of age at start of RSV season, or with history of premature birth 29-32 weeks gestational age who are less than six months of age at start of RSV season.
   -Palivizumab (Synagis) 15 mg/kg IM once a month throughout RSV season (usually October-March)
   -RSV-IVIG (RespiGam) 750 mg/kg IV once a month throughout RSV season (usually from October to March).

Influenza A:
   -Oseltamivir (Tamiflu)

   ≥1 yr and <15 kg: 30 mg PO bid
   15-23 kg: 45 mg PO bid
   >23 - 40 kg: 60 mg PO bid
   >40 kg: 75 mg PO bid
   >18 yr: 75 mg PO bid
   [cap: 75 mg; susp: 12 mg/mL]
   Approved for treatment of uncomplicated influenza A or B when patient has been symptomatic no longer than 48 hrs. **OR**
   -Rimantadine (Flumadine)
   <10 yr: 5 mg/kg/day PO qd, max 150 mg/day
   >10 yr: 100 mg PO bid
   [syrup: 50 mg/5 mL; tab: 100 mg].
   Approved for treatment or prophylaxis of Influenza A. Not effective against Influenza B. **OR**
   -Amantadine (Symmetrel)
   1-9 yr: 5 mg/kg/day PO qd-bid, max 150 mg/day
   >9 yr: 5 mg/kg/day PO qd-bid, max 200 mg/day
   [cap: 100 mg; syr: 50 mg/5 mL].
   Approved for treatment or prophylaxis of Influenza A. Not effective against Influenza B.

Pertussis:
The estolate salt is preferred due to greater penetration.

-Erythromycin estolate 50 mg/kg/day PO q8-12h, max 2 gm/day
[caps: 125, 250 mg; drops: 100 mg/1 mL; susp: 125 mg/5 mL, 250 mg/5 mL;
tab: 500 mg; tabs, chew: 125,250 mg]
-Erythromycin lactobionate (Erythrocin) 20-40 mg/kg/day IV q6h, max 4
gm/day
[inj: 500 mg, 1 gm].
Oral Beta 2 Agonists and Acetaminophen:
-Albuterol liquid (Proventil, Ventolin)
2-6 years: 0.1-0.2 mg/kg/dose PO q6-8h
6-12 years: 2 mg PO tid-qid
>12 years: 2-4 mg PO tid-qid
[soln: 2 mg/5 mL; tabs: 2,4 mg; tabs, SR: 4, 8 mg]
-Acetaminophen (Tylenol) 10-15 mg/kg PO/PR q4-6h prn temp >38°.
10. **Extras and X-rays:** CXR.
11. **Labs:** CBC, SMA 7, CBG/ABG, UA. Urine antigen screen. Nasopharyngeal
washings for direct fluorescent antibody (RSV, adenovirus, parainfluenza,
influenza virus, chlamydia), viral culture.

Viral Laryngotracheitis (Croup)

1. **Admit to:**
2. **Diagnosis:** Croup
3. **Condition:**
4. **Vital signs:** Call MD if:
5. **Activity:**
6. **Nursing:** Pulse oximeter, laryngoscope and endotracheal tube at bedside.
Respiratory isolation, inputs and outputs.
7. **Diet:**
8. **IV Fluids:**
9. **Special Medications:**
-Oxygen, cool mist, 1-2 L/min by NC or 40-60% by mask, keep sat >92%.
-Racemic epinephrine (2.25% sln) 0.05 mL/kg/dose (max 0.5 mL) in 2-3 mL
saline nebulized q1-6h.
-Dexamethasone (Decadron) 0.25-0.5 mg/kg/dose IM/IV q6h prn, max dose
10 mg **OR**
-Prednisone 1-2 mg/kg/day PO q12-24h x 3-5 days [syr: 1mg/mL, 5 mg/mL;
tabs: 1, 2.5, 5, 10, 20, 50 mg]
-Prednisolone 1-2 mg/kg/day PO q12-24h x 3-5 days [5 mg/5 mL, Orapred
20.2mg/5mL, Prelone 15 mg/5 mL].
10. **Extras and X-rays:** CXR PA and LAT, posteroanterior x-ray of neck.
11. **Labs:** CBC, CBG/ABG, blood culture and sensitivity; UA, culture and
sensitivity. Urine antigen screen.

Varicella Zoster Infections

Immunocompetent Patient
A. Therapy with oral acyclovir is not recommended routinely for the treatment
of uncomplicated varicella in the otherwise healthy child <12 years of age.
B. Oral acyclovir may be given within 24 hours of the onset of rash. Adminis-
tration results in a modest decrease in the duration and magnitude of fever
and a decrease in the number and duration of skin lesions.
C. Acyclovir (Zovirax) 80 mg/kg/day PO q6h for five days, max 3200 mg/day
[cap: 200 mg; susp: 200 mg/5 mL; tabs: 400, 800 mg]
Immunocompromised Patient
A. Intravenous acyclovir should be initiated early in the course of the illness.
Therapy within 24 hours of rash onset maximizes efficacy. Oral acyclovir
should not be used because of unreliable oral bioavailability.
Dose: 500 mg/m^2/dose IV q8h x 7-10 days
B. Varicella zoster immune globulin (VZIG) may be given shortly after

exposure to prevent or modify the course of the disease. It is not effective once disease is established.
Dose: 125 U per 10 kg body weight, round up to nearest vial size to max of 625 U [vial: 125 U/1.25ml]. Must be administered IM.

Appendicitis

1. **Admit to:**
2. **Diagnosis:** Appendicitis.
3. **Condition:** Guarded.
4. **Vital signs:** Call MD if:
5. **Activity:**
6. **Nursing:** Inputs and outputs, daily weights; cooling measures prn temp >38°C. Age appropriate pain scale.
7. **Diet:**
8. **IV Fluids:** Isotonic fluids at maintenance rate.
9. **Special Medications:**
   -Ampicillin 100 mg/kg/day IV/IM q6h, max 12 gm/day **AND**
   -Gentamicin (Garamycin):
      30 days-5 yr: 7.5 mg/kg/day IV/IM q8h.
      5-10 yr: 6.0 mg/kg/day IV/IM q8h.
      >10 yr: 5.0 mg/kg/day IV/IM q8h AND
   -Metronidazole (Flagyl) 30 mg/kg/day q6h, max 4 gm/day
   OR (non-perforated)
   -Cefotetan (Cefotan) 40-80 mg/kg/day IM/IV q12h, max 6 gm/day **OR**
   -Cefoxitin (Mefoxin) 100 mg/kg/day IM/IV q6-8h, max 12 gm/day
10. **Symptomatic Medications:**
   -Ibuprofen 5-10 mg/kg/dose PO q6-8h prn **OR**
   -Acetaminophen 15 mg/kg PO/PR q4h prn temp >38°C or pain.
11. **Extras and X-rays:** Abdominal ultrasound, abdominal x-ray series.
12. **Labs:** CBC, SMA 7, blood culture and sensitivity, antibiotic levels.

Lower Urinary Tract Infection

1. **Admit to:**
2. **Diagnosis:** UTI
3. **Condition:**
4. **Vital signs:** Call MD if:
5. **Activity:**
6. **Nursing:** Inputs and outputs
7. **Diet:**
8. **IV Fluids:**
9. **Special Medications:**
Lower Urinary Tract Infection:
   -Trimethoprim/sulfamethoxazole (Bactrim, Septra) 6-10 mg/kg/day TMP PO q12h, max 320 mg TMP/day [susp per 5 mL: TMP 40 mg, SMX 200 mg; tab, SS: 80 mg/400 mg; tab, DS: 160 mg/800 mg] **OR**
   -Cefpodoxime (Vantin) 10 mg/kg/day PO q12h, max 800 mg/day [susp: 50 mg/5 mL, 100 mg/5 mL; tabs: 100, 200 mg] **OR**
   -Cefprozil (Cefzil) 30 mg/kg/day PO q12h, max 1 gm/day [susp: 125 mg/5 mL, 250 mg/5 mL; tabs: 250, 500 mg] **OR**
Prophylactic Therapy:
   -Trimethoprim/Sulfamethoxazole (Bactrim, Septra) 2 mg TMP/kg/day and 10 mg SMX/kg/day PO qhs [susp per 5 mL: TMP 40 mg/SMX 200 mg; tab DS: TMP 160 mg/SMX 800 mg; tab SS: TMP 80mg/SMX 400 mg] **OR**
   -Sulfisoxazole (Gantrisin) 10-20 mg/kg/day PO q12h [syr: 500 mg/5 mL; tab: 500 mg].
10. **Symptomatic Medications:**
   -Phenazopyridine (Pyridium), children 6-12 yrs: 12 mg/kg/day PO tid (max

200 mg/dose); >12 yrs: 100-200 mg PO tid x 2 days prn dysuria [tabs: 100, 200 mg]. Does not treat infection; acts only as an analgesic.

11. **Extras and X-rays:** Renal ultrasound. Voiding cystourethrogram 3 weeks after infection. Radiological work up on all children <1 year of age.

12. **Labs:** CBC, SMA 7. UA with micro, urine Gram stain, culture and sensitivity. Repeat urine culture and sensitivity 24-48 hours after therapy; blood culture and sensitivity.

Pyelonephritis

1. **Admit to:**
2. **Diagnosis:** Pyelonephritis
3. **Condition:**
4. **Vital signs:** Call MD if:
5. **Activity:**
6. **Nursing:** Inputs and outputs, daily weights
7. **Diet:**
8. **IV Fluids:**
9. **Special Medications:**
   -If less than 1 week old, see suspected sepsis, pages 117, 171.
   -Ampicillin 100 mg/kg/day IV/IM q6h, max 12 gm/day **AND**
   -Gentamicin (Garamycin) or Tobramycin (Nebcin):
      30 days-5 yr: 7.5 mg/kg/day IV/IM q8h.
      5-10 yr: 6.0 mg/kg/day IV/IM q8h.
      >10 yr: 5.0 mg/kg/day IV/IM q8h **OR**
   -Cefotaxime (Claforan) 100 mg/kg/day IV/IM q8h, max 12 gm/day.
10. **Symptomatic Medications:**
   -Acetaminophen (Tylenol) 10-15 mg/kg PO/PR q4-6h prn temp >38°.
11. **Extras and X-rays:** Renal ultrasound.
12. **Labs:** CBC, SMA-7. UA with micro, urine culture and sensitivity. Repeat urine culture and sensitivity 24-48 hours after initiation of therapy; blood culture and sensitivity x 2; drug levels.

Osteomyelitis

1. **Admit to:**
2. **Diagnosis:** Osteomyelitis
3. **Condition:**
4. **Vital signs:** Call MD if:
5. **Activity:**
6. **Nursing:** Keep involved extremity elevated. Consent for osteotomy.
7. **Diet:**
8. **IV Fluids:**
9. **Special Medications:**

Children ≤3 yrs (H flu, strep, staph):
   -Cefuroxime (Zinacef) 100-150 mg/kg/day IV/IM q8h, max 9 gm/day.
Children >3 yrs (staph, strep, H flu):
   -Nafcillin (Nafcil) or oxacillin (Bactophill) 100-150 mg/kg/day IV/IM q6h, max 12 gm/day **OR**
   -Cefotaxime (Claforan) 100-150 mg/kg/day IV/IM q8h, max 12 gm/day **OR**
   -Cefazolin (Ancef) 100 mg/kg/day IV/IM q6-8h, max 6 gm/day **OR**
   -Cefuroxime (Zinacef) 100-150 mg/kg/day IV/IM q8h, max 9 gm/day.
Postoperative or Traumatic (staph, gram neg, Pseudomonas):
   -Ticarcillin/clavulanate (Timentin) 200-300 mg/kg/day of ticarcillin IV/IM q6-8h, max 24 gm/day **OR**
   -Vancomycin (Vancocin) 40-60 mg/kg/day IV q6-8h, max 4 gm/day **AND**
   -Ceftazidime (Fortaz) 150 mg/kg/day IV/IM q8h, max 12 gm/day **OR**
   -Nafcillin (Nafcil) or oxacillin (Bactocill) 150 mg/kg/day IV/IM q6h, max 12

gm/day **AND**
-Tobramycin (Nebcin)
  30 days-5 yr: 7.5 mg/kg/day IV/IM q8h.
  5-10 yr: 6.0 mg/kg/day IV/IM q8h.
  >10 yr: 5.0 mg/kg/day IV q8h.
Chronic Osteomyelitis (staphylococcal):
-Dicloxacillin (Dycill, Dynapen, Pathocil) 75-100 mg/kg/day PO q6h, max 2 gm/day [caps: 125, 250, 500 mg; susp: 62.5 mg/5 mL] **OR**
-Cephalexin (Keflex) 50-100 mg/kg/day PO q6-12h, max 4 gm/day [caps: 250, 500 mg; drops 100 mg/mL; susp 125 mg/5 mL, 250 mg/5 mL; tabs: 500 mg, 1 gm].
10. Symptomatic Medications:
-Acetaminophen (Tylenol) 10-15 mg/kg PO/PR q4-6h prn temp >38°.
11. Extras and X-rays: Bone scan, multiple X-ray views, CT. Orthopedic and infectious disease consultations.
12. Labs: CBC, SMA 7, blood culture and sensitivity x 3, ESR, sickle prep, UA, culture and sensitivity, antibiotic levels, serum bacteriocidal titers.

Otitis Media

Acute Otitis Media (S pneumoniae, non-typable H flu, M catarrhalis, Staph a, group A strep):
-Amoxicillin (Amoxil) 25-50 mg/kg/day PO q8h, max 3 gm/day
  [caps: 250, 500 mg; drops: 50 mg/mL; susp; 125 mg/5mL, 200 mg/5mL, 250 mg/5mL, 400 mg/5mL; tabs: 500, 875 mg; tabs, chew: 125, 200, 250, 400 mg] **OR**
-Trimethoprim/Sulfamethoxazole (Bactrim, Septra) 6-8 mg/kg/day of TMP PO bid, max 320 mg TMP/day
  [susp per 5 mL: TMP 40 mg/SMX 200 mg; tab DS: TMP 160 mg/SMX 800 mg; tab SS: TMP 80mg/SMX 400 mg] **OR**
-Erythromycin/sulfisoxazole (Pediazole) 1 mL/kg/day PO qid or 40 mg/kg/day of erythromycin PO qid, max 50 mL/day
  [susp per 5 mL: erythromycin 200 mg/sulfisoxazole 600 mg] **OR**
-Amoxicillin/clavulanate (Augmentin) 40 mg/kg/day of amoxicillin PO q8h x 7-10d, max 500 mg/dose
  [susp per 5 mL: 125, 250 mg; tabs: 250, 500 mg; tab, chew: 125, 250 mg] **OR**
-Amoxicillin/clavulanate (Augmentin BID)
  40 mg/kg/day PO q12h, max 875 mg of amoxicillin/dose
  [susp: 200 mg/5mL, 400 mg/5mL; tab: 875 mg; tab, chew: 200, 400 mg]
-Azithromycin (Zithromax)

  Children ≥2 yrs: 12 mg/kg/day PO qd x 5 days, max 500 mg/day

  ≥16 yrs: 500 mg PO on day 1, 250 mg PO qd on days 2-5
  [cap: 250 mg; susp: 100 mg/5mL, 200 mg/5mL; tabs: 250, 600 mg] **OR**
-Clarithromycin (Biaxin) 15-30 mg/kg/day PO bid, max 1 gm/day
  [susp: 125 mg/5 mL, 250 mg/5 mL; tabs: 250, 500 mg] **OR**
-Cefixime (Suprax) 8 mg/kg/day PO bid-qd, max 400 mg/day
  [susp: 100 mg/5 mL; tabs: 200, 400 mg] **OR**
-Cefuroxime axetil (Ceftin) tab: child: 125-250 mg PO bid; adult: 250-500 mg PO bid; susp: 30 mg/kg/day PO q12h, max 500 mg/day
  [susp: 125 mg/5 mL; tabs 125, 250, 500 mg] **OR**
-Loracarbef (Lorabid) 30 mg/kg/day PO bid, max 400 mg/day
  [caps: 200, 400 mg; susp: 100 mg/5 mL, 200 mg/5mL] **OR**
-Cefpodoxime (Vantin) 10 mg/kg/day PO bid, max 800 mg/day
  [susp: 50 mg/5 mL, 100 mg 5 mL; tabs: 100, 200 mg] **OR**
-Cefprozil (Cefzil) 30 mg/kg/day PO bid, max 1gm/day
  [susp: 125 mg/5 mL, 250 mg/5 mL; tabs: 250 mg, 500 mg] **OR**
-Ceftriaxone (Rocephin) 50 mg/kg IM x one dose, max 2000 mg

Acute Otitis Media (resistant strains of Strep pneumoniae):
-Amoxicillin (Amoxil) 80-90 mg/kg/day PO q12h, max 3 gm/day
[caps: 250, 500 mg; drops: 50 mg/mL; susp; 125 mg/5mL, 200 mg/5mL, 250 mg/5mL, 400 mg/5mL; tabs: 500, 875 mg; tabs, chew: 125, 200, 250, 400mg]
-Amoxicillin/clavulanate (Augmentin BID) 80-90 mg/kg/day PO q12h.
[susp 200 mg/5 mL, 400 mg/5 mL; tab: 875 mg; tab, chew: 200, 400 mg]

Prophylactic Therapy (≥3 episodes in 6 months):
Therapy reserved for control of recurrent acute otitis media, defined as three or more episodes per 6 months or 4 or more episodes per 12 months.
-Sulfisoxazole (Gantrisin) 50 mg/kg/day PO qhs
[tab 500 mg; susp 500 mg/5 mL] **OR**
-Amoxicillin (Amoxil) 20 mg/kg/day PO qhs
[caps: 250,500 mg; drops: 50 mg/mL; susp; 125 mg/5mL, 200 mg/5mL, 250 mg/5mL, 400 mg/5mL; tabs: 500, 875 mg; tabs, chew: 125, 200, 250, 400mg] **OR**
-Trimethoprim/Sulfamethoxazole (Bactrim, Septra) 4 mg/kg/day of TMP PO qhs
[susp per 5 mL: TMP 40 mg/SMX 200 mg; tab DS: TMP 160 mg/SMX 800 mg; tab SS: TMP 80mg/SMX 400 mg]

Symptomatic Therapy:
-Ibuprofen (Advil) 5-10 mg/kg/dose PO q6-8 hrs prn fever
[suspension: 100 mg/5 mL, tabs: 200, 300, 400, 600, 800 mg] **AND/OR**
-Acetaminophen (Tylenol) 10-15 mg/kg/dose PO/PR q4-6h prn fever
[tabs: 325, 500 mg; chewable tabs: 80 mg; caplets: 160 mg, 500 mg; drops: 80 mg/0.8 mL; elixir: 120 mg/5 mL, 130 mg/5 mL, 160 mg/5 mL, 325 mg/5 mL; caplet, ER: 650 mg; suppositories: 120, 325, 650 mg].
-Benzocaine/antipyrine (Auralgan otic): fill ear canal with 2-4 drops; moisten cotton pledget and place in external ear; repeat every 1-2 hours prn pain
[soln, otic: Antipyrine 5.4%, benzocaine 1.4% in 10 mL and 15 mL bottles]
Extras and X rays: Aspiration tympanocentesis, tympanogram; audiometry.

Otitis Externa

Otitis Externa (Pseudomonas, gram negatives, proteus):
-Polymyxin B/neomycin/hydrocortisone (Cortisporin otic susp or solution) 2-4 drops in ear canal tid-qid x 5-7 days.
[otic soln or susp per mL: neomycin sulfate 5 mg; polymyxin B sulfate 10,000 units; hydrocortisone 10 mg in 10 mL bottles)].
The suspension is preferred. The solution should not be used if the eardrum is perforated.

Malignant Otitis Externa in Diabetes (Pseudomonas):
-Ceftazidime (Fortaz) 100-150 mg/kg/day IV/IM q8h, max 12gm/day **OR**
-Piperacillin (Pipracil) or ticarcillin (Ticar) 200-300 mg/kg/day IV/IM q4-6h, max 24gm/day **OR**
-Tobramycin (Nebcin)
30 days-5 yr: 7.5 mg/kg/day IV/IM q8h.
5-10 yr: 6.0 mg/kg/day IV/IM q8h.
>10 yr: 5.0 mg/kg/day IV q8h.

Tonsillopharyngitis

Streptococcal Pharyngitis:
-Penicillin V (Pen Vee K) 25-50 mg/kg/day PO qid x 10 days, max 3 gm/day
[susp: 125 mg/5 mL, 250 mg/5 mL; tabs: 125, 250, 500 mg] **OR**
-Penicillin G benzathine (Bicillin LA) 25,000-50,000 U/kg (max 1.2 MU) IM x 1 dose **OR**
-Azithromycin (Zithromax) 12 mg/kg/day PO qd x 5 days, max 500 mg/day

    [cap: 250 mg; susp: 100 mg/5mL, 200 mg/5mL; tabs: 250, 600 mg] **OR**
-Clarithromycin (Biaxin)15 mg/kg/day PO bid, max 1 gm/day
    [susp 125 mg/5 mL, 250 mg/5 mL; tabs: 250, 500 mg] **OR**
  -Erythromycin (penicillin allergic patients) 40 mg/kg/day PO qid x 10 days,
    max 2 gm/day
    Erythromycin ethylsuccinate (EryPed, EES)
      [susp: 200 mg/5 mL, 400 mg/5 mL; tab: 400 mg; tab, chew: 200 mg]
    Erythromycin base (E-Mycin, Ery-Tab, Eryc)
      [cap, DR: 250 mg; tabs: 250, 333, 500 mg]

Refractory Pharyngitis:
  -Amoxicillin/clavulanate (Augmentin)
    40 mg/kg/day of amoxicillin PO q8h x 7-10d, max 500 mg/dose
    [susp: 125 mg/5 mL, 250 mg/5 mL; tabs: 250, 500 mg; tabs, chew: 125,
    250 mg] **OR**
  -Dicloxacillin (Dycill, Dynapen, Pathocil)
    50 mg/kg/day PO qid, max 2 gm/day
    [caps 125, 250, 500; elixir 62.5 mg/5 mL] **OR**
  -Cephalexin (Keflex)
    50 mg/kg/day PO qid-tid, max 4 gm/day
    [caps: 250, 500 mg; drops 100 mg/mL; susp 125 mg/5 mL, 250 mg/5 mL;
    tabs: 500 mg, 1 gm].

Prophylaxis (5 strep infections in 6 months):
  -Penicillin V Potassium (Pen Vee K)
    40 mg/kg/day PO bid, max 3 gm/day
    [susp 125 mg/5 mL, 250 mg/5 mL; tabs: 125, 250, 500 mg].

Retropharyngeal Abscess (strep, anaerobes, E corrodens):
  -Clindamycin (Cleocin) 25-40 mg/kg/day IV/IM q6-8h, max 4.8 gm/day **OR**
  -Nafcillin (Nafcil) or oxacillin (Bactocill, Prostaphlin) 100-150 mg/kg/day IV/IM
    q6h, max 12 gm/day **AND**
  -Cefuroxime (Zinacef) 75-100 mg/kg/day IV/IM q8h, max 9 gm/day

Labs: Throat culture, rapid antigen test; PA lateral and neck films; CXR.
  Otolaryngology consult for incision and drainage.

Epiglottitis

1. **Admit to:** Pediatric intensive care unit.
2. **Diagnosis:** Epiglottitis
3. **Condition:**
4. **Vital Signs:** Call MD if:
5. **Activity:**
6. **Nursing:** Pulse oximeter. Keep head of bed elevated, allow patient to sit;
   curved blade laryngoscope, tracheostomy tray and oropharyngeal tube at
   bedside. Avoid excessive manipulation or agitation. Respiratory isolation.
7. **Diet:** NPO
8. **IV Fluids:**
9. **Special Medications:**
  -Oxygen, humidified, blow-by; keep sat >92%.
Antibiotics:
Most common causative organism is Haemophilus influenzae.
  -Ceftriaxone (Rocephin) 50 mg/kg/day IV/IM qd, max 2 gm/day **OR**
  -Cefuroxime (Zinacef) 100-150 mg/kg/day IV/IM q8h, max 9 gm/day **OR**
  -Cefotaxime (Claforan) 100-150 mg/kg/day IV/IM q6-8h, max 12 gm/day
10. **Extras and X-rays:** CXR PA and LAT, lateral neck. Otolaryngology
    consult.
11. **Labs:** CBC, CBG/ABG. Blood culture and sensitivity, latex agglutination;
    UA, urine antigen screen.

Sinusitis

Treatment of Sinusitis (S. pneumoniae, H flu, M catarrhalis, group A strep, anaerobes):
  -Treat for 14-21 days.
  -Amoxicillin (Amoxil) 40 mg/kg/day PO tid, max 3 gm/day [caps: 250,500 mg; drops: 50 mg/mL; susp: 125 mg/5mL, 200 mg/5mL, 200 mg/5mL, 400 mg/5mL; tabs: 500, 875 mg; tabs, chew: 125, 200, 250 , 400mg] **OR**
  -Azithromycin (Zithromax)

   Children ≥2 yrs: 12 mg/kg/day PO qd x 5 days, max 500 mg/day

   ≥16 yrs: 500 mg PO on day 1, 250 mg PO qd on days 2-5
   [cap: 250 mg; susp: 100 mg/5mL; tab: 250, 600 mg] **OR**
  -Trimethoprim/sulfamethoxazole (Bactrim, Septra) 6-8 mg/kg/day of TMP PO bid, max 320 mg TMP/day
   [susp per 5 mL: TMP 40 mg/SMX 200 mg; tab DS: TMP 160 mg/SMX 800 mg; tab SS: TMP 80mg/SMX 400 mg] **OR**
  -Erythromycin/sulfisoxazole (Pediazole) 1 mL/kg/day PO qid or 40-50 mg/kg/day of erythromycin PO qid, max 2 gm erythromycin/day
   [susp per 5 mL: Erythromycin 200 mg, sulfisoxazole 600 mg] **OR**
  -Amoxicillin/clavulanate (Augmentin) 40 mg/kg/day of amoxicillin PO tid, max 500 mg/dose
   [elixir 125 mg/5 mL, 250 mg/5 mL; tabs: 250, 500 mg; tabs, chew: 125, 250 mg] **OR**
  -Amoxicillin/clavulanate (Augmentin BID)
   40 mg/kg/day PO bid, max 875 mg (amoxicillin)/dose
   [susp: 200 mg/5 mL, 400 mg/5 mL; tab: 875 mg; tabs, chew: 200, 400 mg] **OR**
  -Cefuroxime axetil (Ceftin)
   tab: child: 125-250 mg PO bid; adult: 250-500 mg PO bid
   susp: 30 mg/kg/day PO qid, max 500 mg/day
   [susp: 125 mg/5 mL; tabs: 125, 250, 500 mg]
Labs: Sinus x-rays, MRI scan.

Helicobacter Pylori

1. **Admit to:**
2. **Diagnosis:** Helicobacter pylori.
3. **Condition:** Guarded.
4. **Vital signs:** Call MD if:
5. **Activity:**
6. **Nursing:**
7. **Diet:**
8. **IV Fluids:** Isotonic fluids at maintenance rate.
9. **Special Medications:**
   Triple drug regimens are more effective for eradication than are two drug regimens.
Antimicrobial Agents
  -Amoxicillin (Amoxil) 25-50 mg/kg/day PO bid-tid (max 3 gm/day)
   [caps: 250,500 mg; drops: 50 mg/mL; susp: 125 mg/5mL, 200 mg/5mL, 250 mg/5mL, 400 mg/5mL; tabs: 500, 875 mg; tabs, chew: 125, 200, 250mg , 400mg]
  -Tetracycline (Achromycin) **>8 yrs only**
   25-50 mg/kg/day PO q6h, max 2 gm/day
   [caps: 100, 250, 500 mg; susp: 125 mg/5 mL; tabs: 250, 500 mg]
  -Metronidazole (Flagyl): 35-50 mg/kg/day PO q8h, max 2250 mg/day [tabs: 250, 500 mg; extemporaneous suspension]
  -Clarithromycin (Biaxin)15 mg/kg/day PO bid, max 1 gm/day
   [susp 125 mg/5 mL, 250 mg/5 mL; tabs: 250, 500 mg]
H-2 Blockers
  -Ranitidine (Zantac) 4-6 mg/kg/day PO q12h [liquid: 15 mg/mL; tabs: 75, 150, 300 mg]

Proton Pump Inhibitors
  -Lansoprazole (Prevacid)
    <10 kg: 7.5 mg PO qd
    10-20 kg: 15 mg PO qd
    > 20 kg: 30 mg PO qd
    Adolescents: 15-30 mg PO qd
    [caps: 15, 30 mg; simplified lansoprazole suspension (SLS) can be made by dissolving the capsules in sodium bicarbonate. The capsule may also be opened and mixed with applesauce].
  -Omeprazole (Prilosec)
    0.3-3 mg/kg/day PO qd (max 20 mg/day)
    [caps: 10, 20, 40 mg; simplified omeprazole suspension (SOS) is made by dissolving the capsule in sodium bicarbonate]
Bismuth subsalicylate (Pepto-Bismol)
  ≤10 yrs: 262 mg PO qid
  >10 yrs: 524 mg PO qid
  [cap: 262 mg; liquid: 262 mg/15 mL, 525 mg/15 mL; tab, chew: 262 mg]
10. Symptomatic Medications:
  -Acetaminophen 15 mg/kg PO/PR q4h prn temp >38°C or pain.
11. Extras and X-rays: Endoscopy, gastric biopsy.
12. Labs: Culture on gastric biopsy tissue.

Active Pulmonary Tuberculosis

1. **Admit to:**
2. **Diagnosis:** Active Pulmonary Tuberculosis
3. **Condition:**
4. **Vital signs:**
5. **Activity:**
6. **Nursing:** Respiratory isolation.
7. **Diet:**
8. **Special Medications:**
Pulmonary Infection:
Six Month Regimen: Two months of isoniazid, rifampin and pyrazinamide daily, followed by 4 months of isoniazid and rifampin daily **OR**
Two months of isoniazid, rifampin and pyrazinamide daily, followed by 4 months of isoniazid and rifampin twice weekly.
Nine Month Regimen (for hilar adenopathy only): Nine months of isoniazid and rifampin daily **OR** one month of isoniazid and rifampin daily, followed by 8 months of isoniazid and rifampin twice weekly.

Anti-tuberculosis Agents			
Drug	**Daily Dose**	**Twice Weekly Dose**	**Dosage Forms**
Isoniazid (Laniazid)	10-15 mg/kg/day PO qd, max 300 mg	20-30 mg/kg PO, max 900 mg	Tab: 50, 100, 300 mg Syr: 10 mg/mL
Rifampin (Rifadin)	10-20 mg/kg/day PO qd, max 600 mg	10-20 mg/kg, max 600 mg	Cap: 150, 300 mg Extemporaneous suspension
Pyrazinamide	20-40 mg/kg PO qd, max 2000 mg	50 mg/kg PO, max 2000 mg	Tab: 500 mg Extemporaneous suspension

Drug	Daily Dose	Twice Weekly Dose	Dosage Forms
Ethambutol (Myambutol)	15-25 mg/kg/day PO qd, max 2500 mg	50 mg/kg PO, max 2500 mg	Tab: 100, 400 mg
Streptomycin	20-40 mg/kg IM qd, max 1 gm	20-40 mg/kg IM, max 1 gm	Inj: 400 mg/mL, IM only

-Directly observed therapy should be considered for all patients. All household contacts should be tested.

Tuberculosis Prophylaxis for Skin Test Conversion:
   -Isoniazid-susceptible: Isoniazid (Laniazid) 10 mg/kg/day (max 300 mg) PO qd x 6-9 months.
   -Isoniazid-resistant: Rifampin (Rifadin) 10 mg/kg/day (max 600 mg) PO qd for 9 months.
9. **Extras and X-rays:** CXR PA, LAT, spinal series.
10. **Labs:** CBC, SMA7, liver panel, HIV antibody, ABG. First AM sputum for AFB x 3 (drug sensitivity tests on first isolate). Gastric aspirates for AFB qAM x 3. UA, urine AFB.

Cellulitis

1. **Admit to:**
2. **Diagnosis:** Cellulitis
3. **Condition:**
4. **Vital signs:** Call MD if:
5. **Activity:**
6. **Nursing:** Keep affected extremity elevated; warm compresses tid prn. Monitor area of infection.
7. **Diet:**
8. **IV Fluids:**
9. **Special Medications:**
Empiric Therapy for Extremity Cellulitis:
   -Nafcillin (Nafcil) or oxacillin (Bactocill, Prostaphlin) 100-200 mg/kg/day/IV/IM q4-6h, max 12gm/day **OR**
   -Cefazolin (Ancef) 75-100 mg/kg/day IV/IM q6-8h, max 6 gm/day **OR**
   -Cefoxitin (Mefoxin) 100-160 mg/kg/day IV/IM q6h, max 12 gm/day **OR**
   -Ticarcillin/clavulanate (Timentin) 200-300 mg/kg/day IV/IM q6-8h, max 24 gm/day **OR**
   -Dicloxacillin (Dycill, Dynapen, Pathocil) 50-100 mg/kg/day PO qid, max 2 gm/day [caps: 125, 250, 500 mg; susp: 62.5 mg/5 mL].
Cheek/Buccal Cellulitis (H flu):
   -Cefuroxime (Zinacef) 100-150 mg/kg/day IV/IM q8h, max 9 gm/day **OR**
   -Cefotaxime (Claforan) 100-150 mg/kg/day IV/IM q6-8h, max 12 gm/day
Periorbital Cellulitis (H. flu, pneumococcus):
   -Cefuroxime (Zinacef) 100-150 mg/kg/day IV/IM q8h, max 9 gm/day **OR**
   -Cefuroxime axetil (Ceftin)
      tab: child: 125-250 mg PO bid; adult: 250-500 mg PO bid
      susp: 30 mg/kg/day PO qid, max 500 mg/day
      [susp: 125 mg/5 mL; tabs: 125, 250, 500 mg]
10. **Symptomatic Medications:**
   -Acetaminophen and codeine, 0.5-1 mg codeine/kg/dose PO q4-6h prn pain [elixir per 5 mL: codeine 12 mg, acetaminophen 120 mg].
11. **Extras and X-rays:** X-ray views of site.
12. **Labs:** CBC, SMA 7, blood culture and sensitivity. Leading edge aspirate, Gram stain, culture and sensitivity; UA, urine culture.

Impetigo, Scalded Skin Syndrome, and Staphylo-coccal Scarlet Fever

1. **Admit to:**
2. **Diagnosis:** Impetigo, scalded skin syndrome or staphylococcal scarlet fever
3. **Condition:**
4. **Vital signs:** Call MD if:
5. **Activity:**
6. **Nursing:** Warm compresses tid prn.
7. **Diet:**
8. **IV Fluids:**
9. **Special Medications:**
   -Nafcillin (Nafcil) or oxacillin (Bactocill, Prostaphlin) 100-200 mg/kg/day IV/IM q4-6h, max 12 gm/day **OR**
   -Dicloxacillin (Dycill, Dynapen, Pathocil) 25-50 mg/kg/day PO qid x 5-7days, max 2 gm/day [caps 125, 250, 500 mg; elixir 62.5 mg/5 mL] **OR**
   -Cephalexin (Keflex) 25-50 mg/kg/day PO qid, max 4 gm/day [caps: 250, 500 mg; drops 100 mg/mL; susp 125 mg/5 mL, 250 mg/5 mL; tabs: 500 mg, 1 gm] **OR**
   -Loracarbef (Lorabid) 30 mg/kg/day PO bid, max 800 mg/day [caps: 200, 400 mg; susp: 100 mg/5 mL, 200 mg/5mL] **OR**
   -Cefpodoxime (Vantin) 10 mg/kg/day PO bid, max 800 mg/day [susp: 50 mg/5 mL, 100 mg/5 mL; tabs: 100 mg, 200 mg] **OR**
   -Cefprozil (Cefzil) 30 mg/kg/day PO bid, max 1 gm/day [susp 125 mg/5 mL, 250 mg/5 mL; tabs: 250, 500 mg] **OR**
   -Vancomycin (Vancocin) 40 mg/kg/day IV q6-8h, max 4 gm/day
   -Mupirocin (Bactroban) ointment or cream, apply topically tid (cream/oint: 2% 15 gm). Extensive involvement requires systemic antibiotics.
10. **Symptomatic Medications:**
    -Acetaminophen and codeine, 0.5-1 mg codeine/kg/dose PO q4-6h prn pain [elixir per 5 mL: codeine 12 mg, acetaminophen 120 mg].
11. **Labs:** CBC, SMA 7, blood culture and sensitivity. Drainage fluid for Gram stain, culture and sensitivity; UA.

Tetanus

History of One or Two Primary Immunizations or Unknown:
  Low risk wound - Tetanus toxoid 0.5 mL IM.
  Tetanus prone - Tetanus toxoid 0.5 mL IM, plus tetanus immunoglobulin (TIG) 250 U IM.
Three Primary Immunizations and 10 yrs or more Since Last Booster:
  Low risk wound - Tetanus toxoid, 0.5 mL IM.
  Tetanus prone - Tetanus toxoid, 0.5 mL IM.
Three Primary Immunizations and 5-10 yrs Since Last Booster:
  Low risk wound - None
  Tetanus prone - Tetanus toxoid 0.5 mL IM.

Three Primary Immunizations and ≤5 yrs Since Last Booster:
  Low risk wound - None
  Tetanus prone - None
Treatment of Clostridium Tetani Infection:
  -Tetanus immune globulin (TIG): single dose of 3,000 to 6,000 U IM (consider immune globulin intravenous if TIG is not available). Part of the TIG dose may be infiltrated locally around the wound. Keep wound clean and débrided.
  -Penicillin G 100,000 U/kg/day IV q4-6h, max 24 MU/day x 10-14 days **OR**
  -Metronidazole (Flagyl) 30 mg/kg/day PO/IV q6h, max 4 gm/day x 10-14 days

Pelvic Inflammatory Disease

1. **Admit to:**
2. **Diagnosis:** Pelvic Inflammatory Disease (PID)
3. **Condition:**
4. **Vital signs:** Call MD if:
5. **Activity:**
6. **Nursing:**
7. **Diet:**
8. **IV Fluids:**
9. **Special Medications:**

Adolescent Outpatients

Regimen A:
-Ofloxacin (Floxin) 400 mg PO bid x 14 days
[tab: 200, 300, 400 mg] **AND**
-Metronidazole (Flagyl) 500 mg PO bid x 14 days
[tab: 250, 500 mg; extemporaneous suspension]

Regimen B:
-Ceftriaxone (Rocephin) 250 mg IM x 1 dose and doxycycline (Vibramycin) 100 mg PO bid [caps: 50, 100 mg; syr: 50 mg/5 mL; tabs: 50, 100 mg] for 14 days **OR**
-Cefoxitin (Mefoxin) 2 gm IM x 1 dose concurrent with probenecid (Probalan) 1 gm PO 1 dose [tab: 500 mg] and doxycycline (Vibramycin) 100 mg PO bid [caps: 50, 100 mg; susp: 25 mg/5mL; syr: 50 mg/5 mL; tabs: 50, 100 mg] x 14 days.

Adolescent Inpatients

Regimen A:
-Cefoxitin (Mefoxin) 2 gm IV q6h **OR**
-Cefotetan (Cefotan) 2 gm IV q12h **AND**
-Doxycycline (Vibramycin) 100 mg IV/PO q12h (IV until afebrile for at least 48h, then complete total of 14 days of doxycycline 100 mg PO bid [caps: 50,100 mg; susp: 25 mg/5mL; syr: 50 mg/5mL; tabs: 50,100 mg]

Regimen B:
-Clindamycin (Cleocin) 900 mg IV q8h plus gentamicin (Garamycin) 2 mg/kg IV loading dose followed by 1.5 mg/kg IV q8h. Continue for 48h after clinical improvement, followed by clindamycin (Cleocin) 600 mg PO tid (caps: 75, 150, 300 mg; soln: 75 mg/5 mL) to complete total of 14 days of treatment.

Gonorrhea in Children less than 45 kg:
Uncomplicated Vulvovaginitis, Cervicitis, Urethritis, Proctitis, or Pharyngitis:
-Ceftriaxone (Rocephin) 125 mg IM x 1 dose (uncomplicated disease only) **AND**
-Erythromycin 50 mg/kg/day PO q6h, max 2gm/day x 7 days **OR**
-Azithromycin (Zithromax) 20 mg/kg PO x 1 dose, max 1 gm

Disseminated Gonococcal Infection:
-Ceftriaxone (Rocephin) 50 mg/kg/day (max 2gm/day) IV/IM q24h x 7 days **AND**
-Azithromycin (Zithromax) 20 mg/kg (max 1gm) PO x 1 dose **OR**
-Erythromycin 40 mg/kg/day PO q6h (max 2gm/day) x 7 days **OR**
-Doxycycline 100 mg PO bid.

Gonorrhea in Children ≥ 45 kg and ≥8 yrs:
Uncomplicated Vulvovaginitis, Cervicitis, Urethritis, Proctitis, or Pharyngitis:
-Ceftriaxone (Rocephin) 125 mg IM x 1 dose **OR** cefixime (Suprax) 400 mg PO x 1 dose or ofloxacin (Floxin) 400 mg PO x 1 **dose AND**
-Azithromycin (Zithromax) 1000 mg PO x 1 dose **OR**
-Doxycycline 100 mg PO bid x 7 days.

Disseminated Gonococcal Infection:
-Ceftriaxone (Rocephin) 1000 mg/day IV/IM q24h x 7 days OR cefotaxime (Claforan) 1000 mg IV q8h x 7 days **AND**
-Azithromycin (Zithromax) 1000 mg PO x 1 dose **OR**
-Doxycycline 100mg PO bid x 7 days.

10. Symptomatic Medications:
-Acetaminophen (Tylenol) 10-15 mg/kg/dose PO/PR q4-6h prn.
11. Extras and X-rays: Pelvic ultrasound; social services consult.
12. Labs: CBC, SMA 7 and 12. GC culture and chlamydia test, RPR or VDRL. UA with micro; urine pregnancy test.

Pediculosis

Pediculosis Capitis (head lice):
-Permethrin (Nix) is the preferred treatment. Available in a 1% cream rinse that is applied to the scalp and hair for 10 minutes. A single treatment is adequate, but a second treatment may be applied 7-10 days after the first treatment [cream rinse: 1% 60 mL].
-Pyrethrin (Rid, A-2000, R&C). Available as a shampoo that is applied to the scalp and hair for 10 minutes. A repeat application 7-10 days later may sometimes be necessary [shampoo (0.3% pyrethrins, 3% piperonyl butoxide): 60, 120, 240 mL].
-For infestation of eyelashes, apply petrolatum ointment tid-qid for 8-10 days and mechanically remove the lice.
Pediculosis Corporis (body lice):
-Treatment consists of improving hygiene and cleaning clothes. Infested clothing should be washed and dried at hot temperatures to kill the lice. Pediculicides are not necessary.
Pediculosis Pubis (pubic lice, "crabs"): Permethrin (Nix) or pyrethrin-based products may be used as described above for pediculosis capitis. Retreatment is recommended 7-10 days later.

Scabies

Treatment:
Bathe with soap and water; scrub and remove scaling or crusted detritus; towel dry. All clothing and bed linen contaminated within past 2 days should be washed in hot water for 20 min.
Permethrin (Elimite) - 5% cream: Adults and children: Massage cream into skin from head to soles of feet. Remove by washing after 8 to 14 hours. Treat infants on scalp, temple and forehead. One application is curative. [cream: 5% 60 gm]
Lindane (Kwell, Gamma benzene) - available as 1% cream or lotion: Use 1% lindane for adults and older children; not recommended in pregnancy, infants, or on excoriated skin. 1-2 treatments are effective. Massage a thin layer from neck to toes (including soles). In adults, 20-30 gm of cream or lotion is sufficient for 1 application. Bathe after 8 hours. May be repeated in one week if mites remain or if new lesions appear. Contraindicated in children <2 years of age. [lotion: 1% 60, 473 mL; shampoo:1%: 60, 473 mL].

Dermatophytoses

Diagnostic procedures:
(1) KOH prep of scales and skin scrapings for hyphae.
(2) Fungal cultures are used for uncertain cases.
Treat for at least 4 weeks.
Tinea corporis (ringworm), cruris (jock itch), pedis (athlete's foot):
-Ketoconazole (Nizoral) cream qd [2%: 15, 30, 60 gm].
-Clotrimazole (Lotrimin) cream bid [1%: 15, 30, 45 gm].
-Miconazole (Micatin) cream bid [2%: 15, 30 gm].
-Econazole (Spectazole) cream bid [1%: 15, 30, 85 gm].
-Oxiconazole (Oxistat) cream or lotion qd-bid [1% cream: 15, 30, 60 gm; 1%

lotion: 30 mL].
-Sulconazole (Exelderm) cream or lotion qd-bid [1% cream: 15, 30, 60 gm; 1% lotion: 30 mL].
-Naftifine (Naftin) cream or gel applied bid [1%: 15, 30 gm].
-Terbinafine (Lamisil) cream or applied bid [1% cream: 15, 30 gm; 1% gel: 5, 15, 30 gm].

Tinea capitis:
-Griseofulvin Microsize (Grisactin, Grifulvin V) 15-20 mg/kg/day PO qd, max 1000 mg/day [caps: 125, 250 mg; susp: 125 mg/5 mL; tabs: 250, 500 mg]
-Griseofulvin Ultramicrosize (Fulvicin P/G, Grisactin Ultra, Gris-PEG) 5-10 mg/kg/day PO qd, max 750 mg/day [tabs: 125, 165, 250, 330 mg].
-Give griseofulvin with whole-milk or fatty foods to increase absorption. May require 4-6 weeks of therapy and should be continued for two weeks beyond clinical resolution.

Tinea Unguium (Fungal Nail Infection):
-Griseofulvin (see dosage above) is effective, but may require up to 4 months of therapy.

Tinea Versicolor:
-Cover body surface from face to knees with selenium sulfide 2.5% lotion or selenium sulfide 1% shampoo daily for 30 minutes for 1 week, then monthly x 3 to help prevent recurrences.

Bite Wounds

1. **Admit to:**
2. **Diagnosis:** Bite Wound.
3. **Condition:** Guarded.
4. **Vital signs:** Call MD if:
5. **Activity:**
6. **Nursing:** Cooling measures prn temp >38° C, age appropriate pain scale.
7. **Diet:**
8. **IV Fluids:** D5 NS at maintenance rate.
9. **Special Medications:**
-Initiate antimicrobial therapy for: moderate/severe bite wounds, especially if edema or crush injury is present; puncture wounds, especially if bone, tendon sheath, or joint penetration may have occurred; facial bites; hand and foot bites; genital area bites; wounds in immunocompromised or asplenic patients.

Dog Bites and Cat Bites:
Oral: amoxicillin/clavulanate
Oral, penicillin allergic: extended-spectrum cephalosporins or trimethoprim-sulfamethoxazole PLUS clindamycin
IV: ampicillin-sulbactam
IV, penicillin allergic: extended spectrum cephalosporins or trimethoprim-sulfamethoxazole PLUS clindamycin

Reptile Bites:
Oral: amoxicillin-clavulanate
Oral, penicillin allergic: extended-spectrum cephalosporins or trimethoprim-sulfamethoxazole PLUS clindamycin
IV: ampicillin-sulbactam PLUS gentamicin
IV, penicillin allergic: clindamycin PLUS gentamicin

Human Bites:
Oral: amoxicillin-clavulanate
Oral, penicillin allergic: trimethoprim-sulfamethoxazole PLUS clindamycin
IV: ampicillin-sulbactam
IV, penicillin allergic: extended-spectrum cephalosporins or trimethoprim-sulfamethoxazole PLUS clindamycin

Antibiotic Dosages:
-Amoxicillin/clavulanate (Augmentin)
40 mg/kg/day of amoxicillin PO tid, max 500 mg/dose

    [elixir 125 mg/5 mL, 250 mg/5 mL; tabs: 250, 500 mg; tabs, chew: 125, 250 mg] **OR**
-Amoxicillin/clavulanate (Augmentin BID)
    40 mg/kg/day PO bid, max 875 mg (amoxicillin)/dose
    [susp: 200 mg/5 mL, 400 mg/5 mL; tab: 875 mg; tabs, chew: 200, 400 mg]
-Cefpodoxime (Vantin)
    10 mg/kg/day PO bid, max 800 mg/day
    [susp: 50 mg/5 mL, 100 mg/5 mL; tabs: 100 mg, 200 mg] **OR**
-Cefprozil (Cefzil)
    30 mg/kg/day PO bid, max 1 gm/day
    [susp 125 mg/5 mL, 250 mg/5 mL; tabs: 250, 500 mg] **OR**
-Cefixime (Suprax)
    8 mg/kg/day PO bid-qd, max 400 mg/day
    [susp: 100 mg/5 mL; tabs: 200, 400 mg]
-Trimethoprim/Sulfamethoxazole (Bactrim, Septra)
    6-8 mg/kg/day of TMP PO/IV bid, max 320 mg TMP/day
    [inj per mL: TMP 16 mg/SMX 80 mg; susp per 5 mL: TMP 40 mg/SMX 200 mg; tab DS: TMP 160 mg/SMX 800 mg; tab SS: TMP 80mg/SMX 400 mg]
-Clindamycin (Cleocin) 10-30 mg/kg/day PO q6-8h, max 1800 mg/day or 25-40 mg/kg/day IV/IM q6-8h, max 4.8 gm/day [cap: 75, 150, 300 mg; soln: 75 mg/5mL]
-Ampicillin-sulbactam (Unasyn) 100-200 mg/kg/day ampicillin IV/IM a6h, max 12 gm ampicillin/day
    [1.5 gm (ampicillin 1 gm and sulbactam 0.5 gm; 3 gm (ampicillin 2 gm and sulbactam 1 gm)]
-Cefotaxime (Claforan) 100-150 mg/kg/day IV/IM q6-8h, max 12 gm/day
-Ceftriaxone (Rocephin) 50 mg/kg/day IV/IM qd, max 2 gm/day
-Gentamicin (Garamycin) (normal renal function):
    <5 yr (except neonates): 7.5 mg/kg/day IV/IM q8h.
    5-10 yr: 6.0 mg/kg/day IV/IM q8h.
    >10 yr: 5.0 mg/kg/day IV/IM q8h.

Additional Considerations:
-Sponge away visible dirt. Irrigate with a copious volume of sterile saline by high-pressure syringe irrigation. Debride any devitalized tissue.
-Tetanus immunization if not up-to-date.
-Assess risk of rabies from animal bites and risk of hepatitis and HIV from human bites.

10. Symptomatic Medications:
-Ibuprofen (Motrin) 5-10 mg/kg/dose PO q6-8h prn **OR**
-Acetaminophen (Tylenol) 15 mg/kg PO/PR q4h prn temp >38°C or pain.

11. Extras and X-rays: X-ray views of site of injury.

12. Labs: CBC, SMA 7, wound culture.

Lyme Disease

1. **Admit to:**
2. **Diagnosis:** Lyme disease.
3. **Condition:**
4. **Vital signs:** Call MD if:
5. **Activity:**
6. **Nursing:**
7. **Diet:**
8. **IV Fluids:** Isotonic fluids at maintenance rate.
9. **Special Medications:**
Early Localized Disease:

    Age ≥8 yrs: doxycycline 100 mg PO bid x 14-21 days [caps: 50, 100 mg; susp: 25 mg/5mL; syrup: 50 mg/5mL; tabs 50, 100 mg]
    All ages: amoxicillin 25-50 mg/kg/day PO bid (max 3 gm/day) x 14-21 days [caps: 250,500 mg; drops: 50 mg/mL; susp: 125 mg/5mL, 200 mg/5mL, 250 mg/5mL, 400 mg/5mL; tabs: 500, 875 mg; tabs, chew: 125, 200, 250 ,

400mg]
Early Disseminated and Late Disease:
> **Multiple Erythema Migrans:** Take same oral regimen as for early disease but for 21 days.
> **Isolated Facial Palsy:** Take same oral regimen as for early disease but for 21-28 days.
> **Arthritis:** Take same oral regimen as for early disease but for 28 days.
> **Persistent or Recurrent Arthritis:**
>> -Ceftriaxone (Rocephin) 75-100 mg/kg/day IM/IV 12-24h (max 2 gm/dose) for 14-21 days **OR**
>> -Penicillin G 300,000 U/kg/day IV q4h (max 20 million units/day) x 14-21 days.

Carditis or Meningitis or Encephalitis:
> -Ceftriaxone (Rocephin) 75-100 mg/kg/day IM/IV q12-24h (max 2 gm/dose) for 14-21 days **OR**
> -Penicillin G 300,000 U/kg/day IV q4h (max 20 million units/day) x 14-21 days.

Lyme disease vaccine is available for children ≥15 years of age.

10. Symptomatic Medications:
> -Ibuprofen (Advil) 5-10 mg/kg/dose PO q6-8h prn temp >38° C **OR**
> -Acetaminophen (Tylenol) 15 mg/kg PO/PR q4h prn temp >38° C.

11. Extras and X-rays: CXR, MRI.

12. Labs: IgM-specific antibody titer usually peaks between weeks 3 and 6 after the onset of infection. Enzyme immunoassay (EIA) is the most commonly used test for detection of antibodies. The Western immunoblot test is the most useful for corroborating a positive or equivocal EIA test.

Gastrointestinal Disorders

Gastroenteritis

1. **Admit to:**
2. **Diagnosis:** Acute Gastroenteritis
3. **Condition:**
4. **Vital signs:** Call MD if:
5. **Activity:**
6. **Nursing:** Inputs and outputs, daily weights, urine specific gravity.
7. **Diet:** Rehydralyte, Pedialyte or soy formula (Isomil DF), bland diet.
8. **IV Fluids:** See Dehydration, page 163.
9. **Special Medications:**

Severe Gastroenteritis with Fever, Gross Blood and Neutrophils in Stool (E coli, Shigella, Salmonella):
-Ceftriaxone (Rocephin) 50-75 mg/kg/day IV/IM q 12-24h, max 4 gm/day **OR**
-Cefixime (Suprax) 8 mg/kg/day PO bid-qd, max 400 mg/day [susp: 100 mg/5 mL; tabs: 200, 400 mg] **OR**
-Trimethoprim/Sulfamethoxazole (Bactrim, Septra) 10 mg of TMP component/kg/day PO bid x 5-7d, max 320 mg TMP/day [susp per 5 mL: TMP 40 mg/SMX 200 mg; tab DS: TMP 160 mg/SMX 800 mg; tab SS: TMP 80mg/SMX 400 mg].

Salmonella (treat infants and patients with septicemia):
-Ceftriaxone (Rocephin) 50-75 mg/kg/day IV/IM q12-24h, max 4 gm/day **OR**
-Cefixime (Suprax) 8 mg/kg/day PO bid-qd, max 400 mg/day [susp: 100 mg/5 mL; tabs: 200, 400 mg] **OR**
-Ampicillin 100-200 mg/kg/day IV q6h, max 12 gm/day or 50-100 mg/kg/day PO qid x 5-7d, max 4 gm/day [caps: 250, 500 mg; drops: 100 mg/mL; susp: 125 mg/5 mL, 250 mg/5 mL, 500 mg/5 mL] **OR**
-Trimethoprim/Sulfamethoxazole (Bactrim, Septra) 10 mg TMP/kg/day PO bid x 5-7d, max 320 mg TMP/day [susp per 5 mL: TMP 40 mg/SMX 200 mg; tab DS: TMP 160 mg/SMX 800 mg; tab SS: TMP 80mg/SMX 400 mg] OR
-If >18 yrs: Ciprofloxacin (Cipro) 250-750 mg PO q12h or 200-400 mg IV q12h [inj: 200, 400 mg; susp: 100 mg/mL; tabs: 100, 250, 500, 750 mg]

Antibiotic Associated Diarrhea and Pseudomembranous Colitis (Clostridium difficile):
-Treat for 7-10 days. Do not give antidiarrheal drugs.
-Metronidazole (Flagyl) 30 mg/kg/day PO/IV (PO preferred) q8h x 7 days, max 4 gm/day. [inj: 500 mg; tabs: 250, 500 mg; extemporaneous suspension] **OR**
-Vancomycin (Vancocin) 40 mg/kg/day PO qid x 7 days, max 2 gm/day [caps: 125, 250 mg; oral soln: 250 mg/5 mL, 500 mg/6 mL]. Vancomycin therapy is reserved for patients who are allergic to metronidazole or who have not responded to metronidazole therapy.

Rotavirus supportive treatment, see Dehydration page 163.
10. **Extras and X-rays:** Upright abdomen
11. **Labs:** SMA7, CBC; stool Wright stain for leukocytes, Rotazyme. Stool culture and sensitivity for enteric pathogens; C difficile toxin and culture, ova and parasites; occult blood. Urine specific gravity, UA, blood culture and sensitivity.

Specific Therapy for Gastroenteritis

Shigella Sonnei:
-Treat x 5 days. Oral therapy is acceptable except for seriously ill patients. For resistant strains, ciprofloxacin should be considered but is not recommended for use for persons younger than 18 years of age except in exceptional circumstances.
-Ampicillin (preferred over amoxicillin) 50-100 mg/kg/day PO q6h, max 3 gm/day [caps: 250, 500 mg; drops: 100 mg/mL; susp: 125 mg/5 mL, 250

mg/5 mL; 500 mg/5 mL] **OR**
-Trimethoprim/Sulfamethoxazole (Bactrim, Septra) 10 mg TMP/kg/day PO/IV q12h x 5 days [inj per mL: TMP 16mg/SMX 80mg; susp per 5 mL: TMP 40 mg/SMX 200 mg; tab DS: TMP 160 mg/SMX 800 mg; tab SS: TMP 80mg/SMX 400 mg] **OR**
-Ampicillin 50-80 mg/kg/day PO q6h, max 4 gm/day; or 100 mg/kg/day IV/IM q6h for 5-7 days, max 12 gm/day [caps: 250, 500 mg; susp: 125 mg/5 mL, 250 mg/5 mL] **OR**
-Ceftriaxone (Rocephin) 50-75 mg/kg/day IV/IM q 12-24h, max 4 gm/day **OR**
-Cefixime (Suprax) 8 mg/kg/day PO bid-qd, max 400 mg/day [susp: 100 mg/5 mL; tabs: 200, 400 mg]

Yersinia (sepsis):
-Most isolates are resistant to first-generation cephalosporins and penicillins.
-Trimethoprim/sulfamethoxazole (Bactrim, Septra) 10 mg/kg/day TMP PO q12h x 5-7days [susp per 5 mL: TMP 40 mg/SMX 200 mg; tab DS: TMP 160 mg/SMX 800 mg; tab SS: TMP 80mg/SMX 400 mg]

Campylobacter jejuni:
-Erythromycin 40 mg/kg/day PO q6h x 5-7 days, max 2 gm/day
   Erythromycin ethylsuccinate (EryPed, EES)
      [susp: 200 mg/5 mL, 400 mg/5 mL; tab: 400 mg; tab, chew: 200 mg]
   Erythromycin base (E-Mycin, Ery-Tab, Eryc)
      [cap, DR: 250 mg; tabs: 250, 333, 500 mg] **OR**
-Azithromycin (Zithromax)
   10 mg/kg PO x 1 on day 1 (max 500 mg) followed by 5 mg/kg/day PO qd on days 2-5 (max 250 mg)
   [cap: 250 mg; susp: 100 mg/5mL, 200 mg/5mL; tabs: 250, 600 mg]

Enteropathogenic E coli (Travelers Diarrhea):
-Trimethoprim/Sulfamethoxazole (Bactrim, Septra) 10 mg/kg/day TMP PO/IV bid [inj per mL: TMP 16 mg/SMX 80 mg; susp per 5 mL: TMP 40 mg/SMX 200 mg; tab DS: TMP 160 mg/SMX 800 mg; tab SS: TMP 80mg/SMX 400 mg].
-Patients older than 8 years old: Doxycycline (Vibramycin) 2-4 mg/kg/day PO q12-24h, max 200 mg/day [caps: 50, 100 mg; susp: 25 mg/5mL; syrup: 50 mg/5mL; tabs 50, 100 mg].

Enteroinvasive E coli:
-Antibiotic selection should be based on susceptibility testing of the isolate. If systemic infection is suspected, parenteral antimicrobial therapy should be given.

Giardia Lamblia:
-Metronidazole is the drug of choice. A 5-7 day course of therapy has a cure rate of 80-95%. Furazolidone is 72-100% effective when given for 7-10 days. Albendazole is also an acceptable alternative when given for 5 days.
-Metronidazole (Flagyl) 15 mg/kg/day PO q8h x 5-7 days (max 4 gm/day) [tabs: 250, 500 mg; extemporaneous suspension] **OR**
-Furazolidone (Furoxone) 5-8.8 mg/kg/day PO qid for 7-10 days, max 400 mg/day [susp: 50 mg/15 mL; tab: 100 mg] **OR**
-Albendazole (Albenza): if > 2 yrs, 400 mg PO qd x 5 days [tab: 200mg; extemporaneous suspension]

Entamoeba Histolytica:
Asymptomatic cyst carriers:
-Iodoquinol (Yodoxin) 30-40 mg/kg/day PO q8h (max 1.95 gm/day) x 20 days [tabs: 210, 650 mg; powder for reconstitution] **OR**
-Paromomycin (Humatin) 25-35 mg/kg/day PO q8h x 7 days [cap: 250 mg] **OR**
-Diloxanide: 20 mg/kg/day PO q8h x 10 days, max 1500 mg/day. (Available only through CDC).
Mild-to-moderate intestinal symptoms with no dysentery:
-Metronidazole (Flagyl): 35-50 mg/kg/day PO q8h x 10 days, max 2250 mg/day [tabs: 250, 500 mg; extemporaneous suspension] followed by:
-Iodoquinol (Yodoxin) 30-40 mg/kg/day PO q8h (max 1.95 gm/day) x 20 days [tabs: 210, 650 mg; powder for reconstitution] **OR**
-Paromomycin (Humatin) 25-35 mg/kg/day PO q8h x 7 days [cap: 250 mg]

OR
-Diloxanide: 20 mg/kg/day PO q8h x 10 days, max 1500 mg/day. (Available only through CDC).
Dysentery or extraintestinal disease (including liver abscess):
-Metronidazole (Flagyl): 35-50 mg/kg/day PO q8h x 10 days, max 2250 mg/day [tabs: 250, 500 mg; extemporaneous suspension] followed by:
-Iodoquinol (Yodoxin) 30-40 mg/kg/day PO q8h x 20 days [tabs: 210, 650 mg; powder for reconstitution] **OR**
-Paromomycin (Humatin) 25-35 mg/kg/day PO q8h x 7 days [cap: 250 mg] **OR**
-Diloxanide: 20 mg/kg/day PO q8h x 10 days, max 1500 mg/day. (Available only through CDC).

Hepatitis A

1. **Admit to:**
2. **Diagnosis:** Hepatitis A
3. **Condition:**
4. **Vital signs:** Call MD if:
5. **Activity:** Up ad lib
6. **Nursing:** Contact precautions.
7. **Diet:**
8. **IV Fluids:** D5NS IV at maintenance rate.
9. **Symptomatic Medications:**
   -Trimethobenzamide (Tigan)
      15 mg/kg/day IM/PO/PR q6-8h, max 100 mg/dose if <13.6 kg or 200 mg/dose if 13.6-41kg.
      [caps: 100, 250 mg; inj: 100 mg/mL; supp: 100, 200 mg].
   -Acetaminophen (Tylenol) 15 mg/kg PO/PR q4h prn temp >38° C or pain.
   -Meperidine (Demerol) 1 mg/kg IV/IM q2-3h prn pain.
10. **Special Medications:**
    -Hepatitis A immune globulin, 0.02 mL/kg IM (usually requires multiple injections at different sites), when given within 2 weeks after exposure to HAV, is 85% effective in preventing symptomatic infection.

    -Hepatitis A vaccine (Havrix) if ≥2 yrs: 0.5 mL IM, repeat in 6-12 months.
11. **Extras and X-rays:** Abdominal x-ray series.
12. **Labs:** IgM anti-HAV antibody, HAV IgG, liver function tests, INR, PTT, stool culture for enteric pathogens.

Hepatitis B

1. **Admit to:**
2. **Diagnosis:** Hepatitis B.
3. **Condition:** Guarded.
4. **Vital signs:** Call MD if:
5. **Activity:**
6. **Nursing:** Standard precautions.
7. **Diet:** Low fat diet.
8. **IV Fluids:** Isotonic fluids at maintenance rate.
9. **Symptomatic Medications:**
   -Trimethobenzamide (Tigan)
      15 mg/kg/day IM/PO/PR q6-8h, max 100 mg/dose if <13.6 kg or 200 mg/dose if 13.6-41kg.
      [caps: 100, 250 mg; inj: 100 mg/mL; supp: 100, 200 mg].
   -Diphenhydramine (Benadryl) 1 mg/kg/dose IV/IM/IO/PO q6h prn pruritus or nausea, max 50 mg/dose **OR**
   -Acetaminophen (Tylenol)15 mg/kg PO/PR q4h prn temp >38° C or pain.
   -Meperidine (Demerol) 1 mg/kg IV/IM q2-3h prn pain.

Post exposure prophylaxis for previously unimmunized persons:
  -Hepatitis B immune globulin 0.06 mL/kg (minimum 0.5 mL) IM x1 AND
  -Hepatitis B vaccine 0.5 mL IM (complete three dose series with second dose in one month and third dose in six months)
10. Extras and X-rays:
11. Labs: IgM anti-HAV, IgM anti-HBc, HBsAg, anti-HCV; alpha-1-antitrypsin, ANA, ferritin, ceruloplasmin, urine copper, liver function tests, INR, PTT.

Ulcerative Colitis

1. Admit to:
2. Diagnosis: Ulcerative colitis.
3. Condition:
4. Vital signs: Call MD if:
5. Activity:
6. Nursing: Daily weights, inputs and outputs.
7. Diet: NPO except for ice chips, no milk products.
8. IV Fluids:
9. Special Medications:
  -Mesalamine (Asacol): 50 mg/kg/day PO q8-12h, max 800 mg PO TID [tab, EC: 400 mg] **OR**
  -Mesalamine (Pentasa) 50 mg/kg/day PO q6-12h, max 1000 mg PO qid [cap, CR: 250 mg] **OR**
  -Mesalamine (Rowasa) >12 yrs: 60 mL (4 gm) retention enema at bedtime retained overnight for approximately 8 hrs [4 gm/60 mL] OR > 12 yrs: mesalamine (Rowasa) 1 suppository PR bid [supp: 500 mg] **OR**
  -Olsalazine sodium (Dipentum) >12 yrs: 500 mg PO with food bid [cap: 250 mg] **OR**
  -Sulfasalazine (Azulfidine), children >2 yrs:
    Mild exacerbation: 40-50 mg/kg/day PO q6h
    Moderate to severe exacerbation: 50-75 mg/kg/day PO q4-6h, max 6 gm/day.
    Maintenance therapy: 30-50 mg/kg/day PO q4-8h, max 2 gm/day.
    [susp: 50 mg/mL; tab, EC: 500 mg] **OR**
  -Hydrocortisone retention enema 100 mg PR qhs **OR**
  -Hydrocortisone acetate 90 mg aerosol foam PR qd-bid or 25 mg supp PR bid.
  -Prednisone 1-2 mg/kg/day PO qAM or bid (max 40-60 mg/day).
Other Medications:
  -Vitamin B_{12} 100 mcg IM qd x 5 days, then 100-200 mcg IM q month.
  -Multivitamin PO qAM or 1 ampule IV qAM.
  -Folic acid 1 mg PO qd.
10. Extras and X-rays: Upright abdomen, GI consult.
11. Labs: CBC, platelets, SMA 7, Mg, ionized calcium; liver panel, blood culture and sensitivity x 2. Stool culture and sensitivity for enteric pathogens, ova and parasites, C. difficile toxin and culture, Wright's stain.

Parenteral Nutrition

1. Admit to:
2. Diagnosis:
3. Condition:
4. Vital signs: Call MD if:
5. Nursing: Daily weights, inputs and outputs; measure head circumference and height. Finger stick glucose bid.
6. Diet:
Total Parenteral Nutrition:
  -Calculate daily protein solution fluid requirement less fluid from lipid and other sources. Calculate total amino acid requirement.
  -Protein: Neonates and infants start with 0.5 gm/kg/day and increase to 2-3

gm/kg/day. For children and young adults, start with 1 gm/kg/day, and increase by 1.0 gm/kg/day (max 2-3 gm/kg/day). Calculate percent amino acid to be infused: amino acid requirement in grams divided by the volume of fluid from the dextrose/protein solution in mL x 100.
-Advance daily dextrose concentration as tolerated, while following blood glucose levels. Usual maximum concentration is D35W.

Total Parenteral Nutrition Requirements			
	Infants-25 kg	**25-45 kg**	**>45 kg**
Calories	90-120 kcal/kg/day	60-105 kcal/kg/day	40-75 kcal/kg/day
Fluid	120-180 mL/kg/day	120-150 mL/kg/day	50-75 mL/kg/day
Dextrose	4-6 mg/kg/min	7-8 mg/kg/min	7-8 mg/kg/min
Protein	2-3 gm/kg/day	1.5-2.5 gm/kg/day	0.8-2.0 gm/kg/day
Sodium	2-6 mEq/kg/day	2-6 mEq/kg/day	60-150 mEq/kg/day
Potassium	2-5 mEq/kg/day	2-5 mEq/kg/day	70-150 mEq/kg/day
Chloride	2-3 mEq/kg/day	2-3 mEq/kg/day	2-3 mEq/kg/day
Calcium	1-2 mEq/kg/day	1 mEq/kg/day	0.2-0.3 mEq/kg/day
Phosphate	0.5-1 mM/kg/day	0.5 mM/kg/day	7-10 mM/1000 cal
Magnesium	1-2 mEq/kg/day	1 mEq/kg/day	0.35-0.45 mEq/kg/day
Multi-Trace Element Formula	1 mL/day	1 mL/day	1 mL/day

Multivitamin (Peds MVI or MVC 9+3)	
<2.5 kg	2 mL/kg Peds MVI
2.5 kg -11 yr	5 mL/day Peds MVI
≥ 11 yrs	MVC 9+3 10 mL/day

Dextrose Infusion:
    -Dextrose mg/kg/min = [% dextrose x rate (mL/hr) x 0.167] ÷ kg
    -Normal Starting Rate: 6-8 mg/kg/min
Lipid Solution:
    -Minimum of 5% of total calories should be from fat emulsion. Max of 40% of calories as fat (10% soln = 1 gm/10 mL = 1.1 kcal/mL; 20% soln = 2 gm/10 mL = 2.0 kcal/mL). 20% Intralipid is preferred in most patients.
    -For neonates, begin fat emulsion at 0.5 gm/kg/day and advance to 0.5-1 gm/kg/day.

-For infants, children and young adults, begin at 1 gm/kg/day, advance as tolerated by 0.5-1 gm/kg/day; max 3 gm/kg/day or 40% of calories/day.
-Neonates - infuse over 20-24h; children and infants - infuse over 16-24h, max 0.15 gm/kg/hr.
-Check serum triglyceride 6h after infusion (maintain <200 mg/dL)

Peripheral Parenteral Supplementation:
-Calculate daily fluid requirement less fluid from lipid and other sources. Then calculate protein requirements: Begin with 1 gm/kg/day. Advance daily protein by 0.5-0.6 gm/kg/day to maximum of 3 gm/kg/day.
-Protein requirement in grams ÷ fluid requirement in mL x 100 = % amino acids.
-Begin with maximum tolerated dextrose concentration. (Dextrose concentration >12.5% requires a central line.)
-Calculate max fat emulsion intake (3 gm/kg/day), and calculate volume of 20% fat required (20 gm/100 mL = 20 %):
[weight (kg) x gm/kg/day] ÷ 20 x 100 = mL of 20% fat emulsion.
Start with 0.5-1.0 gm/kg/day lipid, and increase by 0.5-1.0 gm/kg/day until 3 gm/kg/day. Deliver over 18-24 hours.
-Draw blood 4-6h after end of infusion for triglyceride level.

8. Extras and X-rays: CXR, plain film for line placement, dietitian consult.

9. Labs:
Daily labs: Glucose, Na, K, Cl, HCO_3, BUN, creatinine, osmolarity, CBC, cholesterol, triglyceride, urine glucose and specific gravity.
Twice weekly Labs: Calcium, phosphate, Mg, SMA-12
Weekly Labs: Protein, albumin, prealbumin, Mg, direct and indirect bilirubin, AST, GGT, alkaline phosphatase, iron, TIBC, transferrin, retinol-binding protein, PT/PTT, zinc, copper, B12, folate, 24h urine nitrogen and creatinine.

Gastroesophageal Reflux

A. Treatment:
-Thicken feedings; give small volume feedings; keep head of bed elevated 30 degrees.
-Metoclopramide (Reglan) 0.1-0.2 mg/kg/dose PO qid 20-30 minutes prior to feedings, max 1 mg/kg/day [concentrated soln: 10 mg/mL; syrup: 1 mg/mL; tab: 10 mg]
-Cimetidine (Tagamet) 20-40 mg/kg/day IV/PO q6h (20-30 min before feeding) [inj: 150 mg/mL; oral soln: 60 mg/mL; tabs: 200, 300, 400, 800 mg]
-Ranitidine (Zantac) 2-4 mg/kg/day IV q8h or 4-6 mg/kg/day PO q12h [inj: 25 mg/mL; liquid: 15 mg/mL; tabs: 75, 150, 300 mg]
-Erythromycin (used as a prokinetic agent not as an antibiotic) 2-3 mg/kg/dose PO q6-8h. [ethylsuccinate susp: 200 mg/5mL, 400 mg/5mL] Concomitant cisapride is contraindicated due to potentially fatal drug interaction.
-Cisapride (Propulsid) 0.15-0.3 mg/kg/dose PO tid-qid [susp: 1 mg/mL; tab, scored: 10 mg]. Available via limited-access protocol only (Janssen, 1-800-Janssen) due to risk of serious cardiac arrhythmias.

B. Extras and X-rays: Upper GI series, pH probe, gastroesophageal nuclear scintigraphy (milk scan), endoscopy.

Constipation

I. Management of Constipation in Infants
A. Glycerin suppositories are effective up to 6 months of age: 1 suppository rectally prn. Barley malt extract, 1-2 teaspoons, can be added to a feeding two to three times daily. Four to six ounces prune juice are often effective. After 6 months of age, lactulose 1 to 2 mL/kg/day is useful.
B. Infants that do not respond may be treated with emulsified mineral oil (Haley's MO) 2 mL/kg/dose PO bid, increasing as needed to 6-8 oz per day.

II. Management of Constipation in Children >2 years of Age
   A. The distal impaction should be removed with hypertonic phosphate enemas (Fleet enema). Usually three enemas are administered during a 36 to 48 hour period.
   B. Lactulose may also be used at 5 to 10 mL PO bid, increasing as required up to 45 mL PO bid.
   C. Emulsified mineral oil (Haley's MO) may be begun at 2 mL/kg/dose PO bid and increased as needed up to 6 to 8 oz per day. Concerns about mineral oil interfering with absorption of fat-soluble vitamins have not been substantiated.
   D. Milk of magnesia: Preschoolers are begun at 2 tsp PO bid, with adjustments made to reach a goal of one to three substantial stools a day over 1 to 2 weeks. Older children: 1-3 tablets (311mg magnesium hydroxide/chewable tablet) PO bid prn.
   E. A bulk-type stool softener (e.g., Metamucil) should be initiated. Increase intake of high-residue foods (e.g. fruits, vegetables), bran, and whole grain products. Water intake should be increased.

III. Stool Softeners and Laxatives:
   A. Docusate sodium (Colace):

<3y	20-40 mg/day PO q6-24h
3-6y	20-60 mg/day PO q6-24h
6-12y	40-150 mg/day PO q6-24h
≥12y	50-400 mg/day PO q6-24h

   [caps: 50,100, 250 mg; oral soln: 10 mg/mL, 50 mg/mL]
   B. Magnesium hydroxide (Milk of Magnesia) 0.5 mL/kg/dose or 2-5 yr: 5-15 mL; 6-12y: 15-30 mL; >12y: 30-60 mL PO prn.
   C. Hyperosmotic soln (CoLyte or GoLytely) 15-20 mL/kg/hr PO/NG.
   D. Polyethylene glycol (MiraLax)
      3-6 yr: 1 tsp powder dissolved in 3 ounces fluid PO qd-tid
      6-12 yr: ½ tablespoon powder dissolved in 4 ounces fluid PO qd-tid

      ≥12 yr: one tablespoon powder dissolved in 8 ounces fluid PO qd-tid
   E. Senna (Senokot, Senna-Gen) 10-20 mg/kg PO/PR qhs prn (max 872 mg/day) [granules: 362 mg/teaspoon; supp: 652 mg; syrup: 218 mg/5mL; tabs: 187, 217, 600 mg]
   F. Sennosides (Agoral, Senokot, Senna-Gen), 2-6 yrs: 3-8.6 mg/dose PO qd-bid; 6-12 yrs: 7.15-15 mg/dose PO qd-bid; > 12 yrs: 12-25 mg/dose PO qd-bid [granules per 5 mL: 8.3, 15, 20 mg; liquid: 33 mg/mL; syrup: 8.8 mg/5 mL; tabs: 6, 8.6, 15, 17, 25 mg]

IV. Diagnostic Evaluation: Anorectal manometry, anteroposterior and lateral abdominal radiographs, lower GI study of unprepared colon.

150 Constipation

Toxicology

Poisonings

Gastric Decontamination:
Ipecac Syrup:
    <6 mos: not recommended
    6-12 mos: 5-10 mL PO followed by 10-20 mL/kg of water
    1-12 yrs: 15 mL PO followed by 10-20 mL/kg of water
    >12 yrs: 30 mL PO followed by 240 mL of water
    May repeat dose one time if vomiting does not occur within 20-30 minutes. Syrup of ipecac is contraindicated in corrosive or hydrocarbon ingestions or in patients without or soon to lose gag reflex.
Activated Charcoal: 1 gm/kg/dose (max 50 gm) PO/NG; the first dose should be given using product containing sorbitol as a cathartic. Repeat ½ of initial dose q4h if indicated.
Gastric Lavage: Left side down, with head slightly lower than body; place large-bore orogastric tube and check position by injecting air and auscultating. Normal saline lavage: 15 mL/kg boluses until clear (max 400 mL), then give activated charcoal or other antidote. Save initial aspirate for toxicological exam. Gastric lavage is contraindicated if corrosives, hydrocarbons, or sharp objects were ingested.
Cathartics:
    -Magnesium citrate 6% sln:
        <6 yrs: 2-4 mL/kg/dose PO/NG
        6-12 yrs: 100-150 mL PO/NG
        >12 yrs: 150-300 mL PO/NG

Antidotes to Common Poisonings

Narcotic or Propoxyphene Overdose:
    -Naloxone (Narcan) 0.1 mg/kg/dose (max 4 mg) IV/IO/ET/IM, may repeat q2min.
Methanol or Ethylene Glycol Overdose:
    -Ethanol 8-10 mL/kg (10% inj soln) IV in D5W over 30min, then 0.8-1.4 mL/kg/hr. Maintain ethanol level at 100-130 mg/dL.
Carbon Monoxide Inhalation:
    -Oxygen 100% or hyperbaric oxygen.
Cyanide Ingestion:
    -Amyl nitrite, break ampule and inhale ampule contents for 30 seconds q1min until sodium nitrite is administered. Use new amp q3min **AND**
    -Sodium nitrite 0.33 mL/kg of 3% inj soln (max 10 mL) IV over 5 minutes. Repeat ½ dose 30 min later if inadequate clinical response.
    Followed By:
    -Sodium thiosulfate 1.65 mL/kg of 25% soln (max 50 mL) IV.
Phenothiazine Reaction (Extrapyramidal Reaction):
    -Diphenhydramine (Benadryl) 1 mg/kg IV/IM q6h x 4 doses (max 50 mg/dose) followed by 5 mg/kg/day PO q6h for 2-3 days.
Digoxin Overdose:
    -Digibind (Digoxin immune Fab). Dose (# vials) = digoxin level in ng/mL x body wt (kg)/100 **OR**
    Dose (# of vials) = mg of digoxin ingested divided by 0.6
Benzodiazepine Overdose:
    -Flumazenil (Romazicon) 0.01 mg/kg IV (max 0.5 mg). Repeat dose if symptoms return.
Alcohol Overdose: Cardiorespiratory support
    -Labs: Blood glucose; CBC, ABG, rapid toxicology screen.
    -Treatment: Dextrose 0.5-1 gm/kg (2-4 mL/kg D25W or 5-10 mL/kg D10W),

max 25 gm.
-Naloxone (Narcan) 0.1 mg/kg (max 2 mg) IV, repeat q2min prn to max dose
8-10 mg if drug overdose suspected. For extreme agitation, give diazepam
0.1-0.5 mg/kg IV (max 5 mg if < 5 yrs, 10 mg if ≥5 yrs).

Organophosphate Toxicity
-Atropine: 0.01-0.02 mg/kg/dose (minimum dose 0.1mg, maximum dose 0.5
mg in children and 1 mg in adolescents) IM/IV/SC. May repeat prn.
-Pralidoxime (2-PAM): 20-50 mg/kg/dose IM/IV. Repeat in 1-2 hrs if muscle
weakness has not been relieved, then at 10-12 hr intervals if cholinergic
signs recur.

Anticholinergic Toxicity
-Physostigmine (Antilirium): 0.01-0.03 mg/kg/dose IV; may repeat after 15-20
minutes to a maximum total dose of 2 mg.

Heparin Overdose
-Protamine sulfate dosage is determined by the most recent dosage of heparin
and the time elapsed since the overdose.

Dosage of Protamine Sulfate	
Time Elapsed	**IV Dose of Protamine (mg) to Neutralize 100 units of Heparin**
Immediate	1-1.5
30-60 minutes	0.5-0.75
> 2 hrs	0.25-0.375

Warfarin Overdose
-Phytonadione (Vitamin K_1)
-If no bleeding and rapid reversal needed and patient will require further oral
anticoagulation therapy, give 0.5-2 mg IV/SC
-If no bleeding and rapid reversal needed and patient will **not** require further
oral anticoagulation therapy, give 2-5 mg IV/SC
-If significant bleeding but not life-threatening, give 0.5-2 mg IV/SC
-If significant bleeding and life-threatening, give 5 mg IV
[inj: 2 mg/mL, 10 mg/mL]

Acetaminophen Overdose

1. **Admit to:**
2. **Diagnosis:** Acetaminophen overdose
3. **Condition:**
4. **Vital signs:** Call MD if
6. **Nursing:** ECG monitoring, inputs and outputs, pulse oximeter, aspiration
precautions.
7. **Diet:**
8. **IV Fluids:**
9. **Special Medications:**
-Gastric lavage with 10 mL/kg (if >5 yrs, use 150-200 mL) of normal saline by
nasogastric tube if < 60 minutes after ingestion.
-Activated charcoal (if recent ingestion) 1 gm/kg PO/ NG q2-4h, remove via
suction prior to acetylcysteine.
-N-Acetylcysteine (Mucomyst, NAC) loading dose 140 mg/kg PO/ NG, then 70
mg/kg PO/NG q4h x 17 doses (20% sln diluted 1:4 in carbonated beverage);
follow acetaminophen levels. Continue for full treatment course even if
serum levels fall below nomogram.

-Phytonadione (Vitamin K) 1-5 mg PO/IV/IM/SQ (if INR >1.5).
-Fresh frozen plasma should be administered if INR >3.
10. **Extras and X-rays:** Portable CXR. Nephrology consult for charcoal hemoperfusion.
11. **Labs:** CBC, SMA 7, liver panel, amylase, INR/PTT; SGOT, SGPT, bilirubin, acetaminophen level now and q4h until nondetectable. Plot serum acetaminophen level on Rumack-Matthew nomogram to assess severity of ingestion unless sustained release Tylenol was ingested. Toxicity is likely with ingestion ≥150 mg/kg (or 7.5 gm in adolescents/adults).

Lead Toxicity

1. **Admit to:**
2. **Diagnosis:** Lead toxicity
3. **Condition:**
4. **Vital signs:** Call MD if
6. **Nursing:** ECG monitoring, inputs and outputs, pulse oximeter
7. **Diet:**
8. **IV Fluids:**
9. **Special Medications:**
Symptoms of lead encephalopathy and/or blood level >70 mcg/DL:
-Treat for five days with edetate calcium disodium and dimercaprol:
-Edetate calcium disodium 250 mg/m^2/dose IM q4h or 50 mg/kg/day continuous IV infusion or 1-1.5 gm/m^2 IV as either an 8hr or 24 hr infusion.
-Dimercaprol (BAL): 4 mg/kg/dose IM q4h
Symptomatic lead poisoning without encephalopathy or asymptomatic with blood level >70 mcg/dL:
-Treat for 3–5 days with edetate calcium disodium and dimercaprol until blood lead level < 50 mcg/dL.
-Edetate calcium disodium 167 mg/m^2 IM q4h or 1 gm/m^2 as a 8-24 hr continuous IV infusion.
-Dimercaprol (BAL): 4 mg/kg IM x 1 then 3 mg/kg/dose IM q4h
Asymptomatic children with blood lead level 45-69 mcg/dL:
-Edetate calcium disodium 25 mg/kg/day as a 8-24 hr IV infusion or IV q12h **OR**
-Succimer (Chemet): 10 mg/kg/dose (or 350 mg/m^2/dose) PO q8h x 5 days followed by 10 mg/kg/dose (or 350 mg/m^2/dose) PO q12h x 14 days [cap: 100 mg]
11. **Labs:** CBC, SMA 7, blood lead level, serum iron level.

Theophylline Overdose

1. **Admit to:**
2. **Diagnosis:** Theophylline overdose
3. **Condition:**
4. **Vital signs:** Call MD if:
5. **Activity:**
6. **Nursing:** ECG monitoring until serum level is less than 20 mcg/mL; inputs and outputs, aspiration and seizure precautions.
7. **Diet:**
8. **IV Fluids:** Give IV fluids at rate to treat dehydration.
9. **Special Medications:**
-No specific antidote is available.
-Activated charcoal 1 gm/kg PO/NG (max 50 gm) q2-4h, followed by cathartic, regardless of time of ingestion. Multiple dose charcoal has been shown to be effective in enhancing elimination.
-Gastric lavage if greater than 20 mg/kg was ingested or if unknown amount ingested or if symptomatic.

-Charcoal hemoperfusion (if serum level >60 mcg/mL or signs of neurotoxicity, seizure, coma).
10. **Extras and X-rays:** Portable CXR, ECG.
11. **Labs:** CBC, SMA 7, theophylline level; INR/PTT, liver panel. Monitor K, Mg, phosphorus, calcium, acid/base balance.

Iron Overdose

1. **Admit to:**
2. **Diagnosis:** Iron overdose
3. **Condition:**
4. **Vital signs:** Call MD if:
5. **Activity:**
6. **Nursing:** Inputs and outputs
7. **Diet:**
8. **IV Fluids:** Maintenance IV fluids
9. **Special Medications:**
    Toxicity likely if >60 mg/kg elemental iron ingested.
    Possibly toxic if 20-60 mg/kg elemental iron ingested.
    Induce emesis with ipecac if recent ingestion (<1 hour ago). Charcoal is not effective. Gastric lavage if greater than 20 mg/kg of elemental iron ingested or if unknown amount ingested.
    If hypotensive, give IV fluids (10-20 mL/kg normal saline) and place the patient in Trendelenburg's position.
    Maintain urine output of >2 mL/kg/h.
    If peak serum iron is greater than 350 mcg/dL or if patient is symptomatic, begin chelation therapy.
       -Deferoxamine (Desferal) 15 mg/kg/hr continuous IV infusion. Continue until serum iron is within normal range.
    Exchange transfusion is recommended in severely symptomatic patients with serum iron >1,000 mcg/dL.
10. **Extras and X-rays:** KUB to determine if tablets are present in intestine.
11. **Labs:** Type and cross, CBC, electrolytes, serum iron, TIBC, INR/PTT, blood glucose, liver function tests, calcium.

Neurologic and Endocrinologic Disorders

Seizure and Status Epilepticus

1. **Admit to:** Pediatric intensive care unit.
2. **Diagnosis:** Seizure
3. **Condition:**
4. **Vital signs:** Neurochecks q2-6h; call MD if:
5. **Activity:**
6. **Nursing:** Seizure and aspiration precautions, ECG and EEG monitoring.
7. **Diet:** NPO
8. **IV Fluids:**
9. **Special Medications:**

Febrile Seizures: Control fever with antipyretics and cooling measures. Anticonvulsive therapy is usually not required.

Status Epilepticus:
1. Maintain airway, 100% O_2 by mask; obtain brief history, fingerstick glucose.
2. Start IV NS. If hypoglycemic, give 1-2 mL/kg D25W IV/IO (0.25-0.5 gm/kg).
3. **Lorazepam (Ativan)** 0.1 mg/kg (max 4 mg) IV/IM. Repeat q15-20 min x 3 prn.
4. **Phenytoin (Dilantin)** 15-18 mg/kg in normal saline at <1 mg/kg/min (max 50 mg/min) IV/IO. Monitor BP and ECG (QT interval).
5. If seizures continue, **intubate** and give **phenobarbital** loading dose of 15-20 mg/kg IV or 5 mg/kg IV every 15 minutes until seizures are controlled or 30 mg/kg is reached.
6. If seizures are refractory, consider midazolam (Versed) infusion (0.1 mg/kg/hr) or general anesthesia with EEG monitoring.
7. Rectal Valium gel formulation
   < 2 yrs: not recommended
   2-5 yrs: 0.5 mg/kg
   6-11 yrs: 0.3 mg/kg
   $\geq$ 12 yrs: 0.2 mg/kg
   Round dose to 2.5, 5, 10, 15, and 20 mg/dose. Dose may be repeated in 4-12 hrs if needed. Do not use more than five times per month or more than once every five days.
   [rectal gel (Diastat): pediatric rectal tip - 5 mg/mL (2.5, 5, 10 mg size); adult rectal tip - 5 mg/mL (10, 15, 20 mg size)]

Generalized Seizures Maintenance Therapy:
-Carbamazepine (Tegretol):
  <6 yr: initially 10-20 mg/kg/day PO bid, then may increase in 5-7 day intervals by 5 mg/kg/day; usual max dose 35 mg/kg/day PO q6-8h
  6-12 yr: initially 100 mg PO bid (10 mg/kg/day PO bid), then may increase by 100 mg/day at weekly intervals; usual maintenance dose 400-800 mg/day PO bid-qid.
  >12 yr: initially 200 mg PO bid, then may increase by 200 mg/day at weekly intervals; usual maintenance dose 800-1200 mg/day PO bid-tid
    Dosing interval depends on product selected. Susp: q6-8h; tab: q8- 12h; tab, chew: q8-12h; tab, ER: q12h
    [susp: 100 mg/5 mL; tab: 200 mg; tab, chewable: 100 mg; tab, ER: 100, 200, 400 mg] **OR**
-Divalproex sodium (Depakote, Valproic acid) PO: Initially 10-15 mg/kg/day bid-tid, then increase by 5-10 mg/kg/day weekly as needed; usual maintenance dose 30-60 mg/kg/day bid-tid. Up to 100 mg/kg/day tid-qid may be required if other enzyme-inducing anticonvulsants are used concomitantly. IV: total daily dose is equivalent to total daily oral dose but divide q6h and switch to oral therapy as soon as possible. PR: dilute syrup 1:1 with water for use as a retention enema, loading dose 17-20 mg/kg x 1 or maintenance 10-15

mg/kg/dose q8h
[cap: 250 mg; cap, sprinkle: 125 mg; inj: 100 mg/mL; syrup: 250 mg/5 mL; tab, DR: 125, 250, 500 mg] **OR**
-Phenobarbital (Luminal): Loading dose 10-20 mg/kg IV/IM/PO, then maintenance dose 3-5 mg/kg/day PO qd-bid
[cap: 16 mg; elixir: 15 mg/5mL, 4 mg/mL; inj: 30 mg/mL, 60 mg/mL, 65 mg/mL, 130 mg/mL; tabs: 8, 15, 16, 30, 32, 60, 65,100 mg] **OR**
-Phenytoin (Dilantin): Loading dose 15-18 mg/kg IV/PO, then maintenance dose 5-7 mg/kg/day PO/IV q8-24h (only sustained release capsules may be dosed q24h)
[caps: 30, 100 mg; elixir: 125 mg/5 mL; inj: 50 mg/mL; tab, chewable: 50 mg]
-Fosphenytoin (Cerebyx): > 5 yrs: loading dose 10-20 mg PE IV/IM, maintenance dose 4-6 mg/kg/day PE IV/IM q12-24h. Fosphenytoin 1.5 mg is equivalent to phenytoin 1 mg which is equivalent to fosphenytoin 1 mg PE (phenytoin equivalent unit). Fosphenytoin is a water-soluble pro-drug of phenytoin and must be ordered as mg of phenytoin equivalent (PE).
[inj: 150 mg (equivalent to phenytoin sodium 100 mg) in 2 mL vial; 750 mg (equivalent to phenytoin sodium 500 mg) in 10 mL vial]

Partial Seizures and Secondary Generalized Seizures:
-Carbamazepine (Tegretol), see above **OR**
-Phenytoin (Dilantin), see above
-Phenobarbital (Luminal), see above **OR**
-Valproic acid (Depacon, Depakote, Depakene), see above.
-Lamotrigine (Lamictal):
  Adding to regimen containing valproic acid: 2-12 yrs: 0.15 mg/kg/day PO qd-bid weeks 1-2, then increase to 0.3 mg/kg/day PO qd-bid weeks 3-4, then increase q1-2 weeks by 0.3 mg/kg/day to maintenance dose 1-5 mg/kg/day (max 200 mg/day)
  >12 yrs: 25 mg PO qOD weeks 1-2, then increase to 25 mg PO qd weeks 3-4, then increase q1-2 weeks by 25-50 mg/day to maintenance dose 100-400 mg/day PO qd-bid
  Adding to regimen without valproic acid: 2-12 yrs: 0.6 mg/kg/day PO bid weeks 1-2, then increase to 1.2 mg/kg/day PO bid weeks 3-4, then increase q1-2 weeks by 1.2 mg/kg/day to maintenance dose 5-15 mg/kg/day PO bid (max 400 mg/day)
  >12 yrs: 50 mg PO qd weeks 1-2, then increase to 50 mg PO bid weeks 3-4, then increase q1-2 weeks by 100 mg/day to maintenance dose 300-500 mg/day PO bid.
  [tabs: 25, 100, 150, 200 mg]
-Primidone (Mysoline) PO: < 8 yrs: 50-125 mg/day qhs, increase by 50-125 mg/day q3-7d; usual dose 10-25 mg/kg/day tid-qid

  ≥ 8 yrs: 125-250 mg qhs; increase by 125-250 mg/day q3-7d, usual dose 750-1500 mg/day tid-qid (max 2 gm/day).
  [susp: 250 mg/5mL; tabs: 50, 250 mg]
10. **Extras and X-rays:** MRI with and without gadolinium, EEG with hyperventilation, CXR, ECG. Neurology consultation.
11. **Labs:** ABG/CBG, CBC, SMA 7, calcium, phosphate, magnesium, liver panel, VDRL, anticonvulsant levels, blood and urine culture. UA, drug and toxin screen.

Therapeutic Serum Levels	
Carbamazepine	4-12 mcg/mL
Clonazepam	20-80 ng/mL
Ethosuximide	40-100 mcg/mL

Phenobarbital	15-40 mcg/mL
Phenytoin	10-20 mcg/mL
Primidone	5-12 mcg/mL
Valproic acid	50-100 mcg/mL

Adjunctive Anticonvulsants

Felbamate (Felbatol)
   2-14 yrs: 15 mg/kg/day PO tid-qid, increase weekly by 15 mg/kg/day if needed to maximum of 45 mg/kg/day or 3600 mg/day (whichever is smaller)

   ≥14 yrs: 1200 mg/day PO tid-qid, increase weekly by 1200 mg/day if needed to maximum of 3600 mg/day
   [susp: 600 mg/5 mL; tabs: 400, 600 mg]
   Warning: due to risk of aplastic anemia and hepatic failure reported with this drug, written informed consent must be obtained from patient/parent prior to initiating therapy. Patients must have CBC, liver enzymes, and bilirubin monitored before starting drug therapy and q1-2 weeks during therapy. Discontinue the drug immediately if bone marrow suppression or elevated liver function tests occur.
Gabapentin (Neurontin)
   2-12 yrs: 5-35 mg/kg/day PO q8h
   > 12 yrs: initially 300 mg PO tid, titrate dose upward if needed; usual dose 900-1800 mg/day, maximum 3600 mg/day
   [caps: 100, 300, 400 mg; soln: 250 mg/5 mL; tabs: 600, 800 mg]
   Adjunctive treatment of partial and secondarily generalized seizures.
Levetiracetam (Keppra)
   ≥ 16 yrs: 500 mg PO bid, may increase by 1000 mg/day q2 weeks to maximum of 3000 mg/day [tabs: 250, 500, 750 mg]
Tiagabine (Gabitril)
   < 12 yrs: dosing guidelines not established
   12-18 yrs: 4 mg PO qd x 1 week, then 4 mg bid x 1 week, then increase weekly by 4-8 mg/day and titrate to response; maximum dose 32 mg/day bid-qid. [tabs: 2, 4, 12, 16, 20 mg]. Lower doses may be effective in patients not receiving enzyme-inducing drugs.
Topiramate (Topamax)
   2-16 yrs with partial onset seizures: 1-3 mg/kg/day PO qhs x 1 week (max 25 mg/day), may increase q1-2 weeks by 1-3 mg/kg/day bid to usual maintenance dose 5-9 mg/kg/day bid
   2-16 yrs with primary generalized tonic clonic seizures: use slower initial titration rate to max of 6 mg/kg/day PO by the end of eight weeks
   > 16 yrs with partial onset seizures: 50 mg/day qhs x 1 week, then 100 mg/day bid x 1 week, then increase by 50 mg/day q week; usual maintenance dose 200 mg bid, max 1600 mg/day
   > 16 yrs with generalized tonic clonic seizures: use slower initial titration rate to usual maintenance dose 200 mg bid, max 1600 mg/day
   [caps, sprinkles: 15, 25, 50 mg; tabs: 25, 100, 200 mg]
Vigabatrin (Sabril) PO
   3-9 yrs: 500 mg bid
   > 9 yrs: 1000 mg bid, may increase if needed to max 4000 mg/day
   [tab: 500 mg]. Most effective in complex partial seizures, with or without generalization. Should be used as add-on therapy in patients with drug-resistant seizures, not as monotherapy. Do not abruptly discontinue therapy; gradually taper off to avoid rebound increase in seizure frequency and possible psychotic-like episodes.

Spasticity

1. **Admit to:**
2. **Diagnosis:** Cerebral palsy, spasticity
3. **Condition:**
4. **Vital signs:**
5. **Activity:** Physical Therapy
6. **Nursing:** Inputs and outputs, daily weights;
7. **Diet:**
8. **IV Fluids:** Isotonic fluids at maintenance rate if NPO
9. **Special Medications:**
   -Baclofen (Lioresal)
   - 2-7 yrs: 10-15 mg/day PO q8h, titrate dose upwards by 5-15 mg/day q3 days to a maximum of 40 mg/day
   - > 7 yrs: 10-15 mg/day PO q8h, titrate dose upwards by 5-15 mg/day q3 days to a maximum of 60 mg/day

   [tabs: 10, 20 mg; extemporaneous suspension]
   -Diazepam (Valium), 0.12-0.8 mg/kg/day PO q6-8h or 0.04-0.3 mg/kg/dose IV/IM q4h prn

   [inj: 5 mg/mL; soln: 1 mg/mL, 5 mg/mL; tabs: 2, 5, 10 mg]
   -Dantrolene (Dantrium), 0.5 mg/kg/dose PO bid, may increase q4-7 days by 0.5 mg/kg/day to maximum of 3 mg/kg/dose PO bid-qid up to 400 mg/day

   [caps: 25, 50, 100 mg; extemporaneous suspension]
10. **Extras and X-rays:** Occupational therapy consult; physical therapy consult; rehab consult.

New Onset Diabetes

1. **Admit to:**
2. **Diagnosis:** New Onset Diabetes Mellitus
3. **Condition:**
4. **Vital signs:** Call MD if:
5. **Activity:**
6. **Nursing:** Record labs on a flow sheet. Fingerstick glucose at 0700, 1200, 1700, 2100, 0200; diabetic and dietetic teaching.
7. **Diet:** Diabetic diet with 1000 kcal + 100 kcal/year of age. 3 meals and 3 snacks (between each meal and qhs.)
8. **IV Fluids:** Hep-lock with flush q shift.
9. **Special Medications:**
   -Goal is preprandial glucose of 100-200 mg/dL

Total Daily Insulin Dosage		
<5 Years (U/kg)	5-11 Years (U/kg)	12-18 Years (U/kg)
0.6-0.8	0.75-0.9	0.8-1.5

   -Divide 2/3 before breakfast and 1/3 before dinner. Give 2/3 of total insulin requirement as NPH and give 1/3 as lispro or regular insulin.
10. **Extras and X-rays:** CXR. Endocrine and dietary consult.
11. **Labs:** CBC, ketones; SMA 7 and 12, antithyroglobulin, antithyroid microsomal, anti-insulin, anti-islet cell antibodies. UA, urine culture and sensitivity; urine pregnancy test; urine ketones.

Diabetic Ketoacidosis

1. **Admit to:** Pediatric intensive care unit.
2. **Diagnosis:** Diabetic ketoacidosis
3. **Condition:** Critical
4. **Vital signs:** Call MD if:
5. **Activity:**
6. **Nursing:** ECG monitoring; capillary glucose checks q1-2h until glucose level is <200 mg/dL, daily weights, inputs and outputs. O_2 at 2-4 L/min by NC. Record labs on flow sheet.
7. **Diet:** NPO
8. **IV Fluids:** 0.9% saline 10-20 mL/kg over 1h, then repeat until hemodynamically stable. Then give 0.45% saline, and replace ½ of calculated deficit plus insensible loss over 8h, replace remaining ½ of deficit plus insensible losses over 16-24h. Keep urine output >1.0 mL/kg/hour.

   Add KCL when potassium is <6.0 mEq/dL

Serum K+	Infusate KCL
<3	40-60 mEq/L
3-4	30
4-5	20
5-6	10
>6	0

   Rate: 0.25-1 mEq KCL/kg/hr, maximum 1 mEq/kg/h or 20 mEq/h.
9. **Special Medications:**
   - Insulin Regular (Humulin) 0.05-0.1 U/kg/hr (50 U in 500 mL NS) continuous IV infusion. Adjust to decrease glucose by 50-100 mg/dL/hr.
   - If glucose decreases at less than 50 mg/dL/hr, increase insulin to 0.14-0.2 U/kg/hr. If glucose decreases faster than 100 mg/dL/hr, continue insulin at 0.05-0.1 U/kg/h and add D5W to IV fluids.
   - When glucose approaches 250-300 mg/dL, add D5W to IV. Change to subcutaneous insulin (lispro or regular) when bicarbonate is >15, and patient is tolerating PO food; do not discontinue insulin drip until one hour after subcutaneous dose of insulin.
10. **Extras and X-rays:** Portable CXR, ECG. Endocrine and dietary consultation.
11. **Labs:** Dextrostixs q1-2h until glucose <200, then q3-6h. Glucose, potassium, phosphate, bicarbonate q3-4h; serum acetone, CBC. UA, urine ketones, culture and sensitivity.

Hematologic and Inflammatory Disorders

Sickle Cell Crisis

1. **Admit to:**
2. **Diagnosis:** Sickle Cell Anemia, Sickle Cell Crisis
3. **Condition:**
4. **Vital signs:** Call MD if
5. **Activity:**
6. **Nursing:** Age appropriate pain scale.
7. **Diet:**
8. **IV Fluids:** D5 ½ NS at 1.5-2.0 x maintenance.
9. **Special Medications:**
   -Oxygen 2-4 L/min by NC.
   -Morphine sulfate 0.1 mg/kg/dose (max 10-15 mg) IV/IM/SC q2-4h prn or follow bolus with infusion of 0.05-0.1 mg/kg/hr prn or 0.3-0.5 mg/kg PO q4h prn **OR**
   -Acetaminophen/codeine 0.5-1 mg/kg/dose (max 60 mg/dose) of codeine PO q4-6h prn [elixir: 12 mg codeine/5 mL; tabs: 15, 30, 60 mg codeine component] **OR**
   -Acetaminophen and hydrocodone [elixir per 5 mL: hydrocodone 2.5 mg, acetaminophen] 167 mg; tabs:
   Hydrocodone 2.5 mg, acetaminophen 500 mg;
   Hydrocodone 5 mg, acetaminophen 500 mg;
   Hydrocodone 7.5 mg, acetaminophen 500 mg,
   Hydrocodone 7.5 mg, acetaminophen 650 mg,
   Hydrocodone 10 mg, acetaminophen 500 mg,
   Hydrocodone 10 mg, acetaminophen 650 mg
   Children: 0.6 mg hydrocodone/kg/day PO q6-8h prn
   <2 yr: do not exceed 1.25 mg/dose
   2-12 yr: do not exceed 5 mg/dose
   >12 yr: do not exceed 10 mg/dose

Patient Controlled Analgesia
   -Morphine
   Basal rate 0.01-0.02 mg/kg/hr
   Intermittent bolus dose 0.01-0.03 mg/kg
   Bolus frequency ("lockout interval") every 6-15 minutes
   -Hydromorphone (Dilaudid)
   Basal rate 0.0015-0.003 mg/kg/hr
   Intermittent bolus dose 0.0015-0.0045 mg/kg
   Bolus frequency ("lockout interval") every 6-15 min

Adjunctive Therapy:
   -Hydroxyzine (Vistaril) 0.5-1 mg/kg/dose PO q6h (max 50 mg/dose)
   -Ibuprofen (Motrin) 10 mg/kg/dose PO q6h (max 800 mg/dose) **OR**
   -Ketorolac (Toradol) 0.4 mg/kg/dose IV/IM q6h (max 30 mg/dose); maximum 3 days, then switch to oral ibuprofen

Maintenance Therapy:
   -Hydroxyurea (Hydrea): 15 mg/kg/day PO qd, may increase by 5 mg/kg/day q12 weeks to a maximum dose of 35 mg/kg/day. Monitor for myelotoxicity. [caps: 200, 300, 400, 500 mg]
   -Folic acid 1 mg PO qd (if >1 yr).
   -Transfusion PRBC 5 mL/kg over 2h, then 10 mL/kg over 2h, then check hemoglobin. If hemoglobin is less than 6-8 gm/dL, give additional 10 mL/kg.
   -Deferoxamine (Desferal) 15 mg/kg/hr x 48 hours (max 12 gm/day) concomitantly with transfusion or 1-2 gm/day SQ over 8-24 hrs
   -Vitamin C 100 mg PO qd while receiving deferoxamine
   -Vitamin E PO qd while receiving deferoxamine
   <1 yr: 100 IU/day

　　　1-6 yr: 200 IU/day
　　　>6 yr: 400 IU/day
　-Penicillin VK (Pen Vee K) (prophylaxis for pneumococcal infections): <3 yrs:
　　125 mg PO bid; ≥3 yrs: 250 mg PO bid [elixir: 125 mg/5 mL, 250 mg/5 mL;
　　tabs: 125, 250, 500 mg]. If compliance with oral antibiotics is poor, use
　　penicillin G benzathine 50,000 U/kg (max 1.2 million units) IM every 3 weeks.
　　Erythromycin is used if penicillin allergic.
10. Extras and X-rays: CXR.
11. Labs: CBC, blood culture and sensitivity, reticulocyte count, type and cross,
　　SMA 7, parvovirus titers, UA, urine culture and sensitivity.

Kawasaki's Syndrome

1. Admit to:
2. Diagnosis:
3. Condition:
4. Vital signs: Call MD if:
5. Activity: Bedrest
6. Nursing: temperature at least q4h
7. Diet:
8. Special Medications:
　-Immunoglobulin (IVIG) 2 gm/kg/dose IV x 1 dose. Administer dose at 0.02
　　mL/kg/min over 30 min; if no adverse reaction, increase to 0.04 mL/kg/min
　　over 30 min; if no adverse reaction, increase to 0.08 mL/kg/min for remain-
　　der of infusion. Defer measles vaccination for 11 months after receiving high
　　dose IVIG. [inj: 50 mg/mL, 100 mg/mL]
　-Aspirin 100 mg/kg/day PO or PR q6h until fever resolves, then 8-10 mg/kg/day
　　PO/PR qd [supp: 60, 120, 125, 130, 195, 200, 300, 325, 600, 650 mg; tabs:
　　325, 500, 650 mg; tab, chew: 81 mg].
　-Ambubag, epinephrine (0.1 mL/kg of 1:10,000), and diphenhydramine 1 mg/kg
　　(max 50 mg) should be available for IV use if an anaphylactic reaction to
　　immunoglobulin occurs.
9. Extras and X-rays: ECG, echocardiogram, chest X-ray. Rheumatology
　　consult.
10. Labs: CBC with differential and platelet count. ESR, CBC, liver function
　　tests, rheumatoid factor, salicylate levels, blood culture and sensitivity x 2,
　　SMA 7.

Fluids and Electrolytes

Dehydration

1. **Admit to:**
2. **Diagnosis:** Dehydration
3. **Condition:**
4. **Vital signs:** Call MD if:
5. **Activity:**
6. **Nursing:** Inputs and outputs, daily weights. Urine specific gravity q void.
7. **Diet:**
8. **IV Fluids:**

Maintenance Fluids:

<10 kg	100 mL/kg/24h
10-20 kg	1000 mL plus 50 mL/kg/24h for each kg >10 kg
>20 kg	1500 mL plus 20 mL/kg/24h for each kg >20 kg.

Electrolyte Requirements:
Sodium: 3-5 mEq/kg/day
Potassium: 2-3 mEq/kg/day
Chloride: 3 mEq/kg/day
Glucose: 5-10 gm/100 mL water required (D5W - D10W)

Estimation of Dehydration			
Degree of Dehydration	**Mild**	**Moderate**	**Severe**
Weight Loss--Infants	5%	10%	15%
Weight Loss--Children	3%-4%	6%-8%	10%
Pulse	Normal	Slightly increased	Very increased
Blood Pressure	Normal	Normal to orthostatic, >10 mm Hg change	Orthostatic to shock
Behavior	Normal	Irritable	Hyperirritable to lethargic
Thirst	Slight	Moderate	Intense
Mucous Membranes	Normal	Dry	Parched
Tears	Present	Decreased	Absent, sunken eyes
Anterior Fontanelle	Normal	Normal to sunken	Sunken
External Jugular Vein	Visible when supine	Not visible except with supraclavicular pressure	Not visible even with supraclavicular pressure
Skin	Capillary refill <2 sec	Delayed capillary refill, 2-4 sec (decreased turgor)	Very delayed capillary refill (>4 sec), tenting; cool skin, acrocyanotic, or mottled

Degree of Dehydration	Mild	Moderate	Severe
Urine Specific Gravity (SG)	>1.020	>1.020; oliguria	Oliguria or anuria
Approximate Fluid Deficit	<50 mL/kg	50-100 mL/kg	≥ 100 mL/kg

Electrolyte Deficit Calculation:
Na^+ deficit = (desired Na - measured Na in mEq/L) x 0.6 x weight in kg
K^+ deficit = (desired K - measured K in mEq/L) x 0.25 x weight in kg
Cl^- deficit= (desired Cl - measured Cl in mEq/L) x 0.45 x weight in kg
Free H_2O deficit in hypernatremic dehydration = 4 mL/kg for every mEq that serum Na >145 mEq/L.

Phase 1, Acute Fluid Resuscitation (Symptomatic Dehydration):
-Give NS 20-30 mL/kg IV at maximum rate; repeat fluid boluses of NS 20-30 mL/kg until adequate circulation.

Phase 2, Deficit and Maintenance Therapy (Asymptomatic dehydration):
Hypotonic Dehydration (Na^+ <125 mEq/L):
-Calculate total maintenance and deficit fluids and sodium deficit for 24h (minus fluids and electrolytes given in phase 1). If isotonic or hyponatremic dehydration, replace 50% over 8h and 50% over next 16h.
-Estimate and replace ongoing losses q6-8h.
-Add potassium to IV solution after first void.
-Usually D5 ½ NS or D5 1/4 NS saline with 10-40 mEq KCL/liter 60 mL/kg over 2 hours. Then infuse at 6-8 mL/kg/h for 12h.
-See hyponatremia, page 166.

Isotonic Dehydration (Na^+ 130-150 mEq/L):
-Calculate total maintenance and replacement fluids for 24h (minus fluids and electrolytes given in phase 1) and give half over first 8h, then remaining half over next 16 hours.
-Add potassium to IV solution after first void.
-Estimate and replace ongoing losses.
-Usually D5 ½ NS or D5 1/4 NS with 10-40 mEq KCL/L.

Hypertonic Dehydration (Na^+ >150 mEq/L):
-Calculate and correct free water deficit and correct slowly. Lower sodium by 10 mEq/L/day; do not reduce sodium by more than 15 mEq/L/24h or by >0.5 mEq/L/hr.
-If volume depleted, give NS 20-40 mL/kg IV until adequate circulation, then give ½-1/4 NS in 5% dextrose to replace half of free water deficit over first 24h. Follow serial serum sodium levels and correct deficit over 48-72h.
-**Free water deficit:** 4 mL/kg x (serum Na^+ -145)
-Also see "hypernatremia" page 166.
-Add potassium to IV solution after first void as KCL.
-Usually D5 1/4 NS or D5W with 10-40 mEq/L KCL. Estimate and replace ongoing losses and maintenance.

Replacement of ongoing losses (usual fluids):
-Nasogastric suction: D5 ½ NS with 20 mEq KCL/L or ½ NS with KCL 20 mEq/L.
-Diarrhea: D5 1/4 NS with 40 mEq KCl/L

Oral Rehydration Therapy (mild-moderate dehydration <10%):
-Oral rehydration electrolyte solution (Rehydralyte, Pedialyte, Ricelyte, Revital Ice) deficit replacement of 60-80 mL/kg PO or via NG tube over 2h. Provide additional fluid requirement over remaining 18-20 hours; add anticipated fluid losses from stools of 10 mL/kg for each diarrheal stool.

Oral Electrolyte Solutions			
Product	Na (mEq/L)	K (mEq/L)	Cl (mEq/L)
Rehydralyte	75	20	65
Ricelyte	50	25	45
Pedialyte	45	20	35

Hyperkalemia

1. **Admit to:** Pediatric ICU
2. **Diagnosis:** Hyperkalemia
3. **Condition:**
4. **Vital signs:** Call MD if:
5. **Activity:**
6. **Nursing:** Continuous ECG monitoring, inputs and outputs, daily weights.
7. **Diet:**
8. **IV Fluids:**
Hyperkalemia (K$^+$ >7 or EKG Changes)
   -Calcium gluconate 50-100 mg/kg (max 1 gm) IV over 5-10 minutes or calcium chloride 10-20 mg/kg (max 1 gm) IV over 10 minutes.
   -Regular insulin 0.1 U/kg plus glucose 0.5 gm/kg IV bolus (as 10% dextrose).
   -Sodium bicarbonate 1-2 mEq/kg IV over 3-5 min (give after calcium in separate IV), repeat in 10-15 min if necessary.
   -Furosemide (Lasix) 1 mg/kg/dose (max 40 mg IV) IV q6-12h prn, may increase to 2 mg/kg/dose IV [inj: 10 mg/mL]
   -Kayexalate resin 0.5-1 gm/kg PO/PR. 1 gm resin binds 1 mEq of potassium.
9. **Extras and X-rays:** ECG, dietetics, nephrology consults.
10. **Labs:** SMA7, Mg, calcium, CBC, platelets. UA; urine potassium.

Hypokalemia

1. **Admit to:** Pediatric ICU
2. **Diagnosis:** Hypokalemia
3. **Condition:**
4. **Vital signs:** Call MD if:
5. **Activity:**
6. **Nursing:** ECG monitoring, inputs and outputs, daily weights.
7. **Diet:**
8. **IV Fluids:**
If serum K >2.5 mEq/L and ECG changes are absent:
   Add 20-40 mEq KCL/L to maintenance IV fluids. May give 1-4 mEq/kg/day to maintain normal serum potassium. May supplement with oral potassium.
K <2.5 mEq/L and ECG abnormalities:
   Give KCL 1-2 mEq/kg IV at 0.5 mEq/kg/hr; max rate 1 mEq/kg/hr or 20 mEq/kg/hr in life-threatening situations (whichever is smaller). Recheck serum potassium, and repeat IV boluses prn; ECG monitoring required.
Oral Potassium Therapy:
   -Potassium chloride (KCl) elixir 1-3 mEq/kg/day PO q8-24h [10% soln = 1.33 mEq/mL].
9. **Extras and X-rays:** ECG, dietetics, nephrology consults.
10. **Labs:** SMA7, Mg, calcium, CBC. UA, urine potassium.

Hypernatremia

1. **Admit to:**
2. **Diagnosis:** Hypernatremia
3. **Condition:**
4. **Vital signs:** Call MD if:
5. **Activity:**
6. **Nursing:** Inputs and outputs, daily weights.
7. **Diet:**
8. **IV Fluids:**

    If volume depleted or hypotensive, give NS 20-40 mL/kg IV until adequate circulation, then give D5 ½ NS IV to replace half of body water deficit over first 24h. Correct serum sodium slowly at 0.5-1 mEq/L/hr. Correct remaining deficit over next 48-72h.

    Body water deficit (liter) = 0.6 x (weight kg) x (serum Na -140)

    Hypernatremia with ECF Volume Excess:

    -Furosemide (Lasix) 1 mg/kg IV.

    -D5 1/4 NS to correct body water deficit.

9. **Extras and X-rays:** ECG.
10. **Labs:** SMA 7, osmolality, triglycerides. UA, urine specific gravity; 24h urine Na, K, creatinine.

Hyponatremia

1. **Admit to:**
2. **Diagnosis:** Hyponatremia
3. **Condition:**
4. **Vital signs:** Call MD if:
5. **Activity:**
6. **Nursing:** Inputs and outputs, daily weights, neurochecks.
7. **Diet:**
8. **IV Fluids:**

Hyponatremia with Edema (Hypervolemia)(low osmolality <280, urine sodium <10 mM/L: nephrosis, CHF, cirrhosis; urine sodium >20: acute/chronic renal failure):

-Water restrict to half maintenance.

-Furosemide (Lasix) 1 mg/kg/dose IV over 1-2 min or 2-3 mg/kg/day PO q8-24h.

Hyponatremia with Normal Volume Status (low osmolality <280, urine sodium <10 mM/L: water intoxication; urine sodium >20 mM/L: SIADH, hypothyroidism, renal failure, Addison's disease, stress, drugs):

-0.9% saline with 20-40 mEq KCL/L infused to correct hyponatremia at rate of <0.5 mEq/L/hr) **OR** use 3% NS in severe hyponatremia [3% NS = 513 mEq/liter].

Hyponatremia with Hypovolemia (low osmolality <280; urine sodium <10 mM/L: vomiting, diarrhea, 3rd space/respiratory/skin loss; urine sodium >20 mM/L: diuretics, renal injury, renal tubular acidosis, adrenal insufficiency, partial obstruction, salt wasting):

-If volume depleted, give NS 20-40 mL/kg IV until adequate circulation.

-Gradually correct sodium deficit in increments of 10 mEq/L. Determine volume deficit clinically, and determine sodium deficit as below.

-Calculate 24 hour fluid and sodium requirement and give half over first 8 hours, then give remainder over 16 hours. 0.9% saline = 154 mEq/L

-Usually D5NS 60 mL/kg IV over 2h (this will increase extracellular sodium by 10 mEq/L), then infuse at 6-8 mL/kg/hr x 12h.

Severe Symptomatic Hyponatremia:

-If volume depleted, give NS 20-40 mL/kg until adequate circulation.

-Determine volume of 3% hypertonic saline (513 mEq/L) to be infused as follows:

Na(mEq) deficit = 0.6 x (wt kg) x (desired Na - actual Na)

Volume of soln (L) = Sodium to be infused (mEq) ÷ mEq/L in solution
-Correct half of sodium deficit slowly over 24h.
-For acute correction, the serum sodium goal is 125 mEq/L; max rate for acute
  replacement is 1 mEq/kg/hr. Serum Na should be adjusted in increments of
  5 mEq/L to reach 125 mEq/L. The first dose is given over 4 hrs. For further
  correction for serum sodium to above 125 mEq/L, calculate mEq dose of
  sodium and administer over 24-48h.
9. **Extras and X-rays:** CXR, ECG.
10. **Labs:** SMA 7, osmolality, triglyceride. UA, urine specific gravity. Urine
  osmolality, Na, K; 24h urine Na, K, creatinine.

Hypophosphatemia

Indications for Intermittent IV Administration:
1. Serum phosphate <1.0 mg/dL or
2. Serum phosphate <2.0 mg/dL and patient symptomatic or
3. Serum phosphate <2.5 mg/dL and patient on ventilator

Treatment of Hypophosphatemia		
Dosage of IV Phosphate		**Serum Phosphate**
Low dose	0.08 mM/kg IV over 6 hrs	>1 mg/dL
Intermediate dose	0.16 mM/kg IV over 6 hrs 0.24 mM/kg IV over 4 hrs	0.5-1 mg/dL
High Dose	0.36 mM/kg IV over 6 hrs	<0.5 mg/dL

IV Phosphate Cations:
  Sodium phosphate: Contains sodium 4 mEq/mL, phosphate 3 mM/mL
  Potassium phosphate: Contains potassium 4.4 mEq/mL, phosphate 3 mM/mL
  Max rate 0.06 mM/kg/hr
Oral Phosphate Replacement
1-3 mM/kg/day PO bid-qid
Potassium Phosphate:
  Powder (Neutra-Phos-K): phosphorus 250 mg [8 mM] and potassium 556 mg
  [14.25 mEq] per packet; Tab (K-Phos Original): phosphorus 114 mg [3.7 mM],
  potassium 144 mg [3.7 mEq]
Sodium Phosphate: Phosphosoda Soln per 100 mL: sodium phosphate 18 gm
  and sodium biphosphate 48 gm [contains phosphate 4 mM/mL]
Sodium and Potassium Phosphate: Powd Packet: phosphorus 250 mg [8 mM],
  potassium 278 mg [7.125 mEq], sodium 164 mg [7.125 mEq];
  Tabs:
  K-Phos MF: phosphorus 125.6 mg [4 mM], potassium 44.5 mg [1.1 mEq],
    sodium 67 mg [2.9 mEq]
  K-Phos Neutral: phosphorus 250 mg [8 mM], potassium 45 mg [1.1 mEq],
    sodium 298 mg [13 mEq]
  K-Phos No 2: phosphorus 250 mg [8 mM], potassium 88 mg [2.3 mEq], sodium
    134 mg [5.8 mEq]
  Uro-KP-Neutral: phosphorus 250 mg [8 mM], potassium 49.4 mg [1.27 mEq],
    sodium 250.5 mg [10.9 mEq]

Hypomagnesemia

Indications for Intermittent IV Administration:
1. Serum magnesium <1.2 mg/dL
2. Serum magnesium <1.6 mg/dL and patient symptomatic
3. Calcium resistant tetany

Magnesium Sulfate, Acute Treatment:
-25-50 mg/kg/dose (0.2-0.4 mEq/kg/dose) IV every 4-6 hrs x 3-4 doses as needed (max 2000 mg = 16 mEq/dose); max rate 1 mEq/kg/hr (125 mg/kg/hr).

Magnesium sulfate IV maintenance dose: 1-2 mEq/kg/day (125-250 mg/kg/day) in maintenance IV solution.

Magnesium PO Maintenance Dose: 10-20 mg/kg/dose **elemental magnesium** PO qid.

Magnesium Chloride (Slow-Mag): mg salt (mEq elemental magnesium; mg elemental magnesium)
Tab, SR: 535 mg (5.2 mEq; 63 mg).

Magnesium Gluconate (Magonate): mg salt (mEq elemental magnesium; mg elemental magnesium)
Liq: 1000 mg/5mL (4.8 mEq/5mL; 54 mg).
Tab: 500 mg (2.4 mEq; 27 mg).

Magnesium Oxide: mg salt (mEq elemental magnesium; mg elemental magnesium)
Tabs: 400 mg (20 mEq; 242 mg), 420 mg (21 mEq; 254 mg), 500 mg (25 mEq; 302 mg).
Caps: 140 mg (7 mEq; 84 mg).

Magnesium Sulfate: mg salt (mEq elemental magnesium; mg elemental magnesium)
Soln: 500 mg/mL (4.1 mEq/mL; 49.3 mg/mL).

Newborn Care

Neonatal Resuscitation

APGAR Score			
Sign	**0**	**1**	**2**
Heart rate per minute	Absent	Slow (<100)	>100
Respirations	Absent	Slow, irregular	Good, crying
Muscle tone	Limp	Some flexion	Active motion
Reflex irritability	No response	Grimace	Cough or sneeze
Color	Blue or pale	Pink body with blue extremities	Completely pink
Assess APGAR score at 1 minute and 5 minutes, then continue assessment at 5 minute intervals until APGAR is greater than 7.			

General Measures:
1. Review history, check equipment, oxygen, masks, laryngoscope, ET tubes, medications.

Vigorous, Crying Infant: Provide routine delivery room care for infants with heart rate >100 beats per minute, spontaneous respirations, and good color and tone: warmth, clearing the airway, and drying.

Meconium in Amniotic Fluid:
1. Deliver the head and suction meconium from the hypopharynx on delivery of the head. If the newly born infant has absent or depressed respirations, heart rate <100 bpm, or poor muscle tone, perform direct tracheal suctioning to remove meconium from the airway.
2. If no improvement occurs or if the clinical condition deteriorates, bag and mask ventilate with intermittent positive pressure using 100% FiO_2; stimulate vigorously by drying. Initial breath pressure: 30-40 cm H_2O for term infants, 20-30 cm H_2O for preterm infants. Ventilate at 15-20 cm H_2O at 30-40 breaths per minute. Monitor bilateral breath sounds and expansion.
3. If spontaneous respirations develop and heart rate is normal, gradually reduce ventilation rate until using only continuous positive airway pressure (CPAP). Wean to blow-by oxygen, but continue blow-by oxygen if the baby remains dusky.
4. Consider intubation if the heart rate remains <100 beats per minute and is not rising, or if respirations are poor and weak.

Resuscitation:
1. Provide assisted ventilation with attention to oxygen delivery, inspiratory time, and effectiveness as judged by chest rise if stimulation does not achieve prompt onset of spontaneous respirations or the heart rate is <100 bpm.
2. Provide chest compressions if the heart rate is absent or remains <60 bpm despite adequate assisted ventilation for 30 seconds. Coordinate chest compressions with ventilations at a ratio of 3:1 and a rate of 120 events per minute to achieve approximately 90 compressions and 30 breaths per minute.

3. Chest compressions should be done by two thumb-encircling hands in newly born infants and older infants. The depth of chest compression should be one third of the anterior-posterior diameter of the chest. Chest compressions should be sufficiently deep to generate a palpable pulse.
4. If condition worsens or if there is no change after 30 seconds, or if mask ventilation is difficult: use laryngoscope to suction oropharynx and trachea and intubate. Apply positive pressure ventilation. Check bilateral breath sounds and chest expansion. Check and adjust ET tube position if necessary. Continue cardiac compressions if heart rate remains depressed. Check CXR for tube placement.

Hypotension or Bradycardia or Asystole: Epinephrine 0.1-0.3 mL/kg [0.01-0.03 mg/kg (0.1 mg/mL = 1:10,000)] IV or ET q3-5min. Dilute ET dose to 2-3 mL in NS. If infant fails to respond, consider increasing dose to 0.1 mg/kg (0.1 mL/kg of 1 mg/mL = 1:1000).

Hypovolemia: Insert umbilical vein catheter and give O negative blood, plasma, 5% albumin, Ringer's lactate, or normal saline 10 mL/kg IV over 5-10 minutes. Repeat as necessary to correct hypovolemia.

Severe Birth Asphyxia, Mixed Respiratory/Metabolic Acidosis (not responding to ventilatory support; pH <7.2): Give sodium Bicarbonate 1 mEq/kg, dilute 1:1 in sterile water IV q5-10min as indicated.

Narcotic-Related Depression:
1. Naloxone (Narcan) 0.1 mg/kg = 0.25 mL/kg (0.4 mg/mL concentration) or 0.1 mL/kg (1 mg/mL concentration) ET/IV/IM/SC, may repeat q2-3 min. May cause drug withdrawal and seizures in the infant if the mother is a drug abuser.
2. Repeat administration may be necessary since the duration of action of naloxone may be shorter than the duration of action of the narcotic.

Endotracheal Tube Sizes			
Weight (gm)	Gestational Age (weeks)	Tube Size (mm)	Depth of Insertion from Upper Lip (cm)
<1000	<28	2.5	6.5-7
1000-2000	28-34	3.0	7-8
2000-3000	34-38	3.5	8-9
>3000	>38	3.5-4.0	>9

Suspected Neonatal Sepsis

1. Admit to:
2. Diagnosis: Suspected sepsis
3. Condition:
4. Vital signs: Call MD if:
5. Activity:
6. Nursing: Inputs and outputs, daily weights, cooling measures prn temp >38°C, consent for lumbar puncture.
7. Diet:
8. IV Fluids: IV fluids at 1-1.5 times maintenance.
9. Special Medications:
Newborn Infants <1 month old (group B strep, E coli, or group D strep, gram negatives, Listeria monocytogenes):
-Ampicillin and gentamicin **OR** ampicillin and cefotaxime as below.
-Add vancomycin as below if >7 days old and a central line is present.
Neonatal Dosage of Ampicillin:
  <1200 gm 0-4 weeks: 100 mg/kg/day IV/IMq12h
  1200-2000 gm:

 ≤7d: 100 mg/kg/day IV/IM q12h
 >7d: 150 mg/kg/day IV/IM q8h
  >2000 gm:

 ≤7d: 150 mg/kg/day IV/IM q8h
 >7d: 200 mg/kg/day IV/IM q6h
Cefotaxime (Claforan):
  <1200 grams: 0-4 wks: 100 mg/kg/day IV/IM q12h

  ≥1200 grams: 0-7 days: 100 mg/kg/day IV/IM q12h
 >7 days: 150 mg/kg/day IV/IM q8h
Gentamicin (Garamycin)/Tobramycin (Nebcin):
  <1200 gm 0-4 weeks: 2.5 mg/kg/dose IV/IMq24h
  1200-2000 gm:

 ≤7d: 2.5 mg/kg/dose IV/IM q12-24h
 >7d: 2.5 mg/kg/dose IV/IM q12-24h
  >2000 gm:

 ≤7d: 2.5 mg/kg/dose IV/IM q12-24h
 >7d: 2.5 mg/kg/dose IV/IM q12h
Neonatal Vancomycin (Vancocin) Dosage:
  <1200 gm 0-4 weeks: 15 mg/kg/dose IV q24h
  1200-2000 gm:

 ≤7d: 10 mg/kg/dose IV q12-18h
 >7d: 10 mg/kg/dose IV q8-12h
  >2000 gm:

 ≤7d: 10 mg/kg/dose IV q12h
 >7d: 10 mg/kg/dose IV q8-12h
Nafcillin (Nafcil):
  <1200 gm:
  0-4 weeks 50 mg/kg/day IV/IM q12h
  1200-2000 gm:

 ≤7 days: 50 mg/kg/day IV/IM q12h
 >7 days: 75 mg/kg/day IV/IM q8h
  >2000 gm:

 ≤7 days: 75 mg/kg/day IV/IM q8h
 >7 days: 100 mg/kg/day IV/IM q6h
Mezlocillin (Mezlin):
  <1200 gm:
  0-4 weeks 150 mg/kg/day IV/IM q12h

1200-2000 gm:

≤7 days: 150 mg/kg/day IV/IM q12h
>7 days: 225 mg/kg/day IV/IM q8h

>2000 gm:

≤7 days: 150 mg/kg/day IV/IM q12h
>7 days: 225 mg/kg/day IV/IM q8h

Amikacin:
<1200 gm 0-4 weeks: 10 mg/kg/dose IV/IM q24h
1200-2000 gm:

≤7d: 10 mg/kg/dose IV/IM q12-24h
>7d: 10 mg/kg/dose IV/IM q12-24h

>2000 gm:

≤7d: 10 mg/kg/dose IV/IM q12-24h
>7d: 10 mg/kg/dose IV/IM q12h

10. **Extras and X-rays:** CXR
11. **Laboratory Studies:** CBC, SMA 7, blood culture and sensitivity; UA, culture and sensitivity, antibiotic levels.
CSF Tube 1 - Gram stain, bacterial culture and sensitivity, antigen screen (1-2 mL).
CSF Tube 2 - Glucose protein (1-2 mL).
CSF Tube 3 - Cell count and differential (1-2 mL).

Respiratory Distress Syndrome

1. **Provide mechanical ventilation** as indicated.
2. **Exogenous surfactant:**
   Prophylactic Therapy: Infants at risk for developing RDS with a birth weight <1250gm.
   Rescue Therapy: Treatment of infants with RDS based on respiratory distress not attributable to any other causes and chest radiographic findings consistent with RDS.
   -Beractant (Survanta): 4 mL/kg of birth weight via endotracheal tube then q6h up to 4 doses total [100 mg (4 mL), 200 mg (8 mL)]
   -Colfosceril (Exosurf): 5 mL/kg of birth weight via endotracheal tube then q12h for 2-3 doses total [108 mg (10 mL)]
   -Poractant alfa (Curosurf): first dose 2.5 mL/kg (200 mg/kg/dose) of birthweight via endotracheal tube, may repeat with 1.25 mL/kg/dose (100 mg/kg/dose) at 12-hour intervals for up to two additional doses [120 mg (1.5 mL), 240 mg (3 mL)]
   -Calfactant (Infasurf): 3 mL/kg via endotracheal tube, may repeat q12h up to a total of 3 doses [6 mL]

Necrotizing Enterocolitis

Treatment:
1. Decompress bowel with a large-bore (10 or 12 French), double lumen nasogastric or orogastric tube and apply intermittent suction.
2. Replace fluid losses with IV fluids; monitor urine output, tissue perfusion and blood pressure; consider central line monitoring.
3. Give blood and blood products for anemia, thrombocytopenia, or coagulopathy. Monitor abdominal X-rays for free air from perforation.
4. **Antibiotics:** Ampicillin and gentamicin or tobramycin or cefotaxime. Add vancomycin if a central line is present
5. **Diagnostic Evaluation:** Serial abdominal X-rays with lateral decubitus, CBC with differential and platelets; DIC panel, blood cultures x 2; Wright's stain of stool; stool cultures.
6. **Monitor** the patient frequently for perforation, electrolyte disturbances, and

radiologic evidence of pneumatosis intestinalis and portal vein gas. Obtain surgical evaluation if perforation is suspected.

Apnea

1. Admit to:
2. Diagnosis: Apnea
3. Condition:
4. Vital signs: Call MD if:
5. Activity:
6. Nursing: Heart rate monitor, impedance apnea monitor, pulse oximeter. Keep bag and mask resuscitation equipment at bed side. Rocker bed or oscillating water bed.
7. Diet: Infant formula ad lib
8. IV Fluids:
9. Special Medications:
Apnea of Prematurity/Central Apnea:
    -Aminophylline: loading dose 5 mg/kg IV, then maintenance 5 mg/kg/day IV q12h [inj: 25 mg/mL] **OR**
    -Theophylline: loading dose 5 mg/kg PO, then 5 mg/kg/day PO q12h. [elixir: 80 mg/15mL].
    -Caffeine citrate: Loading dose 10-20 mg/kg IV/PO, then 5 mg/kg/day PO/IV q12-24h [inj: 20 mg/mL, oral soln: 20 mg/mL, extemporaneously prepared oral suspension: 10 mg/mL].
10. Extras and X-rays: Pneumogram, cranial ultrasound. Upper GI (rule out reflux), EEG.
11. Labs: CBC, SMA 7, glucose, calcium, theophylline level (therapeutic range 6-14 mcg/mL) , caffeine level (therapeutic range 10-20 mcg/mL).

Bronchopulmonary Dysplasia

1. Admit to:
2. Diagnosis: Bronchopulmonary Dysplasia.
4. Vital signs: Call MD if:
5. Activity:
6. Nursing: Inputs and outputs, daily weights
7. Diet:
8. IV Fluids: Isotonic fluids at maintenance rate.
9. Special Medications:
Diuretics:
    -Furosemide (Lasix) 1 mg/kg/dose PO/IV/IM q6-24h prn [inj: 10 mg/mL; oral soln: 10 mg/mL, 40 mg/5mL]
    -Chlorothiazide (Diuril) 2-8 mg/kg/day IV q12-24h or 20-40 mg/kg/day PO q12h [inj: 500 mg; susp: 250 mg/5mL]
    -Spironolactone (Aldactone) 2-3 mg/kg/day PO q12-24h [tabs: 25, 50, 100 mg; extemporaneous suspension]
Steroids:
    -Dexamethasone (Decadron) 0.5-1 mg/kg/day IV/IM q6-12h
    -Prednisone 1-2 mg/kg/day PO q12-24h [soln: 1 mg/mL, 5 mg/mL]
11. Extras and X-rays: CXR
12. Labs: CBC, SMA 7.

Hyperbilirubinemia

1. **Admit to:**
2. **Diagnosis:** Hyperbilirubinemia.
3. **Condition:** Guarded.
4. **Vital signs:** Call MD if:
5. **Activity:**
6. **Nursing:** Inputs and outputs, daily weights, monitor skin color, monitor for lethargy and hypotonia
7. **Diet:**
8. **IV Fluids:** Isotonic fluids at maintenance rate (100-150 mL/kg/day). Encourage enteral feedings if possible.
9. **Special Medications:**
   -Phenobarbital 5 mg/kg/day PO/IV q12-24h [elixir: 15 mg/5mL, 20 mg/5mL; inj: 30 mg/mL, 60 mg/mL, 65 mg/mL, 130 mg/mL]
   -Phototherapy
   -Exchange transfusion for severely elevated bilirubin
10. **Symptomatic Medications:**
11. **Extras and X-rays:**
12. **Labs:** Total bilirubin, indirect bilirubin, albumin, SMA 7. Blood group typing of mother and infant, a direct Coombs' test. Complete blood cell count, reticulocyte count, blood smear. In infants of Asian or Greek descent, glucose-6-phosphate dehydrogenase (G6PD) should be measured.

Congenital Syphilis

Treatment:
-Penicillin G aqueous: 50,000 U/kg/dose IV/IM; 0-7 days of age: q12h; >7 days: q8h. Treat for 10-14 days. If one or more days is missed, restart entire course **OR**
-Procaine penicillin G 50,000 U/kg/day IM qd for 10-14 day. Procaine penicillin does not achieve adequate CSF concentrations and may NOT be administered intravenously.
-Obtain follow-up serology at 3, 6, 12 months until nontreponemal test is nonreactive. Infectious skin precautions should be taken.

Congenital Herpes Simplex Infection

-Acyclovir (Zovirax) 60 mg/kg/day IV q8h. Infuse each dose over 1 hr x 14 days (if disease is limited to skin, eye, and mouth) or 21 days (if disease is disseminated or involves the CNS). Infants with ocular involvement should also receive topical ophthalmic trifluridine.
-Trifluridine ophthalmic solution (Viroptic) 1 drop in each affected eye q2h while awake [ophth soln 1%: 7.5 mL bottle].

Patent Ductus Arteriosus

Treatment:
1. Restrict fluids if the infant is symptomatic.
2. Provide respiratory support and maintain hematocrit at 40%.
3. Furosemide (Lasix) 1-2 mg/kg/dose q6-8h PO.

4. Indomethacin (Indocin):

Three dose course:			
Age at First Dose	Dose 1 (mg/kg/dose)	Dose 2 (mg/kg/dose)	Dose 3 (mg/kg/dose)
<48h	0.2	0.1	0.1
2-7d	0.2	0.2	0.2
>7d	0.2	0.25	0.25
Give q12-24h IV over 20-30 min. Check serum creatinine and urine output prior to each dose.			

Five-dose course: 0.1 mg/kg/dose IV q24h x 5 days. Check serum creatinine and urine output prior to each dose.
5. **Diagnostic Considerations:** ABG, chest X-ray, ECG, CBC, electrolytes. Echocardiogram (to determine if PDA has closed).
6. Consider surgical intervention if two courses of indomethacin fail to close the PDA or if indomethacin therapy is contraindicated (hemodynamically unstable, renal impairment).

Hepatitis Prophylaxis

Infant born to HBs-Ag Positive Mother or Unknown Status Mother:
   -Hepatitis B immune globulin (HBIG) 0.5 mL IM x 1 within 12 hours of birth
   -Hepatitis B vaccine 0.5 mL IM (at separate site) within 12 hours of birth, second dose at age 1-2 months, third dose at age 6 months.

Neonatal HIV Prophylaxis

1. Pregnant women with HIV should be given oral zidovudine (200 mg PO q8h or 300 mg PO q12h) beginning at 14 weeks gestation and continuing throughout the pregnancy.
2. Intravenous zidovudine should be given to the mother during labor until delivery (2 mg/kg during the first hour and then 1 mg/kg/hr until delivery).
3. Oral administration of zidovudine to the newborn should be instituted immediately after birth and continued for at least six weeks (start at 8mg/kg/day PO q6h for the first two weeks, and then follow the dosing regimens on page ?. The mother should not breast feed the infant.

GYNECOLOGY

Surgical Documentation for Gynecology

Gynecologic Surgical History

Identifying Data. Age, gravida (number of pregnancies), para (number of deliveries).

Chief Compliant. Reason given by patient for seeking surgical care.

History of Present Illness (HPI). Describe the course of the patient's illness, including when it began, character of the symptoms; pain onset (gradual or rapid), character of pain (constant, intermittent, cramping, radiating); other factors associated with pain (urination, eating, strenuous activities); aggravating or relieving factors. Other related diseases; past diagnostic testing.

Obstetrical History. Past pregnancies, durations and outcomes, preterm deliveries, operative deliveries.

Gynecologic History: Last menstrual period, length of regular cycle.

Past Medical History (PMH). Past medical problems, previous surgeries, hospitalizations, diabetes, hypertension, asthma, heart disease.

Medications. Cardiac medications, oral contraceptives, estrogen.

Allergies. Penicillin, codeine.

Family History. Medical problems in relatives.

Social History. Alcohol, smoking, drug usage, occupation.

Review of Systems (ROS):

    General: Fever, fatigue, night sweats.

    HEENT: Headaches, masses, dizziness.

    Respiratory: Cough, sputum, dyspnea.

    Cardiovascular: Chest pain, extremity edema.

    Gastrointestinal: Vomiting, abdominal pain, melena (black tarry stools), hematochezia (bright red blood per rectum).

    Genitourinary: Dysuria, hematuria, discharge.

    Skin: Easy bruising, bleeding tendencies.

Gynecologic Physical Examination

General:

Vital Signs: Temperature, respirations, heart rate, blood pressure.

Eyes: Pupils equally round and react to light and accommodation (PERRLA); extraocular movements intact (EOMI).

Neck: Jugular venous distention (JVD), thyromegaly, masses, lymphadenopathy.

Chest: Equal expansion, rales, breath sounds.

Heart: Regular rate and rhythm (RRR), first and second heart sounds, murmurs.

Breast: Skin retractions, masses (mobile, fixed), erythema, axillary or supraclavicular node enlargement.

Abdomen: Scars, bowel sounds, masses, hepatosplenomegaly, guarding, rebound, costovertebral angle tenderness, hernias.

Genitourinary: Urethral discharge, uterus, adnexa, ovaries, cervix.

Extremities: Cyanosis, clubbing, edema.

Neurological: Mental status, strength, tendon reflexes, sensory testing.

Laboratory Evaluation: Electrolytes, glucose, liver function tests, INR/PTT, CBC with differential; X-rays, ECG (if >35 yrs or cardiovascular disease), urinalysis.

Assessment and Plan: Assign a number to each problem. Discuss each problem, and describe surgical plans for each numbered problem, including preoperative testing, laboratory studies, medications, and antibiotics.

Discharge Summary

Patient's Name:
Chart Number:
Date of Admission:
Date of Discharge:
Admitting Diagnosis:
Discharge Diagnosis:
Name of Attending or Ward Service:
Surgical Procedures:
History and Physical Examination and Laboratory Data: Describe the course of the disease up to the time the patient came to the hospital, and describe the physical exam and laboratory data on admission.
Hospital Course: Describe the course of the patient's illness while in the hospital, including evaluation, treatment, outcome of treatment, and medications given.
Discharged Condition: Describe improvement or deterioration in condition.
Disposition: Describe the situation to which the patient will be discharged (home, nursing home).
Discharged Medications: List medications and instructions.
Discharged Instructions and Follow-up Care: Date of return for follow-up care at clinic; diet, exercise instructions.
Problem List: List all active and past problems.
Copies: Send copies to attending physician, clinic, consultants and referring physician.

Discharge Note

The discharge note should be written in the patient's chart prior to discharge.

Discharge Note

Date/time:
Diagnoses:
Treatment: Briefly describe therapy provided during hospitalization, including antibiotic therapy, surgery, and cardiovascular drugs.
Studies Performed: Electrocardiograms, CT scan.
Discharge medications:
Follow-up Arrangements:

General Gynecology

Management of the Abnormal Pap Smear

Cervical cancer has an incidence of about 15,700 new cases each year (representing 6% of all cancers), and 4,900 women die of the disease each year. Those at increased risk of preinvasive disease include patients with human-papilloma virus (HPV) infection, those infected with HIV, cigarette smokers, those with multiple sexual partners, and those with previous preinvasive or invasive disease.

I. **Screening for cervical cancer**
   A. Regular Pap smears are recommended for all women who are or have been sexually active and who have a cervix.
   B. Testing should begin when the woman first engages in sexual intercourse. Adolescents whose sexual history is thought to be unreliable should be presumed to be sexually active at age 18.
   C. Pap smears should be performed at least every 1 to 3 years. Testing is usually discontinued after age 65 in women who have had regular normal screening tests. Women who have had a hysterectomy, including removal of the cervix for reasons other than cervical cancer or its precursors, do not require Pap testing.

II. **Management of minor Pap smear abnormalities**
   A. **Satisfactory, but limited by few (or absent) endocervical cells**
      1. Endocervical cells are absent in up to 10% of Pap smears before menopause and up to 50% postmenopausally.
      2. **Management.** The Pap smear is usually either repeated annually or recall women with previously abnormal Pap smears.
   B. **Unsatisfactory for evaluation**
      1. Repeat Pap smear midcycle in 6-12 weeks.
      2. If atrophic smear, treat with estrogen cream for 6-8 weeks, then repeat Pap smear.
   C. **Benign cellular changes**
      1. **Infection--candida.** Most cases represent asymptomatic colonization. Treatment should be offered for symptomatic cases. The Pap should be repeated at the usual interval.
      2. **Infection--Trichomonas.** If wet preparation is positive, treat with metronidazole (Flagyl), then continue annual Pap smears.
      3. **Infection--predominance of coccobacilli consistent with shift in vaginal flora.** This finding implies bacterial vaginosis, but it is a non-specific finding. Diagnosis should be confirmed by findings of a homogeneous vaginal discharge, positive amine test, and clue cells on saline suspension.
      4. **Infection--herpes simplex virus.** Pap smear has a poor sensitivity, but good specificity, for HSV. Positive smears usually are caused by asymptomatic infection. The patient should be informed of pregnancy risks and the possibility of transmission. Treatment is not necessary, and the Pap should be repeated as for a benign result.
      5. **Inflammation on Pap smear**
         a. **Mild inflammation** on an otherwise normal smear does not need further evaluation.
         b. **Moderate or severe inflammation** should be evaluated with a saline preparation, KOH preparation, and gonorrhea and Chlamydia tests. If the source of infection is found, treatment should be provided, and a repeat Pap smear should be done every 6 to 12 months. If no etiology is found, the Pap smear should be repeated in 6 months.
         c. **Persistent inflammation** may be infrequently the only manifestation of high-grade squamous intraepithelial lesions (HGSIL) or invasive cancer; therefore, persistent inflammation is an indication for

colposcopy.
6. **Atrophy with inflammation** is common in post-menopausal women or in those with estrogen-deficiency states. Atrophy should be treated with vaginal estrogen for 4-6 weeks, then repeat Pap smear.

III. **Managing cellular abnormalities**
   A. **Atypical squamous cells of undetermined significance (ASCUS).** On retesting, 25%-60% of patients will have LSIL or HSIL, and 15% will demonstrate HSIL. In a low-risk patient, it is reasonable to offer the option of repeating the cervical smears every 4 months for the next 2 years--with colposcopy, endocervical curettage (ECC) and directed biopsy if findings show progression or the atypical cells have not resolved. Alternatively, the patient can proceed immediately with colposcopy, ECC, and directed biopsy. In a high-risk patient (particularly when follow-up may be a problem), it is advisable to proceed with colposcopy, ECC, and directed biopsy.
   B. **Low-grade squamous intraepithelial lesion (LSIL).** The smear will revert to normal within 2 years in 30%-60% of patients. Another 25% have, or will progress to, moderate or severe dysplasia (HSIL). With a low-risk patient, cervical smears should be repeated every 4 months for 2 years; colposcopy, ECC, and directed biopsy are indicated for progression or nonresolution. In the high-risk patient, prompt colposcopy, ECC, and directed biopsy are recommended.

The Bethesda system

Adequacy of the specimen
   Satisfactory for evaluation
   Satisfactory for evaluation but limited by... Specify reason
   Unsatisfactory for evaluation: Specify reason
General categorization (optional)
   Within normal limits
   Benign cellular changes: See descriptive diagnoses
   Epithelial cell abnormality: See descriptive diagnoses
Descriptive diagnoses
   Benign cellular changes
   Infection
   Trichomonas vaginalis
   Fungal organisms morphologically consistent with Candida spp
   Predominance of coccobacilli consistent with shift in vaginal flora
   Bacteria morphologically consistent with Actinomyces spp
   Cellular changes associated with herpes simplex virus
   Other
   Reactive changes
   Inflammation (includes typical repair)
   Atrophy with inflammation (atrophic vaginitis)
   Radiation
   Intrauterine contraceptive device
Epithelial cell abnormalities
Squamous cell
   Atypical squamous cells of undetermined significance (ASCUS): Qualify
   Low-grade squamous intraepithelial lesion (LSIL) compassing HPV; mild dysplasia/CIN 1
   High-grade squamous intraepithelial lesions (HSIL) encompassing moderate and severe dysplasia, CIS/CIN 2 and CIN
   Squamous cell carcinoma
Glandular cell
   Endometrial cells, cytologically benign, in a postmenopausal woman
   Atypical glandular cells of undetermined significance (AGUS): Qualify
   Endocervical adenocarcinoma
   Endometrial adenocarcinoma
   Extrauterine adenocarcinoma
   Adenocarcinoma, not otherwise specified
Other malignant neoplasms: Specify

   C. **High-grade squamous intraepithelial lesions (HSIL),** moderate-to-severe dysplasia, CIS 1, CIN 2, and CIN 3 Colposcopy, ECC, and directed biopsies are recommended.

D. **Atypical glandular cells of undetermined significance (AGUS).** One-third of those for whom the report "favors reactive" will actually have dysplasia. For this reason, colposcopy, ECC (or cytobrush), and directed biopsies are recommended. If glandular neoplasia is suspected or persistent AGUS does not correlate with ECC findings, cold-knife conization perhaps with dilatation and curettage (D&C) is indicated. D&C with hysteroscopy is the treatment of choice for AGUS endometrial cells.

E. **Squamous cell carcinoma** should be referred to a gynecologist or oncologist experienced in its treatment.

IV. **Management of glandular cell abnormalities**

A. **Endometrial cells on Pap smear.** When a Pap smear is performed during menstruation, endometrial cells may be present. However, endometrial cells on a Pap smear performed during the second half of the menstrual cycle or in a post-menopausal patient may indicate the presence of polyps, hyperplasia, or endometrial adenocarcinoma. An endometrial biopsy should be considered in these women.

B. **Atypical glandular cells of undetermined significance (AGUS).** Colposcopically directed biopsy and endocervical curettage is recommended in all women with AGUS smears, and abnormal endometrial cells should be investigated by endometrial biopsy, fractional curettage, or hysteroscopy.

C. **Adenocarcinoma.** This diagnosis requires endocervical curettage, cone biopsy, and/or endometrial biopsy.

V. **Colposcopically directed biopsy**

A. Liberally apply a solution of 3-5% acetic acid to cervix, and inspect cervix for abnormal areas (white epithelium, punctation, mosaic cells, atypical vessels). Biopsies of any abnormal areas should be obtained under colposcopic visualization. Record location of each biopsy. Monsel solution may be applied to stop bleeding.

B. **Endocervical curettage** is done routinely during colposcopy, except during pregnancy.

VI. **Treatment based on cervical biopsy findings**

A. **Benign cellular changes (infection, reactive inflammation).** Treat the infection, and repeat the smear every 4-6 months; after 2 negatives, repeat yearly.

B. **Squamous intraepithelial lesions**

1. Women with SIL should be treated on the basis of the histological biopsy diagnosis. Patients with CIN I require no further treatment because the majority of these lesions resolve spontaneously. Patients with CIN II or CIN III require treatment to prevent development of invasive disease.

2. These lesions are treated with cryotherapy, laser vaporization, or loop electric excision procedure (LEEP).

References: See page 290.

Contraception

One-half of unplanned pregnancies occur among the 10 percent of women who do not use contraception. The remainder of unintended pregnancies result from contraceptive failure.

Advantages and Disadvantages of Various Birth Control Methods		
Method	Advantages	Disadvantages
Diaphragm	Inexpensive; some protection against STDs other than HIV	Not to be used with oil-based lubricants; latex allergy; urinary tract infections

Method	Advantages	Disadvantages
Cervical cap (Prentif Cavit)	Inexpensive; some protection against STDs other than HIV	Damaged by oil-based lubricants; latex allergy; toxic shock syndrome; decreased efficacy with increased frequency of intercourse; difficult to use
Oral combination contraceptive	Decreased menstrual flow and cramping; decreased incidence of pelvic inflammatory disease, ovarian and endometrial cancers, ovarian cyst, ectopic pregnancy, fibrocystic breasts, fibroids, endometriosis and toxic shock syndrome; highly effective	Increased risk of benign hepatic adenomas; mildly increased risk of blood pressure elevation or thromboembolism; no protection against HIV and other STDs; nausea
Depot-medroxy-progesterone acetate (Depo-Provera)	Decreased or no menstrual flow or cramps; compatible with breast-feeding; highly effective	Delayed return of fertility; irregular bleeding; decreased libido; no protection against HIV; nausea
Intrauterine device	Long-term use (up to 10 years)	Increased bleeding, spotting or cramping; risk of ectopic pregnancy with failure; risk of infertility; no protection against HIV and other STDs
Progestin-only agent	Compatible with breast-feeding; no estrogenic side effects	Possible amenorrhea; must be taken at the same time every day; no protection against HIV; nausea
Levonorgestrel implant (Norplant)	Decreased menstrual flow, cramping and ovulatory pain; no adherence requirements; highly effective	Costly; surgical procedure required for insertion; no protection against HIV
Tubal ligation	Low failure rate; no adherence requirements	Surgery; no protection against HIV and other STDs
Vasectomy	Low failure rate; no adherence requirements; outpatient procedure	Surgical procedure; postoperative infection; no protection against HIV
Condoms (male and female)	Inexpensive; some protection against HIV infection and other STDs	Poor acceptance by some users; latex allergy; not to be used with oil-based lubricants

I. **Oral contraceptives**
  A. Two types of oral contraceptives are available in the USA: combination oral contraceptives that contain both an estrogen and a progestin, and progestin-only contraceptives, or "mini-pills." All oral contraceptives marketed in the USA are similarly effective in preventing pregnancy.

Oral Contraceptives		
Drug	**Estrogen (ug)**	**Progestin (mg)**
Monophasic Combination		
Ovral 21, 28	ethinyl estradiol (50)	norgestrel (0.5)
Ogestrel-28	ethinyl estradiol (50)	norgestrel (0.5)
Ovcon 50 28	ethinyl estradiol (50)	norethindrone (1)
Zovia 1/50E 21	ethinyl estradiol (50)	ethynodiol diacetate (1)
Genora 1/50 28	mestranol (50)	norethindrone (1)
Necon 1/50 21, 28	mestranol (50)	norethindrone (1)
Nelova 1/50 21, 28	mestranol (50)	norethindrone (1)
Norinyl 1/50 21, 28	mestranol (50)	norethindrone (1)
Ortho-Novum 1/5028	mestranol (50)	norethindrone (1)
Ovcon 35 21, 28	ethinyl estradiol (35)	norethindrone (0.4)
Brevicon 21, 28	ethinyl estradiol (35)	norethindrone (0.5)
Modicon 28	ethinyl estradiol (35)	norethindrone (0.5)
Necon 0.5/35E 21, 28	ethinyl estradiol (35)	norethindrone (0.5)
Nelova 10/11 21	ethinyl estradiol (35)	norethindrone (0.5, 1)
Genora 1/35 21, 28	ethinyl estradiol (35)	norethindrone (1)
Necon 1/35 21	ethinyl estradiol (35)	norethindrone (1)
Nelova 1/35 28	ethinyl estradiol (35)	norethindrone (1)
Norinyl 1/35 21, 28	ethinyl estradiol (35)	norethindrone (1)
Ortho-Novum 1/35 21, 28	ethinyl estradiol (35)	norethindrone (1)
Ortho-Cyclen* 21, 28	ethinyl estradiol (35)	norgestimate (0.25)
Demulen 1/35 21	ethinyl estradiol (35)	ethynodiol diacetate (1)
Zovia 1/35 E	ethinyl estradiol (35)	ethynodiol diacetate (1)
LoEstrin 1.5/30 21, 28	ethinyl estradiol (30)	norethindrone acetate (1.5)
Levlen 21, 28	ethinyl estradiol (30)	levonorgestrel (0.15)
Levora 21, 28	ethinyl estradiol (30)	levonorgestrel (0.15)

Drug	Estrogen (ug)	Progestin (mg)
Nordette 21, 28	ethinyl estradiol (30)	levonorgestrel (0.15)
Lo/Ovral	ethinyl estradiol (30)	norgestrel (0.3)
Low-Ogestrel	ethinyl estradiol (30)	norgestrel (0.3)
Desogen* 28	ethinyl estradiol (30)	desogestrel (0.15)
Ortho-Cept* 21	ethinyl estradiol (30)	desogestrel (0.15)
Alesse** 21, 28	ethinyl estradiol (20)	levonorgestrel (0.1)
Levlite** 21, 28	ethinyl estradiol (20)	levonorgestrel (0.1)
LoEstrin** 1/20 21, 28	ethinyl estradiol (20)	norethindrone acetate (1)
Multiphasic Combination		
Tri-Levlen 21, 28	ethinyl estradiol (30, 40, 30)	levonorgestrel (0.05, 0.075, 0.125)
Triphasil 21	ethinyl estradiol (30, 40, 30)	levonorgestrel (0.05, 0.075, 0.125)
Trivora-28	ethinyl estradiol (30, 40, 30)	levonorgestrel (0.05, 0.075, 0.125)
Estrostep 28	ethinyl estradiol (20, 30, 35)	norethindrone acetate (1)
Ortho Tri-Cyclen* 30	ethinyl estradiol (35)	norgestimate (0.18, 0.215, 0.25)
Tri-Norinyl 21, 28	ethinyl estradiol (35)	norethindrone (0.5, 1, 0.5)
Ortho-Novum 7/7/7 21	ethinyl estradiol (35)	norethindrone (0.5, 0.75, 1)
Jenest-28	ethinyl estradiol (35)	norethindrone (0.5, 1)
Necon 10/11 21, 28	ethinyl estradiol (35)	norethindrone (0.5, 1)
Ortho-Novum 10/11 28	ethinyl estradiol (35)	norethindrone (0.5, 1)
Mircette* 28	ethinyl estradiol (20, 0, 10)	desogestrel (0.15)
Progestin Only		
Ovrette		norgestrel (0.075)
Micronor		norethindrone (0.35)
Nor-QD		norethindrone (0.35)

*Third generation agent
**Very low-dose estrogen agent

B. **Combination oral contraceptives.** Monophasic oral contraceptives contain fixed doses of estrogen and progestin in each active pill. Multiphasic oral contraceptives vary the dose of one or both hormones during the cycle. The rationale for multiphasic oral contraceptives is that they more closely simulate the hormonal changes of a normal menstrual cycle. Multi-phasic pills have a lower total hormone dose per cycle, but there is no convincing evidence that they cause fewer adverse effects or offer any other advantage over monophasic pills, which are simpler to take.

C. **Adverse effects.** Estrogens can cause nausea, breast tenderness and breast enlargement. Progestins can cause unfavorable changes in LDL and HDL cholesterol. Other adverse effects associated with oral contraceptives, such as weight gain or depression, are more difficult to attribute to one component or the other. Women smokers more than 35 years old who use combination oral contraceptives have an increased risk of cardiovascular disease.

D. **Acne.** Use of a combined oral contraceptive containing norgestimate (Ortho Tri-Cyclen) will often significantly improve acne. Combination oral contraceptives containing levonorgestrel or norethindrone acetate also improved acne.

E. **Third-generation progestins** (desogestrel, norgestimate, gestodene) used in combination oral contraceptives have been claimed to be less androgenic. They have been associated with a small increase in the risk of venous thromboembolism.

F. **Very low-dose estrogen.** Combined oral contraceptive products containing 20 µg of ethinyl estradiol may cause less bloating and breast tenderness than those containing higher doses of estrogen. The potential disadvantage of low estrogen doses is more breakthrough bleeding.

G. **Drug interactions.** Macrolide antibiotics, tetracyclines, rifampin, metronidazole (Flagyl), penicillins, trimethoprim-sulfamethoxazole (Bactrim), several anti-HIV agents and many anti-epileptic drugs, can induce the metabolism and decrease the effectiveness of oral contraceptives.

H. A careful personal and family medical history (with particular attention to cardiovascular risk factors) and an accurate blood pressure measurement are recommended before the initiation of oral contraceptive pills. A physical examination and a Papanicolaou smear (with screening genital cultures as indicated) are usually performed at the time oral contraceptive pills are initially prescribed. An initial prescription of OCPs can be written before a physical examination and a Pap test are performed in healthy young women.

Noncontraceptive Benefits of Oral Contraceptive Pills	
Dysmenorrhea Mittelschmerz	Functional ovarian cysts
Metrorrhagia	Benign breast cysts
Premenstrual syndrome	Ectopic pregnancy
Hirsutism	Acne
Ovarian and endometrial cancer	Endometriosis

Factors to Consider in Starting or Switching Oral Contraceptive Pills		
Objective	Action	Products that achieve the objective
To minimize high risk of thrombosis	Select a product with a lower dosage of estrogen.	Alesse, Loestrin 1/20, Levlite, Mircette

To minimize nausea, breast tenderness or vascular headaches	Select a product with a lower dosage of estrogen.	Alesse, Levlite, Loestrin 1/20, Mircette
To minimize spotting or breakthrough bleeding	Select a product with a higher dosage of estrogen or a progestin with greater potency.	Demulen, Desogen, Levlen, Lo/Ovral, Nordette, Ortho-Cept, Ortho-Cyclen, Ortho Tri-Cyclen
To minimize androgenic effects	Select a product containing a third-generation progestin, low-dose norethindrone or ethynodiol diacetate.	Brevicon, Demulen 1/35, Desogen,* Modicon, Ortho-Cept,* Ortho-Cyclen,* Ortho Tri-Cyclen,* Ovcon 35
To avoid dyslipidemia	Select a product containing a third-generation progestin, low-dose norethindrone or ethynodiol diacetate.	Brevicon, Demulen 1/35, Desogen,* Modicon, Ortho-Cept,* Ortho-Cyclen,* Ortho Tri-Cyclen,* Ovcon 35
*--These products contain a third-generation progestin.		

Instructions on the Use of Oral Contraceptive Pills

Initiation of use (choose one):
The patient begins taking the pills on the first day of menstrual bleeding.
The patient begins taking the pills on the first Sunday after menstrual bleeding begins.
The patient begins taking the pills immediately if she is definitely not pregnant and has not had unprotected sex since her last menstrual period.

Missed pill
If it has been less than 24 hours since the last pill was taken, the patient takes a pill right away and then returns to normal pill-taking routine.
If it has been 24 hours since the last pill was taken, the patient takes both the missed pill and the next scheduled pill at the same time.
If it has been more than 24 hours since the last pill was taken (ie, two or more missed pills), the patient takes the last pill that was missed, throws out the other missed pills and takes the next pill on time. Additional contraception is used for the remainder of the cycle.

Additional contraceptive method
The patient uses an additional contraceptive method for the first 7 days after initially starting oral contraceptive pills.
The patient uses an additional contraceptive method for 7 days if she is more than 12 hours late in taking an oral contraceptive pill.
The patient uses an additional contraceptive method while she is taking an interacting drug and for 7 days thereafter.

Contraindications to Use of Hormonal Contraceptive Methods

Method	Contraindications
Oral combination contraceptive	Active liver disease, hepatic adenoma, thrombophlebitis, history of or active thromboembolic disorder, cardiovascular or cerebrovascular disease, known or suspected breast cancer, undiagnosed abnormal vaginal bleeding, jaundice with past pregnancy or hormone use, pregnancy, breast-feeding, smoking in women over age 35

Method	Contraindications
Progestin-only pill	Undiagnosed abnormal vaginal bleeding, known or suspected breast cancer, cholestatic jaundice of pregnancy or jaundice with previous pill use, hepatic adenoma, known or suspected pregnancy
Depot-medroxyprogesterone acetate (Depo-Provera) injection	Acute liver disease or tumor, thrombophlebitis, known or suspected breast cancer, undiagnosed abnormal vaginal bleeding
Levonorgestrel implant (Norplant)	Acute liver disease or tumor, active thrombophlebitis, known or suspected breast cancer, history of idiopathic intracranial hypertension, undiagnosed abnormal vaginal bleeding, pregnancy, hypersensitivity to any component of the implant system

Side Effects of Hormones Used in Contraceptive Agents	
Type of effect	**Symptoms**
Estrogenic	Nausea, breast tenderness, fluid retention
Progestational	Acne, increased appetite, weight gain, depression, fatigue
Androgenic	Weight gain. hirsutism, acne, oily skin, breakthrough bleeding

I. Administration issues

1. **Amenorrhea** may occur with long-term use. Administration of an agent with higher estrogen or lower progestin activity may resolve this problem. A missed menstrual period indicates a need for a pregnancy test.
2. **Breakthrough bleeding** often occurs during the first three months of use. If breakthrough bleeding is a problem, a higher-dose progestin or estrogen agent may be tried. Agents that contain norgestrel are associated with low rates of breakthrough bleeding.

J. Progestin-only agents

1. Progestin-only agents are slightly less effective than combination oral contraceptives. They have failure rates of 0.5 percent compared with the 0.1 percent rate with combination oral contraceptives.
2. Progestin-only oral contraceptives (Micronor, Nor-QD, Ovrette) provide a useful alternative in women who cannot take estrogen and those over age 40. Progestin-only contraception is recommended for nursing mothers. Milk production is unaffected by use of progestin-only agents.
3. If the usual time of ingestion is delayed for more than three hours, an alternative form of birth control should be used for the following 48 hours. Because progestin-only agents are taken continuously, without hormone-free periods, menses may be irregular, infrequent or absent.

II. Medroxyprogesterone acetate injections

A. Depot medroxyprogesterone acetate (Depo-Provera) is an injectable progestin. A 150-mg dose provides 12 weeks of contraception. However, an effective level of contraception is maintained for 14 weeks after an injection. After discontinuation of the injections, resumption of ovulation may require up to nine months.
B. The medication is given IM every 12 weeks. An injection should be administered within five days after the onset of menses or after proof of a negative pregnancy test. Medroxyprogesterone may be administered immediately after childbirth.
C. Medroxyprogesterone injections are a good choice for patients, such as adolescents, who have difficulty remembering to take their oral contracep-

tive or who have a tendency to use other methods inconsistently. Medroxyprogesterone may also be a useful choice for women who have contraindications to estrogen. This method should not be used for women who desire a rapid return to fertility after discontinuing contraception.

D. **Contraindications and side effects**
1. Breakthrough bleeding is common during the first few months of use. Most women experience regular bleeding or amenorrhea within six months after the first injection. If breakthrough bleeding persists beyond this period, nonsteroidal anti-inflammatory agents, combination oral contraceptives or a 10- to 21-day course of oral estrogen may eliminate the problem. About 50% of women who have received the injections for one year experience amenorrhea.
2. Side effects include weight gain, headache and dizziness.

III. **Diaphragm**
A. Diaphragms function as a physical barrier and as a reservoir for spermicide. They are particularly acceptable for patients who have only intermittent intercourse. Diaphragms are available in 5-mm incremental sizes from 55 to 80 mm. They must remain in place for eight hours after intercourse and may be damaged by oil-based lubricants.
B. **Method for fitting a diaphragm**
1. Selecting a diaphragm may begin by inserting a 70-mm diaphragm (the average size) and then determining whether this size is correct or is too large or too small.
2. Another method is to estimate the appropriate size by placing a gloved hand in the vagina and using the index and middle fingers to measure the distance from the introitus to the cervix.

IV. **Levonorgestrel contraceptive implant (Norplant)** is effective for 5 years and consists of six flexible Silastic capsules. Adequate serum levels are obtained within 24 hours after implantation.

V. **Emergency contraception**
A. Emergency contraception may be considered for a patient who reports a contraceptive failure, such as condom breakage, or other circumstances of unprotected sexual intercourse, such as a sexual assault. If menstruation does not occur within 21 days, a pregnancy test should be performed.
B. Emergency contraception is effective for up to 72 hours after intercourse.

Emergency Contraception

1. Consider pretreatment one hour before each oral contraceptive pill dose, using one of the following orally administered antiemetic agents:
   Prochlorperazine (Compazine), 5 to 10 mg
   Promethazine (Phenergan), 12.5 to 25 mg
   Trimethobenzamide (Tigan), 250 mg
2. Administer the first dose of oral contraceptive pill within 72 hours of unprotected coitus, and administer the second dose 12 hours after the first dose. Brand name options for emergency contraception include the following:
   Preven Kit--two pills per dose (0.5 mg of levonorgestrel and 100 µg of ethinyl estradiol per dose) Ovral--two pills per dose (0.5 mg of levonorgestrel and 100 µg of ethinyl estradiol per dose)
   Nordette--four pills per dose (0.6 mg of levonorgestrel and 120 µg of ethinyl estradiol per dose)
   Triphasil--four pills per dose (0.5 mg of levonorgestrel and 120 µg of ethinyl estradiol per dose)
   Plan B--one pill per dose (0.75 mg of levonorgestrel per dose)

C. The major side effect of emergency contraception with oral contraceptives is nausea, which occurs in 50% of women; vomiting occurs in 20%. If the patient vomits within two hours after ingesting a dose, the dose should be repeated. An antiemetic, such as phenothiazine (Compazine), 5-10 mg PO, or trimethobenzamide (Tigan), 100-250 mg, may be taken one hour before administration of the contraceptive.

VI. **Intrauterine devices**
   A. IUDs represent the most commonly used method of reversible contraception worldwide. The Progestasert IUD releases progesterone and must be replaced every 12 months. The Copper-T IUD is a copper-containing device which may be used for 10 years.
   B. IUDs act by causing a localized foreign-body inflammatory reaction that inhibits implantation of the ovum. An IUD may be a good choice for parous women who are in a monogamous relationship and do not have dysmenorrhea.
   C. **Contraindications** include women who are at high risk for STDs and those who have a history of pelvic inflammatory disease, and women at high risk for endocarditis. Oral administration of doxycycline, 200 mg, or azithromycin (Zithromax), 500 mg, one hour before insertion reduces the incidence of insertion-related infections.

References: See page 290.

Ectopic Pregnancy

Ectopic pregnancy causes 15% of all maternal deaths. Once a patient has had an ectopic pregnancy, there is a 7- to 13-fold increase in the risk of recurrence. Factors that have been shown to increase the risk of tubal pregnancy include 1) previous pelvic inflammatory disease, 2) previous tubal surgery, 3) current use of an intrauterine device, and 4) previous ectopic gestation.

I. **Evaluation**
   A. Any pregnancy in which the embryo implants outside the uterine cavity is defined as an ectopic pregnancy (EP). Hemorrhagic shock secondary to EP accounts for 6-7% of all maternal deaths.

Risk Factors for Ectopic Pregnancy
Lesser Risk Previous pelvic or abdominal surgery Cigarette smoking Vaginal douching Age of 1st intercourse <18 years
Greater Risk Previous genital infections (eg, PID) Infertility (In vitro fertilization) Multiple sexual partners
Greatest Risk Previous ectopic pregnancy Previous tubal surgery or sterilization Diethylstilbestrol exposure in utero Documented tubal pathology (scarring) Use of intrauterine contraceptive device

II. **Clinical presentation**
   A. The first symptoms of ectopic pregnancy (EP) are those associated with early pregnancy, including nausea with or without vomiting, breast tenderness, and amenorrhea. Nonspecific abdominal pain or pelvic pain is reported in 80% of patients with EP. Patients may also report having "normal" periods, light periods, or spotting.
   B. As an EP progresses, the greatest danger to the patient is fallopian tube rupture. The symptoms of rupture produce the "classical" presentation of

sudden, severe unilateral abdominal pain, vaginal bleeding, and a history of amenorrhea.

  C. Classical symptoms are uncommon. Loss of blood into the peritoneal cavity usually will produce symptoms of peritoneal irritation. The uterus in a patient with suspected EP should be softened and normal size, or slightly enlarged but smaller than expected by gestational dates. This finding is reported in up to 70% of cases.

Presenting Signs and Symptoms of Ectopic Pregnancy	
Symptom	Percentage of Women with Symptom
Abdominal pain	80-100%
Amenorrhea	75-95%
Vaginal bleeding	50-80%
Dizziness, fainting	20-35%
Urge to defecate	5-15%
Pregnancy symptoms	10-25%
Passage of tissue	5-10%
Sign	Percentage of Women with Sign
Adnexal tenderness	75-90%
Abdominal tenderness	80-95%
Adnexal mass	50%
Uterine enlargement	20-30%
Orthostatic changes	10-15%
Fever	5-10%

III. Diagnostic strategy
  A. Rh status must be verified in every patient with vaginal bleeding to avoid the failure to treat Rh-negative mothers with Rhogam.
  B. Beta-human chorionic gonadotropin
    1. Beta-hCG is a hormone produced by both ectopic and normally implanted trophoblastic cells. Monoclonal antibody assays can detect the presence of beta-hCG as soon as 2-3 days postimplantation. In a normal pregnancy, the level of this protein doubles about every two days up to a value of 10,000 mIU/mL. A urine pregnancy test is ordered to verify the presence of beta-hCG in the urine and, if positive, a serum quantitative level may then be obtained in order to verify if the level is above the discriminatory level for ultrasound.
    2. An intrauterine pregnancy should be seen by transabdominal ultrasound with beta-hCG levels of 6500 mIU/mL, or at 1500 to 2000 mIU/mL using transvaginal ultrasound. Consequently, absence of a gestational sac in a patient whose beta-hCG indicates that a pregnancy should be detectable by these ultrasonographic modalities increases the likelihood for EP. The beta-hCG level can be followed in stable patients in whom the level is too low to expect ultrasound visualization of a normal intrauterine pregnancy. The level should be rechecked in 48 hours.
  C. Progesterone is produced by the corpus luteum in response to the presence of a pregnancy. Progesterone levels change little in the first 8-10 weeks of gestation. Progesterone levels normally fall after 10 weeks gestation. When a pregnancy fails during the first 8-10 weeks, progesterone levels fall. A single progesterone level higher than 25 ng/mL is

consistent with a viable intrauterine pregnancy, and this level excludes EP with a 97.5% sensitivity. Moreover, 25% of viable intrauterine pregnancies have levels below 25 ng/mL. A level below 5 ng/mL is 100% diagnostic of a non-viable pregnancy. However, a low level does not correlate with the location of the pregnancy.

D. Ultrasound
1. Transvaginal ultrasound has become the single most valuable modality for the work-up of patients suspected of having an EP. The beta-hCG level at which signs of pregnancy can first be seen ultrasonographically is called the discriminatory threshold.
2. The discriminatory beta-hCG threshold is between 1000 mIU/mL and 2000 mIU/mL. Transvaginal ultrasound has the capability, assuming sufficiently high and "discriminatory" beta-HCG levels are detected, to identify a pregnancy location as soon as one week after missing a menstrual period.

E. Other diagnostic tests
1. **Uterine curettage** is performed only when serum hormones indicate a non-viable pregnancy (progesterone <5 ng/mL or falling/plateauing beta-hCG). Typically, chorionic villi are identified (by floating tissue obtained in saline) when a failed intrauterine pregnancy is present. When villi are not seen, diagnosis of completed miscarriage can still be made if the beta-hCG falls 15% or more 8-12 hours after the procedure. When no villi are seen and beta-hCG levels do not fall, EP is highly suspected. Ectopic pregnancy is diagnosed in this situation if the beta-hCG plateaus or continues to rise after the procedure.
2. **Laparoscopy** can be both diagnostic and therapeutic for EP. Use of laparoscopy is indicated in patients with peritoneal signs and equivocal results from testing with ultrasound and uterine curettage. It can also used alone for treatment when the diagnosis has been made by other means, although many patients are now managed medically.

IV. Treatment
A. Ectopic pregnancy can be treated medically or surgically.

Criteria for Receiving Methotrexate

Absolute indications
Hemodynamically stable without active bleeding or signs of hemoperitoneum
Nonlaparoscopic diagnosis
Patient desires future fertility
General anesthesia poses a significant risk
Patient is able to return for follow-up care
Patient has no contraindications to methotrexate

Relative indications
Unruptured mass <3.5 cm at its greatest dimension
No fetal cardiac motion detected
Patients whose bet-hCG level does not exceed 6,000-15,000 mIU/mL

Contraindications to Medical Therapy

Absolute contraindications
Breast feeding
Overt or laboratory evidence of immunodeficiency
Alcoholism, alcoholic liver disease, or other chronic liver disease
Preexisting blood dyscrasias, such as bone marrow hypoplasia, leukopenia, thrombocytopenia, or significant anemia
Known sensitivity to methotrexate
Active pulmonary disease
Peptic ulcer disease
Hepatic, renal, or hematologic dysfunction
Relative contraindications
Gestational sac >3.5 cm
Embryonic cardiac motion

   B. Methotrexate
   1. Before methotrexate is injected, blood is drawn to determine baseline laboratory values for renal, liver, bone marrow function, beta-hCG level, and progesterone Blood type, Rh factor, and the presence of antibodies should be determined. Patients who are Rh negative should receive Rh immune globulin.
   2. **The methotrexate dose** is calculated according to estimated body surface area (50 mg/m^2) and is given in one dose. Treatment with a standard 75 mg dose and multiple serial doses with a folinic acid rescue on alternate days (four doses of methotrexate [1.0 mg/kg] on days 0, 2, 4, and 6 and four doses of leucovorin [0.1 mg/kg] on days 1, 3, 5, and 7) also have been successful.
   3. **Follow-up care** continues until beta-hCG levels are nondetectable. Time to resolution is variable and can be protracted, taking a month or longer. With the single-dose regimen, levels of beta-hCG usually increase during the first several days following methotrexate injection and peak 4 days after injection. If a treatment response is observed, hCG levels should decline by 7 days after injection. If the beta-hCG level does not decline by at least 15% from day 4 to day 7, the patient may require either surgery, or a second dose of methotrexate. If there is an adequate treatment response, hCG determinations are reduced to once a week. An additional dose of methotrexate may be given if beta-hCG levels plateau or increase in 7 days.
   4. **Surgical intervention** may be required for patients who do not respond to medical therapy. Ultrasound examination may be repeated to evaluate increased pelvic pain, bleeding, or inadequate declines of beta-hCG levels.

Side Effects Associated with Methotrexate Treatment

Nausea	Vaginal bleeding or spotting
Vomiting	Severe neutropenia (rare)
Stomatitis	Reversible alopecia (rare)
Diarrhea	Pneumonitis
Gastric distress	Treatment effects
Dizziness	Increase in abdominal pain (occurs in up
Increase in beta-hCG levels during first	to two-thirds of patients)
1-3 days of treatment	

Signs of treatment failure and tubal rupture

Significantly worsening abdominal pain, regardless of change in beta-hCG levels
Hemodynamic instability
Levels of beta-hCG that do not decline by at least 15% between day 4 and day 7 postinjection
Increasing or plateauing beta-hCG levels after the first week of treatment

---

5. During treatment, patients should be counseled to discontinue folinic acid supplements, including prenatal vitamins, and avoid the use of nonsteroidal antiinflammatory drugs.
6. An initial increase in beta-hCG levels often occurs by the third day and is not a cause for alarm. Most patients experience at least one episode of increased abdominal pain sometime during treatment. Abdominal pain may also suggest tubal rupture.
7. Medical treatment has failed when beta-hCG levels either increase or plateau by day 7, indicating a continuing ectopic pregnancy, or when the tube ruptures.
C. **Operative management** can be accomplished by either laparoscopy or laparotomy. Linear salpingostomy or segmental resection is the procedure of choice if the fallopian tube is to be retained. Salpingectomy is the procedure of choice if the tube requires removal.

References: See page 290.

Acute Pelvic Pain

I. **Clinical evaluation**
   A. Assessment of acute pelvic pain should determine the patient's age, obstetrical history, menstrual history, characteristics of pain onset, duration, and palliative or aggravating factors.
   B. **Associated symptoms** may include urinary or gastrointestinal symptoms, fever, abnormal bleeding, or vaginal discharge.
   C. **Past medical history.** Contraceptive history, surgical history, gynecologic history, history of pelvic inflammatory disease, ectopic pregnancy, sexually transmitted diseases should be determined. Current sexual activity and practices should be assessed.
   D. **Method of contraception**
      1. Sexual abstinence in the months preceding the onset of pain lessons the likelihood of pregnancy-related etiologies.
      2. The risk of acute PID is reduced by 50% in patients taking oral contraceptives or using a barrier method of contraception. Patients taking oral contraceptives are at decreased risk for an ectopic pregnancy or ovarian cysts.
   E. **Risk factors for acute pelvic inflammatory disease.** Age between 15-25 years, sexual partner with symptoms of urethritis, prior history of PID.
II. **Physical examination**
   A. Fever, abdominal or pelvic tenderness, and peritoneal signs should be sought.
   B. Vaginal discharge, cervical erythema and discharge, cervical and uterine motion tenderness, or adnexal masses or tenderness should be noted.
III. **Laboratory tests**
   A. **Pregnancy testing** will identify pregnancy-related causes of pelvic pain. Serum beta-HCG becomes positive 7 days after conception. A negative test virtually excludes ectopic pregnancy.
   B. **Complete blood count.** Leukocytosis suggest an inflammatory process; however, a normal white blood count occurs in 56% of patients with PID and 37% of patients with appendicitis.
   C. **Urinalysis.** The finding of pyuria suggests urinary tract infection. Pyuria can also occur with an inflamed appendix or from contamination of the urine by

vaginal discharge.
   D. **Testing for Neisseria gonorrhoeae and Chlamydia trachomatis** are necessary if PID is a possibility.
   E. **Pelvic ultrasonography** is of value in excluding the diagnosis of an ectopic pregnancy by demonstrating an intrauterine gestation. Sonography may reveal acute PID, torsion of the adnexa, or acute appendicitis.
   F. **Diagnostic laparoscopy** is indicated when acute pelvic pain has an unclear diagnosis despite comprehensive evaluation.
III. **Differential diagnosis of acute pelvic pain**
   A. **Pregnancy-related causes.** Ectopic pregnancy, spontaneous, threatened or incomplete abortion, intrauterine pregnancy with corpus luteum bleeding.
   B. **Gynecologic disorders.** PID, endometriosis, ovarian cyst hemorrhage or rupture, adnexal torsion, Mittelschmerz, uterine leiomyoma torsion, primary dysmenorrhea, tumor.
   C. **Nonreproductive tract causes**
      1. **Gastrointestinal.** Appendicitis, inflammatory bowel disease, mesenteric adenitis, irritable bowel syndrome, diverticulitis.
      2. **Urinary tract.** Urinary tract infection, renal calculus.
IV. **Approach to acute pelvic pain with a positive pregnancy test**
   A. In a female patient of reproductive age, presenting with acute pelvic pain, the first distinction is whether the pain is pregnancy-related or non-pregnancy-related on the basis of a serum pregnancy test.
   B. In the patient with acute pelvic pain associated with pregnancy, the next step is localization of the tissue responsible for the hCG production. Transvaginal ultrasound should be performed to identify an intrauterine gestation. Ectopic pregnancy is characterized by a noncystic adnexal mass and fluid in the cul-de-sac.
   C. **If a gestational sac is not demonstrated on ultrasonography, the following possibilities exist:**
      1. **Ectopic pregnancy**
      2. **Very early intrauterine pregnancy** not seen on ultrasound
      3. **Recent abortion**
   D. **Management of patients when a gestational sac is not seen with a positive pregnancy test**
      1. **Diagnostic laparoscopy** is the most accurate and rapid method of establishing or excluding the diagnosis of ectopic pregnancy.
      2. **Examination of endometrial tissue.** For pregnant patients desiring termination, and for those patients in whom it can be demonstrated that the pregnancy is nonviable, suction curettage with immediate histologic examination of the curettings is a diagnostic option. The presence of chorionic villi confirms the diagnosis of intrauterine pregnancy, whereas the absence of such villi indicates ectopic pregnancy.
V. **Management of the ectopic gestation**
   A. Two IV catheters of at least 18 gauge should be placed and 1-2 L of normal saline infused.
   B. **Laparoscopy or laparotomy** with linear salpingostomy or salpingectomy should be accomplished in unstable patients. An HCG level should be checked in one week to assure that the level is declining.
   C. **Methotrexate.** Stable patients can be treated with methotrexate in a single intramuscular dose of 50 mg per meter^2. Treatment response should be assessed by serial HCG measurements made until the hormone is undetectable.
VI. **Approach to acute pelvic pain in non-pregnant patients with a negative HCG**
   A. **Acute PID** is the leading diagnostic consideration in patients with acute pelvic pain unrelated to pregnancy. The pain is usually bilateral, but may be unilateral in 10%. Cervical motion tenderness, fever, and cervical discharge are common findings.
   B. **Acute appendicitis** should be considered in all patients presenting with acute pelvic pain and a negative pregnancy test. Appendicitis is character-ized by leukocytosis and a history of a few hours of periumbilical pain followed by migration of the pain to the right lower quadrant. Neutrophilia

occurs in 75%. A slight fever exceeding 37.3°C, nausea, vomiting, anorexia, and rebound tenderness may be present.

C. **Torsion of the adnexa** usually causes unilateral pain, but pain can be bilateral in 25%. Intense, progressive pain combined with a tense, tender adnexal mass is characteristic. There is often a history of repetitive, transitory pain. Pelvic sonography often confirms the diagnosis. Laparoscopic diagnosis and surgical intervention are indicated.

D. **Ruptured or hemorrhagic corpus luteal cyst** usually causes bilateral pain, but it can cause unilateral tenderness in 35%. Ultrasound aids in diagnosis.

E. **Endometriosis** usually causes chronic or recurrent pain, but it can occasionally cause acute pelvic pain. There usually is a history of dysmenorrhea and deep dyspareunia. Pelvic exam reveals fixed uterine retrodisplacement and tender uterosacral and cul-de-sac nodularity. Laparoscopy confirms the diagnosis.

References: See page 290.

Chronic Pelvic Pain

Chronic pelvic pain (CPP) affects approximately one in seven women in the United States (14 percent). Chronic pelvic pain (>6 months in duration) is less likely to be associated with a readily identifiable cause than is acute pain.

I. **Etiology of chronic pelvic pain**

A. **Physical and sexual abuse.** Numerous studies have demonstrated a higher frequency of physical and/or sexual abuse in women with CPP. Between 30 and 50 percent of women with CPP have a history of abuse (physical or sexual, childhood or adult).

B. **Gynecologic problems**

1. **Endometriosis** is present in approximately one-third of women undergoing laparoscopy for CPP and is the most frequent finding in these women. Typically, endometriosis pain is a sharp or "crampy" pain. It starts at the onset of menses, becoming more severe and prolonged over several menstrual cycles. It is frequently accompanied by deep dyspareunia. Uterosacral ligament nodularity is highly specific for endometriosis. Examining the woman during her menstruation may make the nodularity easier to palpate. A more common, but less specific, finding is tenderness in the cul-de-sac or uterosacral ligaments that reproduces the pain of deep dyspareunia.

2. **Pelvic adhesions** are found in approximately one-fourth of women undergoing laparoscopy for CPP. Adhesions form after intra-abdominal inflammation; they should be suspected if the woman has a history of surgery or pelvic inflammatory disease (PID). The pain may be a dull or sharp pulling sensation that occurs at any time during the month. Physical examination is usually nondiagnostic.

3. **Dysmenorrhea** (painful menstruation) and mittelschmerz (midcycle pain) without other organic pathology are seen frequently and may contribute to CPP in more than half of all cases.

4. **Chronic pelvic inflammatory disease** may cause CPP. Therefore, culturing for sexually transmitted agents should be a routine part of the evaluation.

Medical Diagnoses and Chronic Pelvic Pain	
Medical diagnosis/symptom source	Prevalence
Bowel dysmotility disorders	50 to 80%
Musculoskeletal disorders	30 to 70%
Cyclic gynecologic pain	20 to 50%
Urologic diagnoses	5 to 10%
Endometriosis, advanced and/or with dense bowel adhesions	Less than 5%
Unusual medical diagnoses	Less than 2%
Multiple medical diagnoses	30 to 50%
No identifiable medical diagnosis	Less than 5%

C. **Nongynecologic medical problems**
1. **Bowel dysmotility** (eg, irritable bowel syndrome and constipation) may be the primary symptom source in 50 percent of all cases of CPP and may be a contributing factor in up to 80 percent of cases. Pain from irritable bowel syndrome is typically described as a crampy, recurrent pain accompanied by abdominal distention and bloating, alternating diarrhea and constipation, and passage of mucus. The pain is often worse during or near the menstrual period. A highly suggestive sign is exquisite tenderness to palpation which improves with continued pressure.
2. **Musculoskeletal dysfunction,** including abdominal myofascial pain syndromes, can cause or contribute to CPP.

D. **Psychologic problems**
1. **Depressive disorders** contribute to more than half of all cases of CPP. Frequently, the pain becomes part of a cycle of pain, disability, and mood disturbance. The diagnostic criteria for depression include depressed mood, diminished interest in daily activities, weight loss or gain, insomnia or hypersomnia, psychomotor agitation or retardation, fatigue, feelings of worthlessness, loss of concentration, and recurrent thoughts of death.
2. **Somatoform disorders,** including somatization disorder, contribute to 10 to 20 percent of cases of CPP. The essential feature of somatization disorder is a pattern of recurring, multiple, clinically significant somatic complaints.

II. **Clinical evaluation of chronic pelvic pain**
A. **History**
1. The character, intensity, distribution, and location of pain are important. Radiation of pain or should be assessed. The temporal pattern of the pain (onset, duration, changes, cyclicity) and aggravating or relieving factors (eg, posture, meals, bowel movements, voiding, menstruation, intercourse, medications) should be documented.
2. **Associated symptoms.** Anorexia, constipation, or fatigue are often present.
3. **Previous surgeries,** pelvic infections, infertility, or obstetric experiences may provide additional clues.
4. For patients of reproductive age, the timing and characteristics of their last menstrual period, the presence of non-menstrual vaginal bleeding or discharge, and the method of contraception used should be determined.
5. Life situations and events that affect the pain should be sought.
6. Gastrointestinal and urologic symptoms, including the relationship between these systems to the pain should be reviewed.
7. The patient's affect may suggest depression or other mood disorders.
B. **Physical examination**
1. If the woman indicates the location of her pain with a single finger, the pain is more likely caused by a discrete source than if she uses a sweeping motion of her hand.

2. A pelvic examination should be performed. Special attention should be given to the bladder, urethra.

3. The piriformis muscles should be palpated; piriformis spasm can cause pain when climbing stairs, driving a car, or when first arising in the morning. This muscle is responsible for external rotation of the hip and can be palpated posteriolaterally, cephalic to the ischial spine. This examination is most easily performed if the woman externally rotates her hip against the resistance of the examiner's other hand. Piriformis spasm is treated with physical therapy.

4. Abdominal deformity, erythema, edema, scars, hernias, or distension should be noted. Abnormal bowel sounds may suggest a gastrointestinal process.

5. Palpation should include the epigastrium, flanks, and low back, and inguinal areas.

C. **Special tests**
   1. Initial laboratory tests should include cervical cytology, endocervical cultures for *Neisseria gonorrhoeae* and Chlamydia, stool hemoccult, and urinalysis. Other tests may be suggested by the history and examination.
   2. Laparoscopy is helpful when the pelvic examination is abnormal or when initial therapy fails.

III. **Management**

A. Myofascial pain syndrome may be treated by a variety of physical therapy techniques. Trigger points can often be treated with injections of a local anesthetic (eg, bupivacaine [Marcaine]), with or without the addition of a corticosteroid.

B. If the pain is related to the menstrual cycle, treatment aimed at suppressing the cycle may help. Common methods to accomplish this include administration of depot medroxyprogesterone (Depo-Provera) and continuously dosed oral contraceptives.

C. Cognitive-behavioral therapy is appropriate for all women with CPP. Relaxation and distraction techniques are often helpful.

D. When endometriosis or pelvic adhesions are discovered on diagnostic laparoscopy, they are usually treated during the procedure. Hysterectomy may be warranted if the pain has persisted for more than six months, does not respond to analgesics (including anti-inflammatory agents), and impairs the woman's normal function.

E. **Antidepressants or sleeping aids** are useful adjunctive therapies. Amitriptyline (Elavil), in low doses of 25-50 mg qhs, may be of help in improving sleep and reducing the severity of chronic pain complaints.

F. **Muscle relaxants** may prove useful in patients with guarding, splinting, or reactive muscle spasms.

References: See page 290.

Endometriosis

Endometriosis is characterized by the presence of endometrial tissue on the ovaries, fallopian tubes or other abnormal sites, causing pain or infertility. Women are usually 25 to 29 years old at the time of diagnosis. Approximately 24 percent of women who complain of pelvic pain are subsequently found to have endometriosis. The overall prevalence of endometriosis is estimated to be 5 to 10 percent.

I. **Clinical evaluation**

A. Endometriosis should be considered in any woman of reproductive age who has pelvic pain. The most common symptoms are dysmenorrhea, dyspareunia, and low back pain that worsens during menses. Rectal pain and painful defecation may also occur. Other causes of secondary dysmenorrhea and chronic pelvic pain (eg, upper genital tract infections, adenomyosis, adhesions) may produce similar symptoms.

Differential Diagnosis of Endometriosis	

Generalized pelvic pain
    Pelvic inflammatory disease
    Endometritis
    Pelvic adhesions
    Neoplasms, benign or malignant
    Ovarian torsion
    Sexual or physical abuse
    Nongynecologic causes
Dysmenorrhea
    Primary
    Secondary (adenomyosis, myomas, infection, cervical stenosis)
	Dyspareunia
	    Musculoskeletal causes (pelvic relaxation, levator spasm)
	    Gastrointestinal tract (constipation, irritable bowel syndrome)
	    Urinary tract (urethral syndrome, interstitial cystitis)
	    Infection
	    Pelvic vascular congestion
	    Diminished lubrication or vaginal expansion because of insufficient arousal
	Infertility
	    Male factor
	    Tubal disease (infection)
	    Anovulation
	    Cervical factors (mucus, sperm antibodies, stenosis)
	    Luteal phase deficiency

B. Infertility may be the presenting complaint for endometriosis. Infertile patients often have no painful symptoms.

C. **Physical examination.** The physician should palpate for a fixed, retroverted uterus, adnexal and uterine tenderness, pelvic masses or nodularity along the uterosacral ligaments. A rectovaginal examination should identify uterosacral, cul-de-sac or septal nodules. Most women with endometriosis have normal pelvic findings.

II. **Treatment**

A. Confirmatory laparoscopy is usually required before treatment is instituted. In women with few symptoms, an empiric trial of oral contraceptives or progestins may be warranted to assess pain relief.

B. **Medical treatment**

1. Initial therapy also should include a nonsteroidal anti-inflammatory drug.
   a. Naproxen (Naprosyn) 500 mg followed by 250 mg PO tid-qid prn [250, 375,500 mg].
   b. Naproxen sodium (Aleve) 200 mg PO tid prn.
   c. Naproxen sodium (Anaprox) 550 mg, followed by 275 mg PO tid-qid prn.
   d. Ibuprofen (Motrin) 800 mg, then 400 mg PO q4-6h prn.
   e. Mefenamic acid (Ponstel) 500 mg PO followed by 250 mg q6h prn.

2. **Progestational agents.** Progestins are similar to combination OCPs in their effects on FSH, LH and endometrial tissue. They may be associated with more bothersome adverse effects than OCPs. Progestins are effective in reducing the symptoms of endometriosis. Oral progestin regimens may include once-daily administration of medroxyprogesterone at the lowest effective dosage (5 to 20 mg). Depot medroxyprogesterone may be given intramuscularly every two weeks for two months at 100 mg per dose and then once a month for four months at 200 mg per dose.

3. **Oral contraceptive pills (OCPs)** suppress LH and FSH and prevent ovulation. Combination OCPs alleviate symptoms in about three quarters of patients. Oral contraceptives can be taken continuously (with no placebos) or cyclically, with a week of placebo pills between cycles. The OCPs can be discontinued after six months or continued indefinitely.

4. **Danazol (Danocrine)** has been highly effective in relieving the symptoms of endometriosis, but adverse effects may preclude its use. Adverse effects include headache, flushing, sweating and atrophic

vaginitis. Androgenic side effects include acne, edema, hirsutism, deepening of the voice and weight gain. The initial dosage should be 800 mg per day, given in two divided oral doses. The overall response rate is 84 to 92 percent.

Medical Treatment of Endometriosis		
Drug	**Dosage**	**Adverse effects**
Danazol (Danocrine)	800 mg per day in 2 divided doses	Estrogen deficiency, androgenic side effects
Oral contraceptives	1 pill per day (continuous or cyclic)	Headache, nausea, hypertension
Medroxyprogesterone (Provera)	5 to 20 mg orally per day	Same as with other oral progestins
Medroxyprogesterone suspension (Depo-Provera)	100 mg IM every 2 weeks for 2 months; then 200 mg IM every month for 4 months or 150 mg IM every 3 months	Weight gain, depression, irregular menses or amenorrhea
Norethindrone (Aygestin)	5 mg per day orally for 2 weeks; then increase by 2.5 mg per day every 2 weeks up to 15 mg per day	Same as with other oral progestins
Leuprolide (Lupron)	3.75 mg IM every month for 6 months	Decrease in bone density, estrogen deficiency
Goserelin (Zoladex)	3.6 mg SC (in upper abdominal wall) every 28 days	Estrogen deficiency
Nafarelin (Synarel)	400 mg per day: 1 spray in 1 nostril in a.m.; 1 spray in other nostril in p.m.; start treatment on day 2 to 4 of menstrual cycle	Estrogen deficiency, bone density changes, nasal irritation

- C. **GnRH agonists.** These agents (eg, leuprolide [Lupron], goserelin [Zoladex]) inhibit the secretion of gonadotropin. GnRH agonists are contraindicated in pregnancy and have hypoestrogenic side effects. They produce a mild degree of bone loss. Because of concerns about osteopenia, "add-back" therapy with low-dose estrogen has been recommended. The dosage of leuprolide is a single monthly 3.75-mg depot injection given intramuscularly. Goserelin, in a dosage of 3.6 mg, is administered subcutaneously every 28 days. A nasal spray (nafarelin [Synarel]) may be used twice daily. The response rate is similar to that with danazol; about 90 percent of patients experience pain relief.
- D. **Surgical treatment**
  - 1. Surgical treatment is the preferred approach to infertile patients with advanced endometriosis. Laparoscopic ablation of endometriosis lesions may result in a 13 percent increase in the probability of pregnancy.
  - 2. Definitive surgery, which includes hysterectomy and oophorectomy, is reserved for women with intractable pain who no longer desire pregnancy.

References: See page 290.

Amenorrhea

Amenorrhea may be associated with infertility, endometrial hyperplasia, or osteopenia. It may be the presenting sign of an underlying metabolic, endocrine, congenital, or gynecologic disorder.

I. Pathophysiology of amenorrhea
   A. Amenorrhea may be caused by failure of the hypothalamic-pituitary-gonadal axis, by absence of end organs, or by obstruction of the outflow tract.
   B. **Menses** usually occur at intervals of 28 days, with a normal range of 18-40 days.
   C. **Amenorrhea** is defined as the absence of menstruation for 3 or more months in a women with past menses (secondary amenorrhea) or by the absence of menarche by age 16 in girls who have never menstruated (primary amenorrhea). Pregnancy is the most common cause of amenorrhea.

II. Clinical evaluation of amenorrhea
   A. **Menstrual history** should include the age of menarche, last menstrual period, and previous menstrual pattern. Diet, medications, and psychologic stress should be assessed.
   B. **Galactorrhea**, previous radiation therapy, chemotherapy, or recent weight gain or loss may provide important clues.
   C. **Prolonged, intense exercise**, often associated with dieting, can lead to amenorrhea. Symptoms of decreased estrogen include hot flushes and night sweats.
   D. **Physical examination**
      1. **Breast development and pubic hair distribution** should be assessed because they demonstrate exposure to estrogens and sexual maturity. Galactorrhea is a sign of hyperprolactinemia.
      2. **Thyroid gland** should be palpated for enlargement and nodules. Abdominal striae in a nulliparous woman suggests hypercortisolism (Cushing's syndrome).
      3. **Hair distribution** may reveal signs of androgen excess. The absence of both axillary and pubic hair in a phenotypically normal female suggests androgen insensitivity.
      4. **External genitalia and vagina** should be inspected for atrophy from estrogen deficiency or clitoromegaly from androgen excess. An imperforate hymen or vaginal septum can block the outflow tract.
      5. **Palpation of the uterus and ovaries** assures their presence and detects abnormalities.

III. Diagnostic approach to amenorrhea
   A. Menstrual flow requires an intact hypothalamic-pituitary-ovarian axis, a hormonally responsive uterus, and an intact outflow tract. The evaluation should localize the abnormality to either the uterus, ovary, anterior pituitary, or hypothalamus.
   B. **Step one--exclude pregnancy.** Pregnancy is the most common cause of secondary amenorrhea, and it must be excluded with a pregnancy test.
   C. **Step two--exclude hyperthyroidism and hyperprolactinemia**
      1. **Hypothyroidism and hyperprolactinemia** can cause amenorrhea. These disorders are excluded with a serum thyroid-stimulating hormone (TSH) and prolactin.
      2. **Hyperprolactinemia.** Prolactin inhibits the secretion of gonadotropin-releasing hormone. One-third of women with no obvious cause of amenorrhea have hyperprolactinemia. Mildly elevated prolactin levels should be confirmed by repeat testing and review the patient's medications. Hyperprolactinemia requires an MRI to exclude a pituitary tumor.

Drugs Associated with Amenorrhea	
Drugs that Increase Prolactin	Antipsychotics Tricyclic antidepressants Calcium channel blockers
Drugs with Estrogenic Activity	Digoxin, marijuana, oral contraceptives
Drugs with Ovarian Toxicity	Chemotherapeutic agents

D. **Step three--assess estrogen status**
  1. **The progesterone challenge test** is used to determine estrogen status and determine the competence of the uterine outflow tract.
  2. Medroxyprogesterone (Provera) 10 mg is given PO qd for 10 consecutive days. Uterine bleeding within 2-7 days after completion is considered a positive test. A positive result suggests chronic anovulation, rather than hypothalamic-pituitary insufficiency or ovarian failure, and a positive test also confirms the presence of a competent outflow tract.
  3. A negative test indicates either an incompetent outflow tract, nonreactive endometrium, or inadequate estrogen stimulation.
      a. An abnormality of the outflow tract should be excluded with a regimen of conjugated estrogens (Premarin), 1.25 mg daily on days 1 through 21 of the cycle. Medroxyprogesterone (Provera) 10 mg is given on the last 5 days of the 21-day cycle. (A combination oral contraceptive agent can also be used.)
      b. Withdrawal bleeding within 2-7 days of the last dose of progesterone confirms the presence of an unobstructed outflow tract and a normal endometrium, and the problem is localized to the hypothalamic-pituitary axis or ovaries.
  4. In patients who have had prolonged amenorrhea, an endometrial biopsy should be considered before withdrawal bleeding is induced. Biopsy can reveal endometrial hyperplasia.
E. **Step four--evaluation of hypoestrogenic amenorrhea**
  1. Serum follicle-stimulating hormone (FSH) and luteinizing hormone (LH) levels should be measured to localize the problem to the ovary, pituitary or hypothalamus.
  2. **Ovarian failure**
      a. An FSH level greater than 50 mIU/mL indicates ovarian failure.
      b. Ovarian failure is considered "premature" when it occurs in women less than 40 years of age.
  3. **Pituitary or hypothalamic dysfunction**
      a. A normal or low gonadotropin level is indicative of pituitary or hypothalamic failure. An MRI is the most sensitive study to rule out a pituitary tumor.
      b. If MRI does not reveal a tumor, a defect in pulsatile GnRH release from the hypothalamus is the probable cause.
IV. **Management of chronic anovulation**
  A. Adequate estrogen and anovulation is indicated by withdrawal bleeding with the progesterone challenge test.
  B. Often there is a history of weight loss, psychosocial stress, or excessive exercise. Women usually have a normal or low body weight and normal secondary sex characteristics.
      1. Reducing stress and assuring adequate nutrition may induce ovulation. These women are at increased risk for endometrial cancer because of the hyperplastic effect of unopposed estrogen.
      2. Progesterone (10 mg/day for the first 7-10 days of every month) is given to induce withdrawal bleeding. If contraception is desired, a low-dose oral contraceptive should be used.
V. **Management of hypothalamic dysfunction**
  A. Amenorrheic women with a normal prolactin level, a negative progester-

one challenge, with low or normal gonadotropin levels, and with a normal sella turcica imaging are considered to have hypothalamic dysfunction.
   B. Hypothalamic amenorrhea usually results from psychologic stress, depression, severe weight loss, anorexia nervosa, or strenuous exercise.
   C. Hypoestrogenic women are at risk for osteoporosis and cardiovascular disease. Oral contraceptives are appropriate in young women. Women not desiring contraception should take estrogen, 0.625 mg, with medroxyprogesterone (Provera) 2.5 mg, every day of the month. Calcium and vitamin D supplementation are also recommended.
VI. **Management of disorders of the outflow tract or uterus--intrauterine adhesions (Asherman syndrome)**
   A. Asherman syndrome is the most common outflow-tract abnormality that causes amenorrhea. This disorder should be considered if amenorrhea develops following curettage or endometritis.
   B. Hysterosalpingography will detect adhesions. Therapy consists of hysteroscopy and lysis of adhesions.
VII. **Management of disorders of the ovaries**
   A. Ovarian failure is suspected if menopausal symptoms are present. Women with premature ovarian failure who are less than 30 years of age should undergo karyotyping to rule out the presence of a Y chromosome. If a Y chromosome is detected, testicular tissue should be removed.
   B. Patients with ovarian failure should be prescribed estrogen 0.625 mg with progesterone 2.5 mg daily with calcium and vitamin D.
VIII. **Disorders of the anterior pituitary**
   A. Prolactin-secreting adenoma are excluded by MRI of the pituitary.
   B. Cabergoline (Dostinex) or bromocriptine (Parlodel) are used for most adenomas; surgery is considered later.
References: See page 290.

Menopause

The average age of menopause is 51 years, with a range of 41-55. Menopause occurs before age 40 in about 5% of women. Menopause is indicated by an elevated follicle-stimulating hormone (FSH) level greater than 40 mIU/mL.

I. **Pharmacologic therapy for symptoms of menopause**
   A. **Vasomotor instability.** A hot flush is a flushed or blushed feeling of the face, neck and upper chest. The most severe hot flushes usually occur at night. Estrogen therapy can reduce hot flushes.
   B. **Psychologic symptoms.** Mood swings, depression and concentration difficulties are associated with menopause. Estrogen improves mood or dysphoria associated with menopause.
   C. **Urogenital symptoms.** Declining estrogen levels lead to atrophy of the urogenital tissues and vaginal thinning and shortening, resulting in dyspareunia and urethral irritation. Urinary tract infections and urinary incontinence may develop. Estrogen treatment (oral or intravaginal) reduces these problems
II. **Pharmacologic management of long-term risks**
   A. **Coronary artery disease**. Physiologic effects of estrogen, such as arterial vasodilatation, increased high-density lipoprotein (HDL) cholesterol levels and decreased low-density lipoprotein (LDL) cholesterol levels, are likely to reduce cardiovascular risk.
   B. **Osteoporosis**. More than 250,000 hip fractures occur annually. Estrogen deficiency is the primary cause of osteoporosis, although many other secondary causes for osteoporosis exist (eg, poor diet, glucocorticoid excess). Thus, women at risk for osteoporosis should be considered candidates for HRT.

Minimum Effective Dosages of Estrogens for Prevention of Osteoporosis

Formulation	Minimum effective dosage
Conjugated estrogen Premarin (0.3, 0.625, 0.9, 1.25, 2.5 mg)	0.625 mg
Micronized estradiol Estrace (0.5, 1.0, 2.0 mg)	1.0 mg

Esterified estrogen
    Estratab (0.3, 0.625, 2.5 mg)
    Menest (0.3, 0.625, 1.25, 2.5 mg)
	0.625 mg

Estropipate
    Ogen (0.625, 1.25, 2.5 mg)
    Ortho-Est (0.625, 1.25 mg)
	1.25 mg

Transdermal estradiol
    Climara (0.05, 0.1 mg)
    Estraderm (0.05, 0.1 mg)
	0.05 mg

Combination preparations	
Prempro	0.625 mg conjugated estrogen/2.5 mg or 5.0 mg medroxyprogesterone. Take one tab daily.
Premphase	0.625 mg conjugated estrogen (14 tablets) and 0.625 mg conjugated estrogen/5 mg medroxyprogesterone (14 tablets in sequence)
Combipatch	0.05 mg estradiol/0.14 mg norethindrone
Estratest	1.25 mg esterified estrogen/2.5 mg methyltestosterone
Estratest HS	0.625 mg esterified estrogen/1.25 mg methyltestosterone
Vaginal preparations	
Micronized estradiol cream (Estrace)	0.01% or 0.1 mg per g (42.5 g/tube)
Estropipate cream (Ogen)	1.5 mg per g (42.5 g/tube)
Conjugated estrogen cream (Premarin)	0.625 mg per g (42.5 g/tube)
Estradiol vaginal ring (Estring)	7.5 µg per 24 hours every 90 days

III. Hormone replacement therapy administration and regimens

A. HRT should not be a universal recommendation. The benefits and risks associated with HRT must be weighed on an individual basis. A woman with significant risk factors for osteoporosis or CHD may benefit from long-term HRT. A woman with a personal or strong family history of breast cancer may not benefit from long-term HRT.

B. Hormone users have a lower risk of death (relative risk, 0.63) than nonusers. This reduction is largest in women with cardiac risk factors. The benefit decreases with use of more than 10 years (due to breast cancer deaths) but still remains significant. HRT should increase life expectancy for nearly all women. The risk of HRT outweighs the benefit only in women without risk factors for CHD or hip fracture, but who have two first-degree relatives with breast cancer.

C. Effective doses of estrogen for the prevention of osteoporosis are: 0.625 mg of conjugated estrogen, 0.5 mg of micronized estradiol, and 0.3 mg of esterified estrogen.

D. In those women with a uterus, a progestin should be given continuously (2.5 mg of medroxyprogesterone per day) or in a sequential fashion [5-10 mg of medroxyprogesterone (Provera) for 12-14 days each month]. The most common HRT regimen consists of estrogen with or without progestin. The oral route of administration is preferable because of the hepatic effect on HDL cholesterol levels.

Relative and Absolute Contraindications for Hormone Replacement Therapy

Absolute contraindications	Relative contraindications
Estrogen-responsive breast cancer	Chronic liver disease
Endometrial cancer	Severe hypertriglyceridemia
Undiagnosed abnormal vaginal bleeding	Endometriosis
Active thromboembolic disease	Previous thromboembolic disease
History of malignant melanoma	Gallbladder disease

E. **Estrogen cream.** 1/4 of an applicator(0.6 mg) daily for 1-2 weeks, then 2-3 times/week will usually relieve urogenital symptoms. This regimen is used concomitantly with oral estrogen.

F. **Adverse effects** attributed to HRT include breast tenderness, breakthrough bleeding and thromboembolic disorders.

G. **Bisphosphonates** inhibit osteoclast activity. Alendronate (Fosamax) is effective in increasing BMD and reducing fractures by 40 percent. Alendronate should be taken in an upright position with a full glass of water 30 minutes before eating to prevent esophagitis. Alendronate is indicated for osteoporosis in women who have a contraindication to estrogen.

H. **Raloxifene (Evista)**, 60 mg qd, is a selective estrogen receptor modulator, FDA-labeled for prophylactic treatment of osteoporosis. This agent offers an alternative to traditional HRT. The modulator increases bone density (although only one-half as effectively as estrogen) and reduces total and LDL cholesterol levels.

IV. Complementary therapies

A. **Adequate dietary calcium** intake is essential, and supplementation is helpful if dietary sources are inadequate. Total calcium intake should approximate 1,500 mg per day, which usually requires supplementation.

B. **Vitamin D supplementation** (400 to 800 IU per day) is recommended for women who do not spend 30 minutes per day in the sun.

C. **Treatment of low libido** consists of 1% testosterone gel (AndroGel). Testosterone gel is supplied in 2.5- or 5-gram packets that deliver 25 or 50 mg of testosterone to the skin surface. Start with ½ gm/day applied to the inner surface of a forearm daily and increase to 1 gm/day if necessary. Androgens are known to increase libido and protect bone mass.

References: See page 290.

Premenstrual Syndrome

Premenstrual syndrome (PMS) refers to a group of menstrually related disorders and symptoms that includes premenstrual dysphoric disorder (PDD) as well as affective disturbances, alterations in appetite, cognitive disturbance, fluid retention and various types of pain. Premenstrual symptoms affect up to 40 percent of women of reproductive age, with severe impairment occurring in 5 percent. PMS may have an onset at any time during the reproductive years and, once symptoms are established, they tend to remain fairly constant until menopause.

I. Clinical evaluation of premenstrual syndrome

Symptom Clusters Commonly Noted in Patients with PMS	
Affective Symptoms Depression or sadness Irritability Tension Anxiety Tearfulness or crying easily Restlessness or jitteriness Anger Loneliness Appetite change Food cravings Changes in sexual interest Pain Headache or migraine Back pain Breast pain Abdominal cramps General or muscular pain	**Cognitive or performance** Mood instability or mood swings Difficulty in concentrating Decreased efficiency Confusion Forgetfulness Accident-prone Social avoidance Temper outbursts Energetic **Fluid retention** Breast tenderness or swelling Weight gain Abdominal bloating or swelling Swelling of extremities **General somatic** Fatigue or tiredness Dizziness or vertigo Nausea Insomnia

II. Clinical evaluation of premenstrual syndrome

A. PMS involves an assortment of disabling physical and emotional symptoms that appear during the luteal phase and resolve within the first week of the follicular phase. Symptoms of PMS fall into four main categories: mood, somatic, cognitive, and behavioral.

B. No specific serum marker can be used to confirm the diagnosis. Premenstrual dysphoric disorder is diagnosed when mood symptoms predominate symptoms of PMS.

C. The differential diagnosis includes hypothyroidism, anemia, perimenopause, drug and alcohol abuse, and affective disorders. Common alternative diagnoses in patients complaining of PMS include affective or personality disorder, menopausal symptoms, eating disorder, and alcohol or other substance abuse. A medical condition such as diabetes or hypothyroidism, is the cause of the symptoms in 8.4%, and 10.6% have symptoms related to oral contraceptive (OC) use.

D. **Affective symptoms** of PMS strongly resemble major depression, except that PDD differs from major depression in that PDD occurs in the premenstrual phase alone. Selective serotonin reuptake inhibitors have been shown to be effective in the treatment of premenstrual dysphoria.

E. PMS is associated only with ovulatory menstrual cycles. While symptoms may occur with nonovulatory cycles, such as during therapy with oral contraceptives, the symptoms are believed to be hormonally related, because changing the contraceptive formulation usually alters the symptom pattern.

F. **Nutrient abnormalities.** Deficiencies of magnesium, manganese, B vitamins, vitamin E and linoleic acid and its metabolites have been reported in women with PMS. In addition, dietary deficiencies of calcium, magnesium and manganese have been described in women with menstrually related discomforts.

III. Primary treatment strategies

A. **Dietary modification.** The recommended dietary intake for the treatment of PMS consists of low-fat, low cholesterol, balanced diet.

B. **Nonsteroidal anti-inflammatory drugs**(NSAIDs) are effective for treatment of dysmenorrhea, and their use has been recommended for other perimenstrual discomforts.

C. **Antidepressants.** The lower side effect profile and efficacy data for the selective serotonin reuptake inhibitors support their use over other classes of antidepressants. Antidepressant therapy should be prescribed daily in the usual dosages for depression.

D. **Cognitive behavioral therapy.** Patients with expectations of negative symptoms or of impaired performance around menses may respond well to cognitive therapy.

E. **Hormonal contraceptives.** Combined oral contraceptive pills or a progestin-only contraceptive agent may provide relief of PMS.

F. **Diuretics.** Symptoms related to fluid retention can usually be eradicated through dietary measures, most specifically restriction of sodium and simple sugars. However, diuretics may be useful in patients with very troubling edema. Spironolactone has bee demonstrated to be effective in a dosage of 100 mg per day.

IV. Treatments not generally recommended

A. **Progesterone.** Multiple double-blind, placebo-controlled studies of progesterone have failed to show evidence of progesterone efficacy in PMS, and its use is not recommended.

B. **High-dose vitamin B6.** Controlled trials have failed to document its effectiveness. Peripheral neuropathy has been reported with daily dosages of 200 mg or more.

C. **Gonadotropin-Releasing Hormone Agonists or Antagonists.** The expense and side effect profile, including hypoestrogenism and an increase risk of osteoporosis, of these agents would recommend against their us for PMS.

DSM-IV Criteria for Premenstrual Dysphoric Disorder

- Five or more symptoms
- At least one of the following four symptoms:
  Markedly depressed mood, feelings of hopelessness, or self-deprecating thoughts
  Marked anxiety, tension, feeling of being "keyed up" or "on edge"
  Marked affective lability
  Persistent and marked anger or irritability or increase in interpersonal conflicts
- Additional symptoms that may be used to fulfill the criteria:
  Decreased interest in usual activities
  Subjective sense of difficulty in concentrating
  Lethargy, easy fatigability, or marked lack of energy
  Marked change in appetite, overeating, or specific food cravings
  Hypersomnia or insomnia
  Subjective sense of being overwhelmed or out of control
- Other physical symptoms such as breast tenderness or swelling, headaches, joint or muscle pain, a sensation of bloating, or weight gain
- Symptoms occurring during last week of luteal phase
- Symptoms are absent postmenstrually
- Disturbances that interfere with work or school or with usual social activities and relationships
- Disturbances that are not an exacerbation of symptoms of another disorder

V. Treatment of premenstrual syndrome

A. More than 70% of women with PMS will respond to therapy.

B. Symptomatic treatment

1. **Fluid retention and bloating** may be relieved by limiting salty foods. If 5 pounds or more are gained during the luteal phase, diuretic therapy may be effective. Spironolactone (Aldactone) is the drug of choice because of its potassium-sparing effects. The dose ranges from 25-200 mg qd during the luteal phase.

2. **Mastalgia.** Support bras, decreased caffeine intake, nutritional supplements (vitamin E, 400 IU), a low-fat diet, oral contraceptives, or non-steroidal anti-inflammatory drugs (NSAIDs) are effective. Cabergoline (Dostinex), 0.25 mg - 1 mg twice a week during the luteal phase may be effective. Side effects include dizziness and gastrointestinal upset.

3. **Sleep disturbances.** Conservative measures include regulating sleep patterns, avoiding stimulating events before bedtime, and progressive relaxation and biofeedback therapy. Doxepin (Sinequan), 10-25 mg hs, also is effective.

Treatment of Premenstrual Syndrome

Fluoxetine (Prozac) 5-20 mg qd
Sertraline (Zoloft) 25-50 mg qd
Paroxetine (Paxil) 5-20 mg qd
Buspirone (BuSpar) 25 mg qd in divided doses

Alprazolam (Xanax) 0.25-0.50 mg tid

Mefenamic acid (Ponstel) 250 mg tid with meals
Oral contraceptives

Calcium, 600 mg bid, may help decrease negative mood, fluid retention, and pain

Calcium, 600 mg bid, may help decrease negative mood, fluid retention, and pain
Magnesium 100 mg qd may help decrease negative mood, fluid retention, and pain
Manganese 400 mg qd
Vitamin E, 400 IU qd

Other
Cabergoline (Dostinex) 0.25 mg - 1 mg twice a week during the luteal phase for breast pain
Spirolactone (Aldactone) 25-200 mg qd

    4. Menstrual migraines often occur just before and during menses. Menstrual migraines are treated with NSAIDs, sumatriptan (Imitrex), 50 mg po or 30-60 mg intramuscularly (IM) or propranolol (Inderal), 80-240 mg in divided doses; or amitriptyline (Elavil), 25-100 mg, taken before bedtime.

VI. Syndromal treatment
  A. Nonpharmacologic remedies include calcium (600 mg bid) and magnesium (360 mg qd), possibly with the addition of vitamins.
  B. SSRIs are appropriate for women with mood symptoms. Administration of fluoxetine (Prozac), 20 mg, or sertraline (Zoloft), 25-50 mg, has shown efficacy.

Lifestyle Modifications That Help Relieve Premenstrual Syndrome

Moderate, regular, aerobic exercise (1-2 miles of brisk walking 4-5 times/week) may decrease depression and pain symptoms

Reducing or eliminating salt and alcohol, especially in the luteal phase; eating small, frequent meals; increasing complex carbohydrates

  C. Anxiolytics and antidepressants. Alprazolam (Xanax), 0.25-0.5 mg tid, given during the luteal phase only may relieve anxiety.
  D. Surgery. Oophorectomy is reserved for patients whose symptoms have resolved completely for 4-6 months with GnRH agonists, who have completed child bearing, and who require more than 5 years of long-term suppression.
References: See page 290.

Abnormal Vaginal Bleeding

Menorrhagia (excessive bleeding) is most commonly caused by anovulatory menstrual cycles. Occasionally it is caused by thyroid dysfunction, infections or cancer.

I. Pathophysiology of normal menstruation
  A. In response to gonadotropin-releasing hormone from the hypothalamus, the pituitary gland synthesizes follicle-stimulating hormone (FSH) and luteinizing hormone (LH), which induce the ovaries to produce estrogen and progesterone.
  B. During the follicular phase, estrogen stimulation causes an increase in endometrial thickness. After ovulation, progesterone causes endometrial maturation. Menstruation is caused by estrogen and progesterone withdrawal.
  C. Abnormal bleeding is defined as bleeding that occurs at intervals of less than 21 days, more than 36 days, lasting longer than 7 days, or blood loss greater than 80 mL.
II. Clinical evaluation of abnormal vaginal bleeding
  A. A menstrual and reproductive history should include last menstrual period, regularity, duration, frequency; the number of pads used per day, and

intermenstrual bleeding.
- B. Stress, exercise, weight changes and systemic diseases, particularly thyroid, renal or hepatic diseases or coagulopathies, should be sought. The method of birth control should be determined.
- C. Pregnancy complications, such as spontaneous abortion, ectopic pregnancy, placenta previa and abruptio placentae, can cause heavy bleeding. Pregnancy should always be considered as a possible cause of abnormal vaginal bleeding.

III. Puberty and adolescence--menarche to age 16
- A. Irregularity is normal during the first few months of menstruation; however, soaking more than 25 pads or 30 tampons during a menstrual period is abnormal.
- B. Absence of premenstrual symptoms (breast tenderness, bloating, cramping) is associated with anovulatory cycles.
- C. Fever, particularly in association with pelvic or abdominal pain may, indicate pelvic inflammatory disease. A history of easy bruising suggests a coagulation defect. Headaches and visual changes suggest a pituitary tumor.
- D. **Physical findings**
  - 1. Pallor not associated with tachycardia or signs of hypovolemia suggests chronic excessive blood loss secondary to anovulatory bleeding, adenomyosis, uterine myomas, or blood dyscrasia.
  - 2. Fever, leukocytosis, and pelvic tenderness suggests PID.
  - 3. Signs of impending shock indicate that the blood loss is related to pregnancy (including ectopic), trauma, sepsis, or neoplasia.
  - 4. Pelvic masses may represent pregnancy, uterine or ovarian neoplasia, or a pelvic abscess or hematoma.
  - 5. Fine, thinning hair, and hypoactive reflexes suggest hypothyroidism.
  - 6. Ecchymoses or multiple bruises may indicate trauma, coagulation defects, medication use, or dietary extremes.
- E. **Laboratory tests**
  - 1. CBC and platelet count and a urine or serum pregnancy test should be obtained.
  - 2. Screening for sexually transmitted diseases, thyroid function, and coagulation disorders (partial thromboplastin time, INR, bleeding time) should be completed.
  - 3. **Endometrial sampling** is rarely necessary for those under age 20.
- F. **Treatment of infrequent bleeding**
  - 1. Therapy should be directed at the underlying cause when possible. If the CBC and other initial laboratory tests are normal and the history and physical examination are normal, reassurance is usually all that is necessary.
  - 2. Ferrous gluconate, 325 mg bid-tid, should be prescribed.
- G. **Treatment of frequent or heavy bleeding**
  - 1. Treatment with nonsteroidal anti-inflammatory drugs (NSAIDs) improves platelet aggregation and increases uterine vasoconstriction. NSAIDs are the first choice in the treatment of menorrhagia because they are well tolerated and do not have the hormonal effects of oral contraceptives.
    - a. Mefenamic acid (Ponstel) 500 mg tid during the menstrual period.
    - b. Naproxen (Anaprox, Naprosyn) 500 mg loading dose, then 250 mg tid during the menstrual period.
    - c. Ibuprofen (Motrin, Nuprin) 400 mg tid during the menstrual period.
    - d. Gastrointestinal distress is common. NSAIDs are contraindicated in renal failure and peptic ulcer disease.
  - 2. Iron should also be added as ferrous gluconate 325 mg tid.
- H. **Patients with hypovolemia or a hemoglobin level below 7 g/dL** should be hospitalized for hormonal therapy and iron replacement.
  - 1. Hormonal therapy consists of estrogen (Premarin) 25 mg IV q6h until bleeding stops. Thereafter, oral contraceptive pills should be administered q6h x 7 days, then taper slowly to one pill qd.
  - 2. If bleeding continues, IV vasopressin (DDAVP) should be administered. Hysteroscopy may be necessary, and dilation and curettage is a last

resort. Transfusion may be indicated in severe hemorrhage.
3. Iron should also be added as ferrous gluconate 325 mg tid.

IV. Primary childbearing years--ages 16 to early 40s

A. Contraceptive complications and pregnancy are the most common causes of abnormal bleeding in this age group. Anovulation accounts for 20% of cases.

B. Adenomyosis, endometriosis, and fibroids increase in frequency as a woman ages, as do endometrial hyperplasia and endometrial polyps. Pelvic inflammatory disease and endocrine dysfunction may also occur.

C. Laboratory tests
   1. CBC and platelet count, Pap smear, and pregnancy test.
   2. Screening for sexually transmitted diseases, thyroid-stimulating hormone, and coagulation disorders (partial thromboplastin time, INR, bleeding time).
   3. If a non-pregnant woman has a pelvic mass, ultrasonography or hysterosonography (with uterine saline infusion) is required.

D. Endometrial sampling
   1. Long-term unopposed estrogen stimulation in anovulatory patients can result in endometrial hyperplasia, which can progress to adenocarcinoma; therefore, in perimenopausal patients who have been anovulatory for an extended interval, the endometrium should be biopsied.
   2. Biopsy is also recommended before initiation of hormonal therapy for women over age 30 and for those over age 20 who have had prolonged bleeding.
   3. Hysteroscopy and endometrial biopsy with a Pipelle aspirator should be done on the first day of menstruation (to avoid an unexpected pregnancy) or anytime if bleeding is continuous.

E. Treatment
   1. Medical protocols for anovulatory bleeding (dysfunctional uterine bleeding) are similar to those described above for adolescents.
   2. Hormonal therapy
      a. In women who do not desire immediate fertility, hormonal therapy may be used to treat menorrhagia.
      b. A 21-day package of oral contraceptives is used. The patient should take one pill three times a day for 7 days. During the 7 days of therapy, bleeding should subside, and, following treatment, heavy flow will occur. After 7 days off the hormones, another 21-day package is initiated, taking one pill each day for 21 days, then no pills for 7 days.
      c. Alternatively, medroxyprogesterone (Provera), 10-20 mg per day for days 16 through 25 of each month, will result in a reduction of menstrual blood loss. Pregnancy will not be prevented.
      d. Patients with severe bleeding may have hypotension and tachycardia. These patients require hospitalization, and estrogen (Premarin) should be administered IV as 25 mg q4-6h until bleeding slows (up to a maximum of four doses). Oral contraceptives should be initiated concurrently as described above.
   3. Iron should also be added as ferrous gluconate 325 mg tid.
   4. Surgical treatment can be considered if childbearing is completed and medical management fails to provide relief.

V. Premenopausal, perimenopausal, and postmenopausal years--age 40 and over

A. Anovulatory bleeding accounts for about 90% of abnormal vaginal bleeding in this age group. However, bleeding should be considered to be from cancer until proven otherwise.

B. History, physical examination and laboratory testing are indicated as described above. Menopausal symptoms, personal or family history of malignancy and use of estrogen should be sought. A pelvic mass requires an evaluation with ultrasonography.

C. Endometrial carcinoma
   1. In a perimenopausal or postmenopausal woman, amenorrhea preceding abnormal bleeding suggests endometrial cancer. Endometrial evaluation is necessary before treatment of abnormal vaginal bleeding.
   2. Before endometrial sampling, determination of endometrial thickness by transvaginal ultrasonography is useful because biopsy is often not required when the endometrium is less than 5 mm thick.
D. Treatment
   1. Cystic hyperplasia or endometrial hyperplasia without cytologic atypia is treated with depo-medroxyprogesterone, 200 mg IM, then 100 to 200 mg IM every 3 to 4 weeks for 6 to 12 months. Endometrial hyperplasia requires repeat endometrial biopsy every 3 to 6 months.
   2. Atypical hyperplasia requires fractional dilation and curettage, followed by progestin therapy or hysterectomy.
   3. If the patient's endometrium is normal (or atrophic) and contraception is a concern, a low-dose oral contraceptive may be used. If contraception is not needed, estrogen and progesterone therapy should be prescribed.
   4. **Surgical management**
      a. **Vaginal or abdominal hysterectomy** is the most absolute curative treatment.
      b. **Dilatation and curettage** can be used as a temporizing measure to stop bleeding.
      c. **Endometrial ablation and resection** by laser, electrodiathermy "rollerball," or excisional resection are alternatives to hysterectomy.

References: See page 290.

Breast Cancer Screening

Breast cancer is the most common form of cancer in women. There are 200,000 new cases of breast cancer each year, resulting in 47,000 deaths per year. The lifetime risk of breast cancer is one in eight for a woman who is age 20. For patients under age 60, the chance of being diagnosed with breast cancer is 1 in about 400 in a given year.

I. Pathophysiology
   A. The etiology of breast cancer remains unknown, but two breast cancer genes have been cloned–the BRCA-1 and the BRCA-2 genes. Only 10% of all of the breast cancers can be explained by mutations in these genes.
   B. Estrogen stimulation is an important promoter of breast cancer, and, therefore, patients who have a long history of menstruation are at increased risk. Early menarche and late menopause are risk factors for breast cancer. Late age at birth of first child or nulliparity also increase the risk of breast cancer.
   C. Family history of breast cancer in a first degree relative and history of benign breast disease also increase the risk of breast cancer. The use of estrogen replacement therapy or oral contraceptives slightly increases the risk of breast cancer. Radiation exposure and alcoholic beverage consumption also increase the risk of breast cancer.

Recommended Intervals for Breast Cancer Screening Studies			
	Age <40 yr	40-49 yr	50-75 yr
Breast Self-Examination	Monthly by age 30	Monthly	Monthly
Professional Breast Examination	Every 3 yr, ages 20-39	Annually	Annually
Mammography, Low Risk Patient		Annually	Annually
Mammography, High Risk Patient	Begin at 35 yr	Annually	Annually

II. Diagnosis and evaluation
A. **Clinical evaluation of a breast mass** should assess duration of the lesion, associated pain, relationship to the menstrual cycle or exogenous hormone use, and change in size since discovery. The presence of nipple discharge and its character (bloody or tea-colored, unilateral or bilateral, spontaneous or expressed) should be assessed.
B. **Menstrual history.** The date of last menstrual period, age of menarche, age of menopause or surgical removal of the ovaries, regularity of the menstrual cycle, previous pregnancies, age at first pregnancy, and lactation history should be determined.
C. **History of previous breast biopsies,** breast cancer, or cyst aspiration should be investigated. Previous or current oral contraceptive and hormone replacement therapy and dates and results of previous mammograms should be ascertained.
D. **Family history** should document breast cancer in relatives and the age at which family members were diagnosed.

III. Physical examination
A. The breasts should be inspected for asymmetry, deformity, skin retraction, erythema, peau d'orange (indicating breast edema), and nipple retraction, discoloration, or inversion.
B. **Palpation**
1. The breasts should be palpated while the patient is sitting and then supine with the ipsilateral arm extended. The entire breast should be palpated systematically.
2. The mass should be evaluated for size, shape, texture, tenderness, fixation to skin or chest wall. The location of the mass should be documented with a diagram in the patient's chart. The nipples should be expressed to determine whether discharge can be induced. Nipple discharge should be evaluated for single or multiple ducts, color, and any associated mass.
3. The axillae should be palpated for adenopathy, with an assessment of size of the lymph nodes, their number, and fixation. The supraclavicular and cervical nodes should also be assessed.

IV. Breast imaging
A. **Mammography**
1. **Screening mammography** is performed in the asymptomatic patients and consists of two views. Patients are not examined by a mammographer. Screening mammography reduces mortality from breast cancer and should usually be initiated at age 40.
2. **Diagnostic mammography** is performed after a breast mass has been detected. Patients usually are examined by a mammographer, and films are interpreted immediately and additional views of the lesion are completed. Mammographic findings predictive of malignancy include

spiculated masses with architectural distortion and microcalcifications. A normal mammography in the presence of a palpable mass does not exclude malignancy.
- **B. Ultrasonography** is used as an adjunct to mammography to differentiate solid from cystic masses. It is the primary imaging modality in patients younger than 30 years old.

V. Methods of breast biopsy
- **A. Stereotactic core needle biopsy**. Using a computer-driven stereotactic unit, the lesion is localized in three dimensions, and an automated biopsy needle obtains samples. The sensitivity and specificity of this technique are 95-100% and 94-98%, respectively.
- **B. Palpable masses. Fine-needle aspiration biopsy (FNAB)** has a sensitivity ranging from 90-98%. Nondiagnostic aspirates require surgical biopsy.
  - **1.** The skin is prepped with alcohol and the lesion is immobilized with the nonoperating hand. A 10 mL syringe, with a 18 to 22 gauge needle, is introduced in to the central portion of the mass at a 90° angle. When the needle enters the mass, suction is applied by retracting the plunger, and the needle is advanced. The needle is directed into different areas of the mass while maintaining suction on the syringe.
  - **2.** Suction is slowly released before the needle is withdrawn from the mass. The contents of the needle are placed onto glass slides for pathologic examination.
- **C. Impalpable lesions**
  - **1. Needle localized biopsy**
    - **a.** Under mammographic guidance, a needle and hookwire are placed into the breast parenchyma adjacent to the lesion. The patient is taken to the operating room along with mammograms for an excisional breast biopsy.
    - **b.** The skin and underlying tissues are infiltrated with 1% lidocaine with epinephrine. For lesions located within 5 cm of the nipple, a periareolar incision may be used or use a curved incision located over the mass and parallel to the areola. Incise the skin and subcutaneous fat, then palpate the lesion and excise the mass.
    - **c.** After removal of the specimen, a specimen x-ray is performed to confirm that the lesion has been removed. The specimen can then be sent fresh for pathologic analysis.
    - **d.** Close the subcutaneous tissues with a 4-0 chromic catgut suture, and close the skin with 4-0 subcuticular suture.

References: See page 290.

Breast Disorders

I. Nipple Discharge
- **A. Clinical evaluation**
  - **1.** Nipple discharge may be a sign of cancer; therefore, it must be thoroughly evaluated. About 8% of biopsies performed for nipple discharge demonstrate cancer. The duration, bilaterality or unilaterality of the discharge, and the presence of blood should be determined. A history of oral contraceptives, hormone preparations, phenothiazines, nipple or breast stimulation or lactation should be sought. Discharges that flow spontaneously are more likely to be pathologic than discharges that must be manually expressed.
  - **2.** Unilateral, pink colored, bloody or non-milky discharge, or discharges associated with a mass are the discharges of most concern. Milky discharge can be caused by oral contraceptive agents, estrogen replacement therapy, phenothiazines, prolactinoma, or hypothyroidism. Nipple discharge secondary to malignancy is more likely to occur in older patients.
  - **3. Risk factors.** The assessment should identify risk factors, including age

over 50 years, past personal history of breast cancer, history of hyperplasia on previous breast biopsies, and family history of breast cancer in a first-degree relative (mother, sister, daughter).

B. Physical examination should include inspection of the breast for ulceration or contour changes and inspection of the nipple. Palpation should be performed with the patient in both the upright and the supine positions to determine the presence of a mass.

C. Diagnostic evaluation

1. **Bloody discharge.** A mammogram of the involved breast should be obtained if the patient is over 35 years old and has not had a mammogram within the preceding 6 months. Biopsy of any suspicious lesions should be completed.

2. **Watery, unilateral discharge** should be referred to a surgeon for evaluation and possible biopsy.

3. **Non-bloody discharge** should be tested for the presence of blood with a Hemoccult card. Nipple discharge secondary to carcinoma usually contains hemoglobin.

4. **Milky, bilateral discharge** should be evaluated with assays of prolactin and thyroid stimulating hormone to exclude an endocrinologic cause.

   a. A mammogram should also be performed if the patient is due for routine mammographic screening.

   b. If results of the mammogram and the endocrinologic screening studies are normal, the patient should return for a follow-up visit in 6 months to ensure that there has been no specific change in the character of the discharge, such as development of bleeding.

II. Breast Pain

A. Determine the duration and location of the pain, associated trauma, previous breast surgery, associated lumps, or nipple discharge.

B. Pain is an uncommon presenting symptom for breast cancer; however, cancer must be excluded. Cancer is the etiology in 5% of patients with breast pain. Pain that is associated with breast cancer is usually unilateral, intense, and constant.

C. Patients less than 35 years of age without a mass

1. Pain is unlikely to be a symptom of cancer.

2. A follow-up clinical breast examination should be performed in 1-2 months. Diagnostic mammography is usually not helpful but may be considered.

D. Patients 35 years of age or older

1. Obtain diagnostic mammogram, and obtain an ultrasound if a cystic lesion is present.

2. If studies are negative, a follow-up examination in 1-2 months is appropriate. If a suspicious lesion is detected, biopsy is required.

E. Mastodynia

1. Mastodynia is defined as breast pain in the absence of a mass or other pathologic abnormality.

2. **Causes of mastodynia** include menstrually related pain, costochondritis, trauma, and sclerosing adenosis.

III. Fibrocystic Complex

A. Breast changes are usually multifocal, bilateral, and diffuse. One or more isolated fibrocystic lumps or areas of asymmetry may be present. The areas are usually tender.

B. This disorder predominantly occurs in women with premenstrual abnormalities, nulliparous women, and nonusers of oral contraceptives.

C. The disorder usually begins in mid-20's or early 30's. Tenderness is associated with menses and lasts about a week. The upper outer quadrant of the breast is most frequently involved bilaterally. There is no increased risk of cancer for the majority of patients.

D. Suspicious areas may be evaluated by fine needle aspiration (FNA) cytology. If mammography and FNA are negative for cancer, and the clinical examination is benign, open biopsy is generally not needed.

E. **Medical management of fibrocystic complex**
   1. **Oral contraceptives** are effective for severe breast pain in most young women. Start with a pill that contains low amounts of estrogen and relatively high amounts of progesterone (Loestrin, LoOvral, Ortho-Cept).
   2. If oral contraceptives do not provide relief, medroxyprogesterone, 5-10 mg/day from days 15-25 of each cycle, is added.
   3. A professionally fitted support bra often provides significant relief.
   4. A low fat diet, vitamins (E and B complex), evening primrose oil, and stopping smoking may provide relief.
   5. NSAIDs and cabergoline (Dostinex) may also be used.

References: See page 290.

Osteoporosis

Osteoporosis is a common cause of skeletal fractures. Bone loss accelerates during menopause due to a decrease in estrogen production. Approximately 20% of women have osteoporosis in their seventh decade of life, 30% of women in their eighth decade of life, and 70% of women older than 80 years.

I. **Diagnosis**
   A. **Risk factors** for osteoporosis include female gender, increasing age, family history, Caucasian or Asian race, estrogen deficient state, nulliparity, sedentarism, low calcium intake, smoking, excessive alcohol or caffeine consumption, and use of glucocorticoid drugs. Patients who have already sustained a fracture have a markedly increased risk of sustaining further fractures.
   B. **Bone density testing.** Bone density is the strongest predictor of fracture risk. Bone density can be assessed by dual X-ray absorptiometry.

Indications for Bone Density Testing

Estrogen-deficient women at clinical risk for osteoporosis
Individuals with vertebral abnormalities
Individuals receiving, or planning to receive, long-term glucocorticoid therapy
Individuals with primary hyperparathyroidism
Individuals being monitored to assess the response of an osteoporosis drug

II. **Prevention and treatment strategies**
   A. A balanced diet including 1000-1500 mg of calcium, weight bearing exercise, and avoidance of alcohol and tobacco products should be encouraged. Daily calcium supplementation (1000-1500 mg) along with 400-800 IU vitamin D should be recommended.
   B. Estrogen therapy is recommended for most females. Females who are not willing or incapable of receiving estrogen therapy and have osteopenic bone densities may consider alendronate and raloxifene. After the age of 65, a bone density test should be performed to decide if pharmacologic therapy should be considered to prevent or treat osteoporosis.

Drugs for Osteoporosis

Drug	Dosage	Indication	Comments
Estrogen	0.625 mg qd with medroxyprogesterone (Provera), 2.5 mg qd	Prevention and Treatment	Recommended for most menopausal females

Drug	Dosage	Indication	Comments
Raloxifene (Evista)	60 mg PO QD	Prevention	No breast or uterine tissue stimulation. Decrease in cholesterol similar to estrogen.
Alendronate (Fosamax)	5 mg PO QD 10 mg PO QD	Prevention Treatment	Take in the morning with 2-3 glasses of water, at least 30 min before any food, beverages, or medication. Reduction in fracture risk.
Calcitonin	200 IU QD (nasal) 50-100 IU QD SQ	Treatment	Modest analgesic effect. Not indicated in the early post-menopausal years.
Calcium	1000-1500 mg/day	Prevention/ Treatment	Calcium alone may not prevent osteoporosis
Vitamin D	400-800 IU QD	Prevention/ Treatment	May help reduce hip fracture incidence

   C. Estrogen replacement therapy
   1. Postmenopausal women without contraindications should consider ERT. Contraindications include a family or individual history of breast cancer; estrogen dependent neoplasia; undiagnosed genital bleeding or a history of or active thromboembolic disorder.
   2. ERT should be initiated at the onset of menopause. Conjugated estrogens, at a dose of 0.625 mg per day, result in increases in bone density of 5%.
   3. **Bone density assessment** at regular intervals (possibly every 3-5 years) provides density data to help determine if continuation of ERT may be further recommended. If ERT is discontinued and no other therapies are instituted, serial bone density measurements should be continued to monitor bone loss.
   4. ERT doubles the risk of endometrial cancer in women with an intact uterus. This increased risk can be eliminated by the addition of medroxyprogesterone (Provera), either cyclically (12-14 days/month) at a dose of 5-10 mg, or continuously at a dose of 2.5 mg daily.
   5. Other adverse effects related to ERT are breast tenderness, weight gain, headaches, and libido changes.
   D. Selective estrogen receptor modulators
   1. Selective estrogen receptor modulators (SERMs) act as estrogen analogs. Tamoxifen is approved for the prevention of breast cancer in patients with a strong family history of breast cancer. Tamoxifen prevents bone loss at the spine.
   2. **Raloxifene (Evista)**
      a. **Raloxifene** is approved for the prevention of osteoporosis. When used at 60 mg per day, raloxifene demonstrates modest increases (1.5-2% in 24 months) in bone density. This increase in density is half of that seen in those patients receiving ERT. Raloxifene has a beneficial effect on the lipid profile similar to that seen with estrogen.
      b. Raloxifene lacks breast stimulation properties, and it may provide a protective effect against breast cancer, resulting in a 50-70% reduction in breast cancer risk.
      c. Minor side effects include hot flashes and leg cramps. Serious side effects include an increased risk of venous thromboembolism.
   E. Bisphosphonates – alendronate (Fosamax)
   1. Alendronate is an oral bisphosphonate approved for the treatment and

prevention of osteoporosis. Alendronate exerts its effect on bone by inhibiting osteoclasts.

2. The dose for prevention of osteoporosis is 5 mg per day. This dose results in significant increases in densities of 2-3.5%, similar to those observed in ERT. The dose for treatment of osteoporosis is 10 mg per day. Alendronate provides a 50% reduction in fracture risk.

3. Patients should take the pill in the morning with 2-3 glasses of water, at least 30 minutes before any food or beverages. No other medication should be taken at the same time, particularly calcium preparations. Patients should not lie down after taking alendronate to avoid gastroesophageal reflux. Contraindicates include severe renal insufficiency and hypocalcemia.

References: See page 290.

Urinary Incontinence

Urinary incontinence is defined as the involuntary loss of urine in amounts or with sufficient frequency to constitute a social and/or health problem. The prevalence of urinary incontinence is 15 to 35 percent in community-dwelling individuals older than age 60.

I. Clinical evaluation

Urinary Incontinence: Types, Signs and Symptoms, and Causes		
Type	**Signs and symptoms**	**Causes**
Urge incontinence		
Detrusor instability (DI)	With or without urgency, usually large volume loss	Involuntary detrusor contraction, isolated or with cystitis, ureteritis, stones, neoplasia
Detrusor hyperreflexia (DI with neurologic cause)	As above, and may have urinary retention and/or vesicoureteral reflux	Central nervous system disorders: stroke, suprasacral or cord injury, parkinsonism, multiple sclerosis
Detrusor hyperreflexia with impaired contractility	Urge incontinence with elevated postvoid residual volume; must strain to empty bladder; may have symptoms of stress or overflow incontinence; episodic leakage, but frequent, moderate to large volume loss	Central nervous system disorders as above; involuntary detrusor contractions, but need to strain to empty bladder because of impaired contractility
Stress incontinence		
Stress incontinence	Small volume of urine loss with increased abdominal pressure (coughing, laughing, exercise); dry during night	Urethral hypermobility, laxity of pelvic floor muscles (common in women); weakness of urethral sphincter or bladder outlet

Type	Signs and symptoms	Causes
Intrinsic urethral sphincter deficiency	Often leak continuously or with minimal exertion	Intrinsic urethral sphincter deficiency: congenital, myelomeningocele, multiple sclerosis In women: history of surgery for urinary incontinence, estrogen deficiency, aging
Mixed incontinence (urge and stress)	Combination of urge and stress symptoms	As above; common in women
Overflow incontinence	Frequent or constant dribbling, with urge or stress symptoms	Underactive or acontractile detrusor, bladder outlet or urethral obstruction, overdistention, and overflow In women: obstruction is rare; in men: obstruction is common, eg, benign prostatic hypertrophy, neoplasm
Functional incontinence	Functional limitations interfere with ability to use the toilet	Caused by decreased physical or cognitive ability, environmental factors

History and Physical Examination in Patients with Urinary Incontinence

Urinary history
Duration of symptoms, frequency, urgency, severity
Amount of urine loss, dribbling, nocturia, hematuria, dysuria, hesitancy, weak stream, straining to void; precipitating factors (coughing, sneezing, exercise, surgery, injury)
Perineal pain, suprapubic pressure, suprapubic pain
Number of continent voids, incontinence episodes
Any previous treatment for incontinence, outcome
Use of protective devices (eg, pads, briefs)
Bladder record (voiding diary for several days)

Medical history
History of surgery, injury, pelvic radiation therapy, trauma
History of major medical illness, diabetes mellitus, congestive heart failure, peripheral edema, neurologic disease
Medications
Change in bowel habits, constipation, fecal impaction
Fluid intake, diuretic fluids (caffeine or alcohol)

Social history
Functional ability (activities of daily living, instrumental activities of daily living)
Living environment, access to toilet
Cognitive deficits, motivation

Physical examination
Orthostatic hypotension
Presence of edema that may explain nocturia or nocturnal incontinence
Neurologic diseases (eg, stroke, multiple sclerosis, spinal cord lesions; functional ability, mobility, manual dexterity; cognitive status, depression)
Abdominal examination to rule out mass, ascites, or organomegaly that might increase intra-abdominal pressure
Rectal examination to rule out mass, impaction, decreased sphincter tone, impaired sensation
Pelvic examination to evaluate for cystocele, rectocele, uterine prolapse, genital atrophy; examination for urethral diverticulum, inflammation on or carcinoma

Medications that May Contribute to Urinary Incontinence	
Medications	**Effect**
Anticholinergics Antipsychotics Antidepressants Calcium channel blockers Antihistamines Sedative-hypnotics beta-adrenergic agonists	Urinary retention (bladder relaxation)
alpha-adrenergic agonists	Urinary retention (sphincter contraction; stress urinary incontinence symptoms improve in women)
alpha-adrenergic antagonists	Urethral relaxation (urinary incontinence symptoms improve in men with benign prostatic hypertrophy)
Diuretics Alcohol Caffeine	Polyuria

A. **Cough stress test** is performed when the woman's bladder is full, but before she has the urge to void. If there is an instantaneous, involuntary loss of urine with increased intra-abdominal pressure (cough, laugh, sneezing, exercise, Valsalva's maneuver), then stress urinary incontinence (SUI) is likely. If the loss of urine occurs after a delay or continues after the cough, then detrusor instability (DI) is suspected.
B. **Postvoid residual volume.** Portable ultrasound or catheterization can accurately measure postvoid residual (PVR) volume. PVR volume is measured a few minutes after voiding. A PVR volume less than 100 mL indicates adequate bladder emptying. A PVR volume of 100 mL or more is considered to be inadequate.
C. **Urinalysis** is performed to detect hematuria, proteinuria, glucosuria, pyuria, and bacteriuria.
D. **Other testing.** Further evaluation may include urodynamic, endoscopic, and imaging tests.

II. Etiology
  A. Causes of transient incontinence include delirium; restricted mobility, retention; infection, inflammation, impaction (fecal); polyuria, pharmaceuticals).
  B. Patients who have a positive cough test and consistent symptoms probably have SUI. This is the second most common type of urinary incontinence in women. A history of sudden urination of large amounts of urine suggests DI (the most common type of urinary incontinence in women), or urge incontinence. A PVR volume of more than 100 mL suggests a neurogenic bladder, especially in patients with diabetes or neurologic disease.

III. Treatment
  A. Routine, or scheduled, voiding requires urinating at regular intervals (two to four hours) on a fixed schedule. In bladder training, the patient schedules voiding. This method can be very effective for stress, urge (DI) and mixed urinary incontinence.
  B. Pelvic muscle exercises (PMEs), eg, Kegel exercises, are recommended for women with SUI. They may also help urge urinary incontinence. PMEs may be performed alone or with biofeedback, vaginal weights, and electrical stimulation of the pelvic floor. The patient is trained to gradually

increase the duration of sustained pelvic muscle contractions to at least 10 seconds. Gradually, the number of repetitions is increased to 30 to 50 times per day for at least eight weeks.

Treatment of Urinary Incontinence

Urge incontinence
First line: behavioral and biofeedback techniques
    Bladder training
    Pelvic floor muscle exercises
    Pelvic floor electrical stimulation
    Vaginal weights
    Anticholinergic agents
    Agent of choice: Oxybutynin (Ditropan), 2.5 to 5.0 mg orally three to four times per day, or tolterodine (Detrol), 1 to 2 mg orally two times per day
    Second choice: Propantheline (Pro-Banthine), 7.5 to 30.0 mg orally three to five times per day
    Alternate: dicyclomine (eg, Bemote, Benty, Byclomine), 10 to 20 mg orally three times per day
    Imipramine (Tofranil), 10 to 25 mg orally three times per day
Second line: Surgical procedures (rarely used, recommended for intractable cases)
    Augmentation intestinocystoplasty or urinary diversion
    Bladder denervation

Stress incontinence
First line: behavioral and biofeedback techniques
    Pelvic floor muscle exercises
    Bladder training
    Phenylpropanolamine (Entex sustained release), 25 to 100 mg orally two times per day
    Pseudoephedrine (Afrin), 15 to 30 mg orally two times per day
    Estrogen (oral [Premarin] or vaginal [eg, Estrace, Ogen, Premarin]), 0.3 to 1.25 mg orally once per day; 2.0 g vaginally once per day
    Progestin (Provera), 2.5 to 10.0 mg orally once per day continuously or intermittently, used with estrogen in women with an intact uterus
    Imipramine (Tofranil) may be use when above agents have proven unsatisfactory; 10 to 25 mg orally two times per day
Second line: surgical procedures (sometimes first line of treatment for selected women)
    Procedures for hypermobility
        Retropubic suspension
        Needle bladder neck suspension
        Anterior vaginal repair
    Procedures for intrinsic sphincter deficiency
        Sling procedures (intrinsic urethral sphincter deficiency with coexisting hypermobility)
        Periurethral bucking injections (intrinsic urethral sphincter deficiency without hypermobility)
    Placement of artificial sphincter (for intrinsic urethral sphincter deficiency with an inability to perform intermittent catheterization)

Overflow incontinence
Surgical removal of obstruction
Medication adjustments for underactive or a contractile bladder because of medication taken for other medical conditions
Intermittent catheterization for underactive detrusor muscle with or without obstruction
Indwelling catheter for women who are not candidates for surgery and those who have urinary incontinence because of urethral obstruction

---

C. Pharmacologic and surgical therapies
1. Urge incontinence
    a. Oxybutynin (Ditropan) produces a 15-58% percent reduction in episodes of urge incontinence. It is an anticholinergic smooth-muscle relaxant. Bothersome side effects are xerostomia, blurred vision, changes in mental status, nausea, constipation, and urinary retention.
    b. Tolterodine (Detrol) produces a 12-18% reduction in episodes of

urinary incontinence and has fewer side effects than oxybutynin.
  - c. **Propantheline (Pro-Banthine)** is a second-line anticholinergic agent that produces a 13-17% reduction in incontinent episodes. High dosages are required.
2. **Stress urinary incontinence**
  - a. SUI due to sphincter insufficiency is treated with alpha-adrenergic agonists. Phenylpropanolamine or pseudoephedrine is the first line of pharmacologic therapy for women with SUI. Side effects include anxiety, insomnia, agitation, respiratory difficulty, headache, sweating, hypertension, and cardiac arrhythmia. Use caution with arrhythmias, angina, hypertension, or hyperthyroidism.
  - b. **Estrogen replacement** restores urethral tone, and alpha-adrenergic response of urethral muscles. Combined therapy (estrogen and alpha-adrenergic agonists) may be more effective than alpha-adrenergic agonist therapy alone.
  - c. **Imipramine** may be used in patients who do not respond to the above treatment. It has alpha-adrenergic agonist and anticholinergic activities and is reported to benefit women with SUI. Side effects include nausea, postural hypotension, insomnia, weakness, and fatigue.
3. **Overflow incontinence.** If overflow incontinence is caused by an anatomic obstruction, and the patient is an acceptable surgical candidate and has an adequately functioning detrusor muscle, then surgery to relieve the obstruction is the treatment of choice. In women, anatomic obstruction can result from severe pelvic prolapse or previous surgery for incontinence. Intermittent catheterization is the treatment of choice in patients with detrusor muscle underactivity, with or without obstruction.

References: See page 290.

Urinary Tract Infection

An estimated 40 percent of women report having had a urinary tract infections (UTI) at some point in their lives. UTIs are the leading cause of gram-negative bacteremia.

I. **Acute uncomplicated cystitis in young women**
  - A. Sexually active young women have the highest risk for UTIs. Their propensity to develop UTIs is caused by a short urethra, delays in micturition, sexual activity, and the use of diaphragms and spermicides.
  - B. **Symptoms of cystitis** include dysuria, urgency, and frequency without fever or back pain. Lower tract infections are most common in women in their childbearing years. Fever is absent.
  - C. **A microscopic bacterial count** of 100 CFU/mL of urine has a high positive predictive value for cystitis in symptomatic women. Ninety percent of uncomplicated cystitis episodes are caused by *Escherichia coli;* 10 to 20 percent are caused by coagulase-negative *Staphylococcus saprophyticus* and 5 percent are caused by other Enterobacteriaceae organisms or enterococci. Up to one-third of uropathogens are resistant to ampicillin, but the majority are susceptible to trimethoprim-sulfamethoxazole (85 to 95 percent) and fluoroquinolones (95 percent).
  - D. Young women with acute uncomplicated cystitis should receive urinalysis (examination of spun urine) and a dipstick test for leukocyte esterase.
  - E. A positive leukocyte esterase test has a sensitivity of 75 to 90 percent in detecting pyuria associated with a UTI. The dipstick test for nitrite indicates bacteriuria. Enterococci, *S. saprophyticus* and Acinetobacter species produce false-negative results on nitrite testing.
  - F. Three-day antibiotic regimens offer the optimal combination of convenience, low cost and efficacy comparable to seven-day or longer regimens.
  - G. **Trimethoprim-sulfamethoxazole (Bactrim, Septra)**, 1 DS tab bid for 3

224 Urinary Tract Infection

days, remains the antibiotic of choice in the treatment of uncomplicated UTIs in young women.

- H. A fluoroquinolone is recommended for patients who cannot tolerate sulfonamides or trimethoprim, who have a high frequency of antibiotic resistance because of recent antibiotic treatment, or who reside in an area with significant resistance to trimethoprim-sulfamethoxazole. Treatment should consist of a three-day regimen of one of the following:
  1. **Ciprofloxacin (Cipro)**, 250 mg bid.
  2. **Ofloxacin (Floxin)**, 200 mg bid.
- I. A seven-day course should be considered in pregnant women, diabetic women and women who have had symptoms for more than one week and thus are at higher risk for pyelonephritis.

II. Recurrent cystitis in young women

- A. Up to 20 percent of young women with acute cystitis develop recurrent UTIs. The causative organism should be identified by urine culture. Multiple infections caused by the same organism require longer courses of antibiotics and possibly further diagnostic tests. Women who have more than three UTI recurrences within one year can be managed using one of three preventive strategies:
  1. **Acute self-treatment** with a three-day course of standard therapy.
  2. **Postcoital prophylaxis** with one-half of a trimethoprim-sulfamethoxazole double-strength tablet (40/200 mg) if the UTIs have been clearly related to intercourse.
  3. **Continuous daily prophylaxis for six months:** Trimethoprim-sulfamethoxazole, one-half tablet/day (40/200 mg); norfloxacin (Noroxin), 200 mg/day; cephalexin (Keflex), 250 mg/day.

III. Pyelonephritis

- A. Acute uncomplicated pyelonephritis presents with a mild cystitis-like illness and accompanying flank pain; fever, chills, nausea, vomiting, leukocytosis and abdominal pain; or a serious gram-negative bacteremia. The microbiologic features of acute uncomplicated pyelonephritis are the same as cystitis, except that *S. saprophyticus* is a rare cause.
- B. The diagnosis should be confirmed by urinalysis with examination for pyuria and/or white blood cell casts and by urine culture. Urine cultures demonstrate more than 100,000 CFU/mL of urine. Blood cultures are positive in 20%.
- C. Oral therapy should be considered in women with mild to moderate symptoms. Since *E. coli* resistance to ampicillin, amoxicillin and first-generation cephalosporins exceeds 30 percent, these agents should not be used for the treatment of pyelonephritis. Resistance to trimethoprim-sulfamethoxazole exceeds 15 percent; therefore, empiric therapy with ciprofloxacin (Cipro), 250 mg twice daily is recommended.
- D. Patients who are too ill to take oral antibiotics should initially be treated parenterally with a third-generation cephalosporin, a broad-spectrum penicillin, a quinolone or an aminoglycoside. Once these patients have improved clinically, they can be switched to oral therapy.
- E. The total duration of therapy is usually 14 days. Patients with persistent symptoms after three days of appropriate antimicrobial therapy should be evaluated by renal ultrasonography or computed tomography for evidence of urinary obstruction. In the small percentage of patients who relapse after a two-week course, a repeated six-week course is usually curative.

IV. Urinary tract infection in men

- A. Urinary tract infections most commonly occur in older men with prostatic disease, outlet obstruction or urinary tract instrumentation. In men, a urine culture growing more than 1,000 CFU of a pathogen/mL of urine is the best sign of a urinary tract infection, with a sensitivity and specificity of 97 percent. Men with urinary tract infections should receive seven days of antibiotic therapy (trimethoprim-sulfamethoxazole or a fluoroquinolone).
- B. Urologic evaluation should be performed routinely in adolescents and men with pyelonephritis or recurrent infections. When bacterial prostatitis is the source of a urinary tract infection, eradication usually requires antibiotic therapy for six to 12 weeks.

References: See page 290.

Pubic Infections

I. **Human Papilloma Virus**
   A. Infections caused by human papillomavirus (HPV) account for 5.5 million, or more than one-third, of sexually transmitted diseases. More than 100 types of HPV have been identified in humans. HPV infections can cause genital warts and various benign or malignant neoplasias, or they can be entirely asymptomatic.
   B. Genital warts occur on the external genitalia and perianal area and can be visible in the vagina, on the cervix, and inside the urethra and anus. External genital warts (EGWs) are usually caused by HPV type 6 and, less commonly, by HPV type 11, both of which are considered "low-risk types" in that they are unlikely to cause squamous intraepithelial lesions (SIL) or malignancy. Approximately 15% of men and women 15-49 years of age have genital warts that can shed HPV DNA.
   C. EGWs are generally visible with the naked eye and occur both in the area of the genitals and surrounding areas (ie, vulva, penis, scrotum, perianal area, perineum, pubic area, upper thighs, and crural folds). Four types of lesions occur.
      1. Condyloma acuminata that are cauliflower shape and usually occur on moist surfaces.
      2. Papular warts that are dome-shaped, flesh-colored, less than 4 mm in size, and occur on keratinized hair-bearing or non-hair-bearing skin.
      3. Keratotic warts that have a thick, horny layer, can appear similar to common, non-genital warts, and occur on fully keratinized skin.
      4. Flat-topped papules that are macular or slightly raised and occur on both moist partially keratinized or fully keratinized skin.
   D. **Diagnostic approaches**
      1. External warts can be diagnosed clinically with the assistance of bright light and a handheld magnifying glass. In most patients, warts have a typical appearance and are not easily confused with other skin lesions. Biopsy should be used when lesions are indurated, fixed to underlying tissue, or heavily ulcerated. Biopsy should also be considered when individual warts are greater than 1 to 2 cm, are pigmented, or respond poorly to treatment.

Treatment of External Genital Warts		
Modality	**Advantages**	**Disadvantages**
Imiquimod	Patient-applied immune response modifier	Results dependent on patient compliance; safety in pregnancy unproved
Podofilox	Patient-applied	Results dependent on patient compliance; contraindicated > 10 cm² wart area; contraindicated in pregnancy
Cryotherapy	Effective for moist and dry warts	Pain; risk of under- or over-application

Podophyllin	Most effective on moist warts	May contain mutagens; limited value for dry warts; contraindicated in pregnancy; contraindicated for large wart area; may require many applications due to low efficacy
Trichloroacetic acid/Bichloroacetic acid	Inexpensive; most effective for moist warts; safe during pregnancy	Limited value for dry warts; contraindicated for large area of friable warts; can cause burns
Curettage, electrosurgery, scissor excision	Prompt wart removal, usually in one or a few visits	Office visits; local anesthetic is usually necessary; pain is common

2. The workup for a patient presenting with EGWs should include a medical and sexual history and tests for common STDs, such as chlamydia, trichomoniasis, and bacterial vaginosis. Conditions that favor the development of EGWs include diabetes, pregnancy, and immunosuppressed states, including HIV/AIDS, lymphoproliferative disorders, and cancer chemotherapy.

E. **Treatment of external genital warts**
1. Imiquimod is the first-line patient-applied therapy because of its better clearance and lower recurrence rates compared with podofilox gel. Cryotherapy was selected as one of the first-line provider-administered therapies because of its effectiveness on both dry and moist warts found in the genital area. TCA was included as the alternate first-line provider-administered therapy in view of its effectiveness in treating warts on moist skin.
2. **Cryosurgery with liquid nitrogen or cryoprobe** is more effective than topical therapies. Lesions should be frozen until a 2 mm margin of freeze appears, then allowed to thaw, then refrozen. Repeat freeze several times.

II. **Molluscum Contagiosum**
A. This disease is produced by a virus of the pox virus family and is spread by sexual or close personal contact. Lesions are usually asymptomatic and multiple, with a central umbilication. Lesions can be spread by autoinoculation and last from 6 months to many years.
B. **Diagnosis.** The characteristic appearance is adequate for diagnosis, but biopsy may be used to confirm the diagnosis.
C. **Treatment.** Lesions are removed by sharp dermal curette, liquid nitrogen cryosurgery, or electrodesiccation.

III. **Pediculosis Pubis (Crabs)**
A. Phthirus pubis is a blood sucking louse that is unable to survive more than 24 hours off the body. It is often transmitted sexually and is principally found on the pubic hairs. Diagnosis is confirmed by locating nits or adult lice on the hair shafts.
B. **Treatment**
1. **Permethrin cream (Elimite),** 5% is the most effective treatment; it is applied for 10 minutes and washed off.
2. **Kwell shampoo,** lathered for at least 4 minutes, can also be used, but it is contraindicated in pregnancy or lactation.
3. All contaminated clothing and linen should be laundered.

IV. **Pubic Scabies**
A. This highly contagious infestation is caused by the Sarcoptes scabiei (0.2-0.4 mm in length). The infestation is transmitted by intimate contact or by contact with infested clothing. The female mite burrows into the skin, and after 1 month, severe pruritus develops. A multiform eruption may develop, characterized by papules, vesicles, pustules, urticarial wheals, and secondary infections on the hands, wrists, elbows, belt line, buttocks,

genitalia, and outer feet.
B. **Diagnosis** is confirmed by visualization of burrows and observation of parasites, eggs, larvae, or red fecal compactions under microscope.
C. **Treatment.** Permethrin 5% cream (Elimite) is massaged in from the neck down and remove by washing after 8 hours.
References: See page 290.

Sexually Transmissible Infections

Approximately 12 million patients are diagnosed with a sexually transmissible infection (STI) annually in the United States. Sequella of STIs include infertility, chronic pelvic pain, ectopic pregnancy, and other adverse pregnancy outcomes.

Diagnosis and Treatment of Bacterial Sexually Transmissible Infections			
Organism	Diagnostic Methods	Recommended Treatment	Alternative
Chlamydia trachomatis	Direct fluorescent antibody, enzyme immunoassay, DNA probe, cell culture, DNA amplification	Doxycycline 100 mg PO 2 times a day for 7 days or Azithromycin (Zithromax) 1 g PO	Ofloxacin (Floxin) 300 mg PO 2 times a day for 7 days or erythromycin base 500 mg PO 4 times a day for 7 days or erythromycin ethylsuccinate 800 mg PO 4 times a day for 7 days.
Neisseria gonorrhoeae	Culture DNA probe	Ceftriaxone (Rocephin) 125 mg IM or Cefixime 400 mg PO or Ciprofloxacin (Cipro) 500 mg PO or Ofloxacin (Floxin) 400 mg PO plus Doxycycline 100 mg 2 times a day for 7 days or azithromycin 1 g PO	Single IM dose of ceftizoxime 500 mg, cefotaxime 500 mg, cefotetan 1 g, and cefoxitin (Mefoxin) 2 g with probenecid 1 g PO; or enoxacin 400 mg PO, lomefloxacin 400 mg PO, or norfloxacin 800 mg PO
Treponema pallidum	Clinical appearance Dark-field microscopy Nontreponemal test: rapid plasma reagin, VDRL Treponemal test: MHA-TP, FTA-ABS	Primary and secondary syphilis and early latent syphilis (<1 year duration): benzathine penicillin G 2.4 million units IM in a single dose.	Penicillin allergy in patients with primary, secondary, or early latent syphilis (<1 year of duration): doxycycline 100 mg PO 2 times a day for 2 weeks.

Diagnosis and Treatment of Viral Sexually Transmissible Infections

Organism	Diagnostic Methods	Recommended Treatment Regimens
Herpes simplex virus	Clinical appearance Cell culture confirmation	First episode: Acyclovir (Zovirax) 400 mg PO 5 times a day for 7-10 days, or famciclovir (Famvir) 250 mg PO 3 times a day for 7-10 days, or valacyclovir (Valtrex) 1 g PO 2 times a day for 7-10 days. Recurrent episodes: acyclovir 400 mg PO 3 times a day for 5 days, or 800 mg PO 2 times a day for 5 days or famciclovir 125 mg PO 2 times a day for 5 days, or valacyclovir 500 mg PO 2 times a day for 5 days Daily suppressive therapy: acyclovir 400 mg PO 2 times a day, or famciclovir 250 mg PO 2 times a day, or valacyclovir 250 mg PO 2 times a day, 500 mg PO 1 time a day, or 1000 mg PO 1 time a day
Human papilloma virus	Clinical appearance of condyloma papules Cytology	External warts: Patient may apply podofilox 0.5% solution or gel 2 times a day for 3 days, followed by 4 days of no therapy, for a total of up to 4 cycles, or imiquimod 5% cream at bedtime 3 times a week for up to 16 weeks. Cryotherapy with liquid nitrogen or cryoprobe, repeat every1-2 weeks; or podophyllin, repeat weekly; or TCA 80-90%, repeat weekly; or surgical removal. Vaginal warts: cryotherapy with liquid nitrogen, or TCA 80-90%, or podophyllin 10-25%
Human immunodeficiency virus	Enzyme immunoassay Western blot (for confirmation) Polymerase chain reaction	Antiretroviral agents

Treatment of Pelvic Inflammatory Disease

Regimen	Inpatient	Outpatient
A	Cefotetan (Cefotan) 2 g IV q12h; or cefoxitin (Mefoxin) 2 g IV q6h plus doxycycline 100 mg IV or PO q12h.	Ofloxacin (Floxin) 400 mg PO bid for 14 days plus metronidazole 500 mg PO bid for 14 days.
B	Clindamycin 900 mg IV q8h plus gentamicin loading dose IV or IM (2 mg/kg of body weight), followed by a maintenance dose (1.5 mg/kg) q8h.	Ceftriaxone (Rocephin) 250 mg IM once; or cefoxitin 2 g IM plus probenecid 1 g PO; or other parenteral third-generation cephalosporin (eg, ceftizoxime, cefotaxime) plus doxycycline 100 mg PO bid for 14 days.

I. **Chlamydia trachomatis**
   A. Chlamydia trachomatis is the most prevalent STI in the United States. Chlamydial infections are most common in women age 15-19 years.
   B. Routine screening of asymptomatic, sexually active adolescent females undergoing pelvic examination is recommended. Annual screening should be done for women age 20-24 years who are either inconsistent users of barrier contraceptives or who acquired a new sex partner or had more than one sexual partner in the past 3 months.

II. Gonorrhea. Gonorrhea has an incidence of 800,000 cases annually. Routine screening for gonorrhea is recommended among women at high risk of infection, including prostitutes, women with a history of repeated episodes of gonorrhea, women under age 25 years with two or more sex partners in the past year, and women with mucopurulent cervicitis.

III. Syphilis
  A. Syphilis has an incidence of 100,000 cases annually. The rates are highest in the South, among African Americans, and among those in the 20- to 24-year-old age group.
  B. Prostitutes, persons with other STIs, and sexual contacts of persons with active syphilis should be screened.

IV. Herpes simplex virus and human papillomavirus
  A. An estimated 200,000-500,000 new cases of herpes simplex occur annually in the United States. New infections are most common in adolescents and young adults.
  B. Human papillomavirus affects about 30% of young, sexually active individuals.

References: See page 290.

Pelvic Inflammatory Disease

Pelvic inflammatory disease (PID) represents a spectrum of infections and inflammatory disorders of the uterus, fallopian tubes, and adjacent pelvic structures. PID may include any combination of endometritis, salpingitis, tubo-ovarian abscess, oophoritis, and in its more extreme manifestation, pelvic peritonitis. One out of every 10 women will have at least one episode of PID during her reproductive years. At least one-quarter of women with PID will have major complications, including infertility, ectopic pregnancy, chronic pelvic pain, tubo-ovarian abscesses, and/or pelvic adhesions.

I. Etiology and clinical pathogenesis
  A. PID results when pathogenic microorganisms spread from the cervix and vagina to the upper portions of the genital tract to such structures as the salpinx, ovaries, and adjacent structures. Chlamydia has been shown to be responsible for 25-50% of all cases of PID. About 10-20% of female patients who are infected with gonorrhea will progress to PID.
  B. Mixed infections are responsible for up to 70% of cases with PID. These polymicrobial infections typically include both anaerobic and aerobic microorganisms. Anaerobes such as Bacteroides, Peptostreptococcus, and Peptococcus have been reported, as have facultative bacteria, including Gardnerella vaginalis, Streptococcus, E. coli, and Haemophilus influenzae.
  C. PID occurs almost exclusively in sexually active women and is most common in adolescents. Risk factors include sexual activity, particularly with multiple sexual partners, young age, and use of an intrauterine device. Oral contraceptive users have a lower risk for developing PID.

II. Diagnosis and evaluation
  A. Presumptive diagnosis of PID is made in women who are sexually active who present with lower abdominal pain and cervical, uterine, or adnexal tenderness on pelvic examination. The CDC has recommended minimum criteria required for empiric treatment of PID. These major determinants include lower abdominal tenderness, adnexal tenderness, and cervical motion tenderness. Minor determinants (ie, signs that may increase the suspicion of PID) include:
    1. Fever (oral temperature >101°F; >38.3°C)
    2. Vaginal discharge
    3. Documented STD
    4. Erythrocyte sedimentation rate (ESR)
    5. C-reactive protein

6. Systemic signs
7. Dyspareunia

Laboratory Evaluation for Pelvic Inflammatory Disease

- Complete blood count with differential
- Pregnancy test
- Tests for Chlamydia and gonorrhea
- RPR or VDRL tests for syphilis

Differential Diagnosis of Pelvic Inflammatory Disease

Appendicitis	Irritable bowel syndrome
Ectopic pregnancy	Somatization
Hemorrhagic ovarian cyst	Gastroenteritis
Ovarian torsion	Cholecystitis
Endometriosis	Nephrolithiasis
Urinary tract Infection	

III. Management

A. A high index of suspicion and a low threshold for initiating treatment are important for facilitating detection and appropriate management of PID for all women of child-bearing age with pelvic pain. Laparoscopy is seldom practical. Antibiotic therapy is usually initiated on clinical grounds. Lower abdominal tenderness, adnexal tenderness, and pain on manipulation of the cervix mandates treatment.

Antibiotic Treatment of Hospitalized Patients with Pelvic Inflammatory Disease

Inpatient Parenteral Regimen One
Azithromycin (Zithromax) IV (500 mg qd for 1 or 2 days) followed by oral azithromycin 250 mg po once daily to complete a total of 7 days
Plus (as clinically indicated for suspicion for anaerobic infection)
Metronidazole (Flagyl) 500 mg IV every 8 hours

Inpatient Parenteral Regimen Option Two
Cefotetan (Cefotan) 2 g IV every 12 hours
  Plus
Doxycycline 100 mg IV or po every 12 hours
  or
Cefoxitin (Mefoxin) 2 g IV every 6 hours
  Plus
Doxycycline 100 mg IV or PO every 12 hours
Parenteral therapy can be discontinued 24 hours after the patient improves. Oral therapy should be started with doxycycline 100 mg bid and continued for 14 days total therapy. If a tubo-ovarian abscess is present, clindamycin or metronidazole should be used.

Inpatient Parenteral Regimen Option Three
Clindamycin 900 mg IV every 8 hours
  Plus
Gentamicin 2mg/kg loading dose IV or IM (with 1.5 mg/kg maintenance dose every 8 hours)
Parenteral therapy can be discontinued 24 hours after the patient improves. Oral therapy should then be continued for a total of 14 days of therapy. Oral therapy should consist of doxycycline 100 mg bid and clindamycin 450 mg qid.

Alterative Parenteral Regimen Options
Ofloxacin (Floxin) 400 mg IV every 12 hours
   Plus
Metronidazole (Flagyl) 500 mg IV every 8 hours
   or
Ampicillin/sulbactam (Unasyn) 3 g IV every 6 hours
   Plus
Doxycycline 100 mg PO or IV every 12 hours
   or
Ciprofloxacin (Cipro) 200 mg IV every 12 hours
   Plus
Doxycycline 100 mg PO or IV every 12 hours
   Plus
Metronidazole (Flagyl) 500 mg IV every 8 hours

Outpatient Treatment of Pelvic Inflammatory Disease

Azithromycin (Zithromax) 500 mg as a single dose intravenously (2 mg/mL over 1 hour) followed by oral azithromycin 250 mg once daily orally to complete a total of seven days of therapy.
Plus/Minus
Metronidazole (Flagyl) 500 mg orally twice daily for 14 days.

Ceftriaxone (Rocephin) 250 mg IM once
   Plus
Doxycycline 100 mg orally twice daily for 14 days
   Plus/Minus
Metronidazole (Flagyl) 500 mg orally twice daily for 14 days

Cefoxitin (Mefoxin) 2 g IM plus probenecid 1 gram orally concurrently
   Plus
Doxycycline 100 mg orally twice daily for 14 days
   Plus/Minus
Metronidazole (Flagyl) 500 mg orally twice daily for 14 days

Ofloxacin (Floxin) 400 mg orally twice daily for 14 days
   Plus
Metronidazole (Flagyl) 500 mg orally twice daily for 14 days

B. Male sexual partners of patients with PID should be evaluated for sexually transmitted infections, and they must be treated for chlamydial and gonococcal disease.

References: See page 290.

Vaginitis

Vaginitis is the most common gynecologic problem encountered by primary care physicians. It may result from bacterial infections, fungal infection, protozoan infection, contact dermatitis, atrophic vaginitis, or allergic reaction.

I. **Pathophysiology**
   A. Vaginitis results from alterations in the vaginal ecosystem, either by the introduction of an organism or by a disturbance that allows normally present pathogens to proliferate.
   B. Antibiotics may cause the overgrowth of yeast. Douching may alter the pH level or selectively suppress the growth of endogenous bacteria.

II. **Clinical evaluation of vaginal symptoms**
   A. The type and extent of symptoms, such as itching, discharge, odor, or pelvic pain should be determined. A change in sexual partners or sexual activity, changes in contraception method, medications (antibiotics), and history of prior genital infections should be sought.
   B. **Physical examination**
      1. Evaluation of the vagina should include close inspection of the external genitalia for excoriations, ulcerations, blisters, papillary structures, erythema, edema, mucosal thinning, or mucosal pallor.
      2. The color, texture, and odor of vaginal or cervical discharge should be noted.
   C. **Vaginal fluid pH** can be determined by immersing pH paper in the vaginal discharge. A pH level greater than 4.5 often indicates the presence of bacterial vaginosis or Trichomonas vaginalis.
   D. **Saline wet mount**
      1. One swab should be used to obtain a sample from the posterior vaginal fornix, obtaining a "clump" of discharge. Place the sample on a slide, add one drop of normal saline, and apply a coverslip.
      2. Coccoid bacteria and clue cells (bacteria-coated, stippled, epithelial cells) are characteristic of bacterial vaginosis.
      3. Trichomoniasis is confirmed by identification of trichomonads--mobile, oval flagellates. White blood cells are prevalent.
   E. **Potassium hydroxide (KOH) preparation**
      1. Place a second sample on a slide, apply one drop of 10% potassium hydroxide (KOH) and a coverslip. A pungent, fishy odor upon addition of KOH--a positive whiff test--strongly indicates bacterial vaginosis.
      2. The KOH prep may reveal Candida in the form of thread-like hyphae and budding yeast.
   F. **Screening for STDs.** Testing for gonorrhea and chlamydial infection should be completed for women with a new sexual partner, purulent cervical discharge, or cervical motion tenderness.

III. **Differential diagnosis**
   A. The most common cause of vaginitis is bacterial vaginosis, followed by Candida albicans. The prevalence of trichomoniasis has declined in recent years.
   B. Common nonvaginal etiologies include contact dermatitis from spermicidal creams, latex in condoms, or douching. Any STD can produce vaginal discharge.

Clinical Manifestations of Vaginitis	
Candidal Vaginitis	Nonmalodorous, thick, white, "cottage cheese-like" discharge that adheres to vaginal walls Presence of hyphal forms or budding yeast cells on wet-mount Pruritus Normal pH (<4.5)
Bacterial Vaginosis	Thin, dark or dull grey, homogeneous, malodorous discharge that adheres to the vaginal walls Elevated pH level (>4.5) Positive KOH (whiff test) Clue cells on wet-mount microscopic evaluation
Trichomonas Vaginalis	Copious, yellow-gray or green, homogeneous or frothy, malodorous discharge Elevated pH level (>4.5) Mobile, flagellated organisms and leukocytes on wet-mount microscopic evaluation Vulvovaginal irritation, dysuria
Atrophic Vaginitis	Vaginal dryness or burning

IV. Bacterial Vaginosis

A. Bacterial vaginosis develops when a shift in the normal vaginal ecosystem causes replacement of the usually predominant lactobacilli with mixed bacterial flora. Bacterial vaginosis is the most common type of vaginitis. It is found in 10-25% of patients in gynecologic clinics.

B. There is usually little itching, no pain, and the symptoms tend to have an indolent course. A malodorous fishy vaginal discharge is characteristic.

C. There is usually little or no inflammation of the vulva or vaginal epithelium. The vaginal discharge is thin, dark or dull grey, and homogeneous.

D. A wet-mount will reveal clue cells (epithelial cells stippled with bacteria), an abundance of bacteria, and the absence of homogeneous bacilli (lactobacilli).

E. **Diagnostic criteria** (3 of 4 criterial present)
1. pH >4.0
2. Clue cells
3. Positive KOH whiff test
4. Homogeneous discharge.

F. **Treatment regimens**
1. **Topical (intravaginal) regimens**
   a. Metronidazole gel (MetroGel) 0.75%, one applicatorful (5 g) bid 5 days.
   b. Clindamycin cream (Cleocin) 2%, one applicatorful (5 g) qhs for 7 nights. Topical therapies have a 90% cure rate.
2. **Oral metronidazole (Flagyl)**
   a. Oral metronidazole is equally effective as topical therapy, with a 90% cure rate.
   b. Dosage is 500 mg bid or 250 mg tid for 7 days. A single 2-g dose is slightly less effective (69-72%) and causes more gastrointestinal upset. Alcohol products should be avoided because nausea and vomiting (disulfiram reaction) may occur.
3. Routine treatment of sexual partners is not necessary, but it is sometimes helpful for patients with frequent recurrences.
4. **Persistent cases** should be reevaluated and treated with clindamycin, 300 mg PO bid for 7 days along with treatment of sexual partners.
5. **Pregnancy.** Clindamycin is recommended, either intravaginally as a daily application of 2% cream or PO, 300 mg bid for 7 days. After the first trimester, oral or topical therapy with metronidazole is acceptable.

V. Candida Vulvovaginitis

A. Candida is the second most common diagnosis associated with vaginal symptoms. It is found in 25% of asymptomatic women. Fungal infections account for 33% of all vaginal infections.

B. Patients with diabetes mellitus or immunosuppressive conditions such as infection with the HIV are at increased risk for candidal vaginitis. Candidal vaginitis occurs in 25-70% of women after antibiotic therapy.

C. The most common symptom is pruritus. Vulvar burning and an increase or change in consistency of the vaginal discharge may be noted.

D. **Physical examination**
   1. Candidal vaginitis causes a nonmalodorous, thick, adherent, white vaginal discharge that appears "cottage cheese-like."
   2. The vagina is usually hyperemic and edematous. Vulvar erythema may be present.

E. The normal pH level is not usually altered with candidal vaginitis. Microscopic examination of vaginal discharge diluted with saline (wet-mount) and 10% KOH preparations will reveal hyphal forms or budding yeast cells. Some yeast infections are not detected by microscopy because there are relatively few numbers of organisms. Confirmation of candidal vaginitis by culture is not recommended. Candida on Pap smear is not a sensitive finding because the yeast is a constituent of the normal vaginal flora.

F. **Treatment of candida vulvovaginitis**
   1. For severe symptoms and chronic infections, a 7-day course of treatment is used, instead of a 1- or 3-day course. If vulvar involvement is present, a cream should be used instead of a suppository.
   2. Most C. albicans isolates are susceptible to either clotrimazole or miconazole. An increasing number of nonalbicans Candida species are resistant to the OTC antifungal agents and require the use of prescription antifungal agents. Greater activity has been achieved using terconazole, butoconazole, tioconazole, ketoconazole, and fluconazole.

Antifungal Medications

Medication	How Supplied	Dosage
Prescription Agents Oral Agents		
Fluconazole (Diflucan)	150-mg tablet	1 tablet PO 1 time
Ketoconazole (Nizoral)	200 mg	1 tablet PO bid for 5 days
Prescription Topical Agents		
Butoconazole (Femstat)	2% vaginal cream [28 g]	1 vaginally applicatorful qhs for 3 nights
Clotrimazole (Gyne-Lotrimin)	500-mg tablet	1 tablet vaginally qhs 1 time
Miconazole (Monistat 3)	200-mg vaginal suppositories	1 suppository vaginally qhs for 3 nights
Tioconazole (Vagistat)	6.5% cream [5 g]	1 applicatorful vaginally qhs 1 time

Medication	How Supplied	Dosage
Terconazole (Terazol 3)	Cream: 0.4% [45 gm]	One applicatorful intravaginally qhs x 7 days
	Cream: 0.8% [20 gm]	One applicatorful intravaginally qhs x 3 days
	Vag suppository: 80 mg [3]	One suppository intravaginally qhs x 3 days
Over-the-Counter Agents		
Clotrimazole (Gyne-Lotrimin)	1% vaginal cream [45 g] 100-mg vaginal tablets	1 applicatorful vaginally qhs for 7-14 nights 1 tablet vaginally qhs for 7-14 days
Miconazole (Monistat 7)	2% cream [45 g] 100-mg vaginal suppository	1 applicatorful vaginally qhs for 7 days 1 suppository vaginally qhs for 7 days

3. Ketoconazole, 200-mg oral tablets twice daily for 5 days, is effective in treating resistant and recurrent candidal infections. Effectiveness is results from the elimination of the rectal reservoir of yeast.
4. Resistant infections also may respond to vaginal boric acid, 600 mg in size 0 gelatin capsules daily for 14 days.
5. Treatment of male partners is usually not necessary but may be considered if the partner has yeast balanitis or is uncircumcised.
6. **During pregnancy**, butoconazole (Femstat) should be used in the 2nd or 3rd trimester. Miconazole or clotrimazole may also be used.

G. **Resistant or recurrent cases**
1. Recurrent infections should be reevaluated. Repeating topical therapy for a 14- to 21-day course may be effective. Oral regimens have the potential for eradicating rectal reservoirs.
2. Cultures are helpful in determining whether a non-candidal species is present. Patients with recalcitrant disease should be evaluated for diabetes and HIV.

VI. Trichomonas Vaginalis
A. Trichomonas, a flagellated anaerobic protozoan, is a sexually transmitted disease with a high transmission rate. Non-sexual transmission is possible because the organism can survive for a few hours in a moist environment.
B. A copious, yellow-gray or green homogeneous discharge is present. A foul odor, vulvovaginal irritation, and dysuria is common. The pH level is usually greater than 4.5.
C. The diagnosis of trichomonal infection is made by examining a wet-mount preparation for mobile, flagellated organisms and an abundance of leukocytes. Occasionally the diagnosis is reported on a Pap test, and treatment is recommended.
D. **Treatment of Trichomonas vaginalis**
1. Metronidazole (Flagyl), 2 g PO in a single dose for both the patient and sexual partner, or 500 mg PO bid for 7 days.
2. Topical therapy with topical metronidazole is not recommended because the organism may persist in the urethra and Skene's glands. Screening for coexisting sexually transmitted diseases should be completed.
3. **Recurrent or recalcitrant infections**
   a. If patients are compliant but develop recurrent infections, treatment of their sexual partners should be confirmed.
   b. Cultures should be performed. In patients with persistent infection, a resistant trichomonad strain may require high dosages of metronidazole of 2.5 g/d, often combined with intravaginal metronidazole for 10 days.

VII. Other diagnoses causing vaginal symptoms
  A. One-third of patients with vaginal symptoms will not have laboratory evidence of bacterial vaginosis, Candida, or Trichomonas. Other causes of the vaginal symptoms include cervicitis, allergic reactions, and vulvodynia.
  B. Atrophic vaginitis should be considered in postmenopausal patients if the mucosa appears pale and thin and wet-mount findings are negative.
    1. Oral estrogen (Premarin) 0.625 mg qd should provide relief.
    2. Estradiol vaginal cream 0.01% may be effective as 2-4 g daily for 1-2 weeks, then 1 g, one to three times weekly.
    3. Conjugated estrogen vaginal cream (Premarin) may be effective as 2-4 g daily (3 weeks on, 1 week off) for 3-6 months.
  C. Allergy and chemical irritation
    1. Patients should be questioned about use of substances that cause allergic or chemical irritation, such as deodorant soaps, laundry detergent, vaginal contraceptives, bath oils, perfumed or dyed toilet paper, hot tub or swimming pool chemicals, and synthetic clothing.
    2. Topical steroids and systemic antihistamines can help alleviate the symptoms.
References: See page 290.

Obstetrics

Prenatal Care

I. **Prenatal history and physical examination**
   A. **Diagnosis of pregnancy**
      1. **Amenorrhea** is usually the first sign of conception. Other symptoms include breast fullness and tenderness, skin changes, nausea, vomiting, urinary frequency, and fatigue.
      2. **Pregnancy tests.** Urine pregnancy tests may be positive within days of the first missed menstrual period. Serum beta human chorionic gonadotropin (HCG) is accurate up to a few days after implantation.
      3. **Fetal heart tones** can be detected as early as 11-12 weeks from the last menstrual period (LMP) by Doppler. The normal fetal heart rate is 120-160 beats per minute.
      4. **Fetal movements** ("quickening") are first felt by the patient at 17-19 weeks.
      5. **Ultrasound** will visualize a gestational sac at 5-6 weeks and a fetal pole with movement and cardiac activity by 7-8 weeks. Ultrasound can estimate fetal age accurately if completed before 24 weeks.
      6. **Estimated date of confinement.** The mean duration of pregnancy is 40 weeks from the LMP. Estimated date of confinement (EDC) can be calculated by Nägele's rule: Add 7 days to the first day of the LMP, then subtract 3 months.
   B. **Contraceptive history.** Recent oral contraceptive usage often causes postpill amenorrhea, and may cause erroneous pregnancy dating.
   C. **Gynecologic and obstetric history**
      1. Gravidity is the total number of pregnancies. Parity is expressed as the number of term pregnancies, preterm pregnancies, abortions, and live births.
      2. The character and length of previous labors, type of delivery, complications, infant status, and birth weight are recorded.
      3. Assess prior cesarean sections and determine type of C-section (low transverse or classical), and determine reason it was performed.
   D. **Medical and surgical history** and prior hospitalizations are documented.
   E. **Medications** and allergies are recorded.
   F. **Family history** of medical illnesses, hereditary illness, or multiple gestation is sought.
   G. **Social history.** Cigarettes, alcohol, or illicit drug use.
   H. **Review of systems.** Abdominal pain, constipation, headaches, vaginal bleeding, dysuria or urinary frequency, or hemorrhoids.
   I. **Physical examination**
      1. Weight, funduscopic examination, thyroid, breast, lungs, and heart are examined.
      2. An extremity and neurologic exam are completed, and the presence of a cesarean section scar is sought.
      3. **Pelvic examination**
         a. Pap smear and culture for gonorrhea are completed routinely. Chlamydia culture is completed in high-risk patients.
         b. **Estimation of gestational age by uterine size**
            (1) The nongravid uterus is 3 x 4 x 7 cm. The uterus begins to change in size at 5-6 weeks.
            (2) Gestational age is estimated by uterine size: 8 weeks = 2 x normal size; 10 weeks = 3 x normal; 12 weeks = 4 x normal.
            (3) At 12 weeks the fundus becomes palpable at the symphysis pubis.
            (4) At 16 weeks, the uterus is midway between the symphysis pubis and the umbilicus.
            (5) At 20 weeks, the uterus is at the umbilicus. After 20 weeks, there

is a correlation between the number of weeks of gestation and the number of centimeters from the pubic symphysis to the top of the fundus.

    (6) Uterine size that exceeds the gestational dating by 3 or more weeks suggests multiple gestation, molar pregnancy, or (most commonly) an inaccurate date for LMP. Ultrasonography will confirm inaccurate dating or intrauterine growth failure.

  c. Adnexa are palpated for masses.

II. Initial visit laboratory testing

A. CBC, AB blood typing and Rh factor, antibody screen, rubella, VDRL/RPR, hepatitis B surface Ag.

B. Pap smear, urine pregnancy test, urinalysis and urine culture. Cervical culture for gonorrhea and chlamydia.

C. Tuberculosis skin testing, HIV counseling/testing.

D. Hemoglobin electrophoresis is indicated in risks groups, such as sickle hemoglobin in African patients, B-thalassemia in Mediterranean patients, and alpha-thalassemia in Asian patients. Tay-Sachs carrier testing is indicated in Jewish patients.

III. Clinical assessment at first trimester prenatal visits

A. Assessment at each prenatal visit includes maternal weight, blood pressure, uterine size, and evaluation for edema, proteinuria, and glucosuria.

B. First Doppler heart tones should become detectable at 10-12 weeks, and they should be sought thereafter.

C. Routine prenatal vitamins are probably not necessary. Folic acid supplementation preconceptually and throughout the early part of pregnancy has been shown to decrease the incidence of fetal neural tube defects.

Frequency of Prenatal Care Visits in Low-Risk Pregnancies	
<28 weeks	Every month
28-36 weeks	Every 2 weeks
36-delivery	Every 1 week until delivery

D. **First Trimester Education.** Discuss smoking, alcohol, exercise, diet, and sexuality.

E. **Headache and backache.** Acetaminophen (Tylenol) 325-650 mg every 3-4 hours is effective. Aspirin is contraindicated.

F. **Nausea and vomiting.** First-trimester morning sickness may be relieved by eating frequent, small meals, getting out of bed slowly after eating a few crackers, and by avoiding spicy or greasy foods. Promethazine (Phenergan) 12.5-50 mg PO q4-6h prn or diphenhydramine (Benadryl) 25-50 mg tid-qid is useful.

G. **Constipation.** A high-fiber diet with psyllium (Metamucil), increased fluid intake, and regular exercise should be advised. Docusate (Colace) 100 mg bid may provide relief.

IV. Clinical assessment at second trimester visits

A. Questions for each follow-up visit

    1. **First detection of fetal movement (quickening)** should occur at around 17 weeks in a multigravida and at 19 weeks in a primigravida. **Fetal movement** should be documented at each visit after 17 weeks.

    2. **Vaginal bleeding or symptoms of preterm labor** should be sought.

B. **Fetal heart rate** is documented at each visit

C. Maternal serum testing at 15-18 weeks

    1. **Triple screen (multiple marker screening).** In women under age 35 years, screening for fetal Down syndrome is accomplished with a triple screen. Maternal serum alpha-fetoprotein is elevated in 20-25% of all cases of Down syndrome, and it is elevated in fetal neural tube deficits. Levels of hCG are higher in Down syndrome and levels of unconjugated

estriol are lower in Down syndrome.
2. If levels are abnormal, an ultrasound examination is performed and genetic amniocentesis is offered. The triple screen identifies 60% of Down syndrome cases. Low levels of all three serum analytes identifies 60-75% of all cases of fetal trisomy 18.
   D. **At 15-18 weeks, genetic amniocentesis** should be offered to patients ≥35 years old, and it should be offered if a birth defect has occurred in the mother, father, or in previous offspring.
   E. **Screening ultrasound** should usually be obtained at 16-18 weeks.
   F. **At 24-28 weeks**, a one-hour Glucola (blood glucose measurement 1 hour after 50-gm oral glucose) is obtained to screen for gestational diabetes. Those with a particular risk (eg, previous gestational diabetes or fetal macrosomia), require earlier testing. If the 1 hour test result is greater than 140 mg/dL, a 3-hour glucose tolerance test is necessary.
   G. **Second trimester education.** Discomforts include backache, round ligament pain, constipation, and indigestion.
V. **Clinical assessment at third trimester visits**
   A. **Fetal movement** is documented. Vaginal bleeding or symptoms of preterm labor should be sought. Pregnancy induced hypertension symptoms (blurred vision, headache, rapid weight gain, edema) are sought.
   B. **Fetal heart rate** is documented at each visit.
   C. **At 26-30 weeks**, repeat hemoglobin and hematocrit are obtained to determine the need for iron supplementation.
   D. **At 28-30 weeks**, an antibody screen is obtained in Rh-negative women, and D immune globulin (RhoGAM) is administered if negative.
   E. **At 36 weeks**, repeat serologic testing for syphilis is recommended for high risk groups.
   F. **Gonorrhea and chlamydia screening is repeated** in the third-trimester in high-risk patients.
   G. **Screening for group B streptococcus colonization at 35-37 weeks**
      1. Lower vaginal and rectal cultures are recommended; cultures should not be collected by speculum examination. The optimal method for GBS screening is collection of a single standard culture swab of the distal vagina and anorectum.
   H. **Third trimester education**
      1. **Signs of labor.** The patient should call physician when rupture of membranes or contractions have occurred every 5 minutes for one hour.
      2. **Danger signs.** Preterm labor, rupture of membranes, bleeding, edema, signs of preeclampsia.
      3. **Common discomforts.** Cramps, edema, frequent urination.
   I. **At 36 weeks**, a cervical exam may be completed. Fetal position should be assessed by palpation (Leopold's Maneuvers).
References: See page 290.

Normal Labor

Labor consists of the process by which uterine contractions expel the fetus. A term pregnancy is 37 to 42 weeks from the last menstrual period (LMP).

I. **Obstetrical History and Physical Examination**
   A. **History of the present labor**
      1. **Contractions.** The frequency, duration, onset, and intensity of uterine contractions should be determined. Contractions may be accompanied by a "bloody show" (passage of blood-tinged mucus from the dilating cervical os). Braxton Hicks contractions are often felt by patients during the last weeks of pregnancy. They are usually irregular, mild, and do not cause cervical change.
      2. **Rupture of membranes.** Leakage of fluid may occur alone or in conjunction with uterine contractions. The patient may report a large gush of fluid or increased moisture. The color of the liquid should be

determine, including the presence of blood or meconium.

3. **Vaginal bleeding** should be assessed. Spotting or blood-tinged mucus is common in normal labor. Heavy vaginal bleeding may be a sign of placental abruption.

4. **Fetal movement.** A progressive decrease in fetal movement from baseline, should prompt an assessment of fetal well-being with a nonstress test or biophysical profile.

B. **History of present pregnancy**

1. **Estimated date of confinement** (EDC) is calculated as 40 weeks from the first day of the LMP.

2. **Fetal heart tones** are first heard with a Doppler instrument 10-12 weeks from the LMP.

3. **Quickening** (maternal perception of fetal movement) occurs at about 17 weeks.

4. **Uterine size** before 16 weeks is an accurate measure of dates.

5. **Ultrasound** measurement of fetal size before 24 weeks of gestation is an accurate measure of dates.

6. **Prenatal history**. Medical problems during this pregnancy should be reviewed, including urinary tract infections, diabetes, or hypertension.

7. **Review of systems.** Severe headaches, scotomas, hand and facial edema, or epigastric pain (preeclampsia) should be sought. Dysuria, urinary frequency or flank pain may indicate cystitis or pyelonephritis.

C. **Obstetrical history.** Past pregnancies, durations and outcomes, preterm deliveries, operative deliveries, prolonged labors, pregnancy-induced hypertension should be assessed.

D. **Past medical history** of asthma, hypertension, or renal disease should be sought.

II. **Physical Examination**

A. Vital signs are assessed.

B. **Head.** Funduscopy should seek hemorrhages or exudates, which may suggest diabetes or hypertension. Facial, hand and ankle edema suggest preeclampsia.

C. **Chest.** Auscultation of the lungs for wheezes and crackles may indicate asthma or heart failure.

D. **Uterine Size.** Until the middle of the third trimester, the distance in centimeters from the pubic symphysis to the uterine fundus should correlate with the gestational age in weeks. Toward term, the measurement becomes progressively less reliable because of engagement of the presenting part.

E. **Estimation of fetal weight** is completed by palpation of the gravid uterus.

F. **Leopold's maneuvers** are used to determine the position of the fetus.

1. **The first maneuver** determines which fetal pole occupies the uterine fundus. The breech moves with the fetal body. The vertex is rounder and harder, feels more globular than the breech, and can be moved separately from the fetal body.

2. **Second maneuver.** The lateral aspects of the uterus are palpated to determine on which side the fetal back or fetal extremities (the small parts) are located.

3. **Third maneuver.** The presenting part is moved from side to side. If movement is difficult, engagement of the presenting part has occurred.

4. **Fourth maneuver.** With the fetus presenting by vertex, the cephalic prominence may be palpable on the side of the fetal small parts.

G. **Pelvic examination.** The adequacy of the bony pelvis, the integrity of the fetal membranes, the degree of cervical dilatation and effacement, and the station of the presenting part should be determined.

H. **Extremities.** Severe lower extremity or hand edema suggests preeclampsia. Deep-tendon hyperreflexia and clonus may signal impending seizures.

I. **Laboratory tests**

1. Prenatal labs should be documented, including CBC, blood type, Rh, antibody screen, serologic test for syphilis, rubella antibody titer, urinalysis, culture, Pap smear, cervical cultures for gonorrhea and

Chlamydia, and hepatitis B surface antigen (HbsAg).
2. During labor, the CBC, urinalysis and RPR are repeated. The HBSAG is repeated for high-risk patients. A clot of blood is placed on hold.
J. **Fetal heart rate.** The baseline heart rate, variability, accelerations, and decelerations are recorded.

Labor History and Physical

Chief compliant: Contractions, rupture of membranes.
HPI: ___ year old Gravida (number of pregnancies) Para (number of deliveries).
Gestational age, last menstrual period, estimated date of confinement.
Contractions (onset, frequency, intensity), rupture of membranes (time, color). Vaginal bleeding (consistency, quantity, bloody show); fetal movement.
Fetal Heart Rate Strip: Baseline rate, accelerations, reactivity, decelerations, contraction frequency.
Dates: First day of last menstrual period, estimated date of confinement. Ultrasound dating.
Prenatal Care: Date of first exam, number of visits; has size been equal to dates? infections, hypertension, diabetes.
Obstetrical History: Dates of prior pregnancies, gestational age, route (C-section with indications and type of uterine incision), weight, complications, length of labor, hypertension.
Gynecologic History: Menstrual history (menarche, interval, duration), herpes, gonorrhea, chlamydia, abortions; oral contraceptives.
Past Medical History: Illnesses, asthma, hypertension, diabetes, renal disease, surgeries.
Medications: Iron, prenatal vitamins.
Allergies: Penicillin, codeine?
Social History: Smoking, alcohol, drug use.
Family History: Hypertension, diabetes, bleeding disorders.
Review of Systems: Severe headaches, scotomas, blurred vision, hand and face edema, epigastric pain, pruritus, dysuria, fever.

Physical Exam
General Appearance:
Vitals: BP, pulse, respirations, temperature.
HEENT: Funduscopy, facial edema, jugular venous distention.
Chest: Wheezes, rhonchi.
Cardiovascular: Rhythm, S1, S2, murmurs.
Abdomen: Fundal height, Leopold's maneuvers (lie, presentation). Estimated fetal weight (EFW), tenderness, scars.
Cervix: Dilatation, effacement, station, position, status of membranes, presentation. Vulvar herpes lesions.
Extremities: Cyanosis, clubbing, edema.
Neurologic: Deep tender reflexes, clonus.
Prenatal Labs: Obtain results of one hour post glucola, RPR/VDRL, rubella, blood type, Rh, CBC, Pap, PPD, hepatitis BsAg, UA, C and S.
Current Labs: Hemoglobin, hematocrit, glucose, UA; urine dipstick for protein.
Assessment: Intrauterine pregnancy (IUP) at 40 weeks, admitted with the following problems:
Plan: Anticipated type of labor and delivery. List plan for each problem.

III. **Normal labor**
A. Labor is characterized by uterine contractions of sufficient frequency, intensity, and duration to result in effacement and dilatation of the cervix.

- B. **The first stage of labor** starts with the onset of regular contractions and ends with complete dilatation (10 cm). This stage is further subdivided into the latent and an active phases.
  1. The latent phase starts with the onset of regular uterine contractions and is characterized by slow cervical dilatation to 4 cm. The latent phase is variable in length.
  2. The active phase follows and is characterized by more rapid dilatation to 10 cm. During the active phase of labor, the average rate of cervical dilatation is 1.5 cm/hour in the multipara and 1.2 cm/hour in the nullipara.
- C. **The second stage of labor** begins with complete dilatation of the cervix and ends with delivery of the infant. It is characterized by voluntary and involuntary pushing. The average second stage of labor is one-half hour in a multipara and 1 hour in the primipara.
- D. **The third stage of labor** begins with the delivery of the infant and ends with the delivery of the placenta.
- E. **Intravenous fluids**. IV fluid during labor is usually Ringer's lactate or 0.45% normal saline with 5% dextrose. Intravenous fluid infused rapidly or given as a bolus should be dextrose-free because maternal hyperglycemia can occur.
- F. **Activity.** Patients in the latent phase of labor are usually allowed to walk.
- G. **Narcotic and analgesic drugs**
  1. Nalbuphine (Nubain) 5 to 10 mg SC or IV q2-3h.
  2. Butorphanol (Stadol) 2 mg IM q3-4h or 0.5-1.0 mg IV q1.5-2.0h **OR**
  3. Meperidine (Demerol) 50 to 100 mg IM q3-4h or 10 to 25 mg IV q1.5-3.0 h **OR**
  4. Narcotics should be avoided if their peak action will not have diminished by the time of delivery. Respiratory depression is reversed with naloxone (Narcan): Adults, 0.4 mg IV or IM and neonates, 0.01 mg/kg.
- H. **Epidural anesthesia**
  1. Contraindications include infection in the lumbar area, clotting defect, active neurologic disease, sensitivity to the anesthetic, hypovolemia, and septicemia.
  2. Risks include hypotension, respiratory arrest, toxic drug reaction, and rare neurologic complications. An epidural has no significant effect on the progress of labor.
  3. Before the epidural is initiated, the patient is hydrated with 500-1000 mL of dextrose-free intravenous fluid.

Labor and Delivery Admitting Orders

Admit: Labor and Delivery
Diagnoses: Intrauterine pregnancy at _____ weeks.
Condition: Satisfactory
Vitals: q1 hr per routine
Activity: May ambulate as tolerated.
Nursing: I and O. Catheterize prn; external or internal monitors.
Diet: NPO except ice chips.
IV Fluids: Lactated Ringers with 5% dextrose at 125 cc/h.
Medications:
Epidural at 4-5 cm.
Nalbuphine (Nubain) 5-10 mg IV/SC q2-3h prn **OR**
Butorphanol (Stadol) 0.5-1 mg IV q1.5-2h prn **OR**
Meperidine (Demerol) 25-75 mg slow IV q1.5-3h prn pain **AND**
Promethazine (Phenergan) 25-50 mg IV q3-4h prn nausea **OR**
Hydroxyzine (Vistaril) 25-50 mg IV q3-4h prn
Fleet enema PR prn constipation.
Labs: CBC, dipstick urine protein, blood type and Rh, antibody screen, VDRL, HBSAG, rubella, type and screen (C-section).

I. Intrapartum chemoprophylaxis for group B streptococcus infection
   1. Intrapartum chemoprophylaxis is offered to all pregnant women identified as GBS carriers by a culture obtained at 35-37 weeks.
   2. If the result of GBS culture is not known at the time of labor, intrapartum chemoprophylaxis should be administered if one of the following is present: Gestation <37 weeks, duration of membrane rupture ≥ 18 hours, or temperature ≥38°C (100.4°F).
   3. Women found to have GBS bacteriuria during pregnancy should be treated at the time of diagnosis, and they should receive intrapartum chemoprophylaxis. Intrapartum chemoprophylaxis should be given to women with a history of previously giving birth to an infant with GBS disease.
   4. Intrapartum chemoprophylaxis consists of penicillin G, 5 million units, then 2.5 million units IV every 4 hours until delivery. Ampicillin, 2 g initially and then 1 g IV every 4 hours until delivery, is an alternative. Clindamycin or erythromycin may be used for women allergic to penicillin.

IV. Normal spontaneous vaginal delivery
   A. Preparation. As the multiparous patient approaches complete dilatation or as the nulliparous patient begins to crown the fetal scalp, preparations are made for delivery.
   B. Maternal position. The mother is usually placed in the dorsal lithotomy position with left lateral tilt.
   C. Delivery of a fetus in an occiput anterior position
   1. **Delivery of the head**
      a. The fetal head is delivered by extension as the flexed head passes through the vaginal introitus.
      b. Once the fetal head has been delivered, external rotation to the occiput transverse position occurs.
      c. The oropharynx and nose of the fetus are suctioned with the bulb syringe. A finger is passed into the vagina along the fetal neck to check for a nuchal cord. If one is present, it is lifted over the vertex. If this cannot be accomplished, the cord is doubly clamped and divided.
      d. If shoulder dystocia is anticipated, the shoulders should be delivered immediately.
   2. **Episiotomy** consists of incision of the perineum, enlarging the vaginal orifice at the time of delivery. If indicated, an episiotomy should be performed when 3-4 cm of fetal scalp is visible.
      a. With adequate local or spinal anesthetic in place, a medial episiotomy is completed by incising the perineum toward the anus and into the vagina.
      b. Avoid cutting into the anal sphincter or the rectum. A short perineum may require a mediolateral episiotomy.
      c. Application of pressure at the perineal apex with a towel-covered hand helps to prevent extension of the episiotomy.
   3. **Delivery of the anterior shoulder** is accomplished by gentle downward traction on the fetal head. The posterior shoulder is delivered by upward traction.
   4. **Delivery of the body.** The infant is grasped around the back with the left hand, and the right hand is placed, near the vagina, under the baby's buttocks, supporting the infant's body. The infant's body is rotated toward the operator and supported by the operator's forearm, freeing the right hand to suction the mouth and nose. The baby's head should be kept lower than the body to facilitate drainage of secretions.
   5. **Suctioning** of the nose and oropharynx is repeated.
   6. **The umbilical cord** is doubly clamped and cut, leaving 2-3 cm of cord.
   D. Delivery of the placenta
   1. The placenta usually separates spontaneously from the uterine wall within 5 minutes of delivery. Gentle fundal massage and gentle traction on the cord facilitates delivery of the placenta.

2. The placenta should be examined for missing cotyledons or blind vessels. The cut end of the cord should be examined for 2 arteries and a vein. The absence of one umbilical artery suggests a congenital anomaly.
3. Prophylaxis against excessive postpartum blood loss consists of external fundal massage and oxytocin (Pitocin), 20 units in 1000 mL of IV fluid at 100 drops/minute after delivery of the placenta. Oxytocin can cause marked hypotension if administered as a IV bolus.
4. After delivery of the placenta, the birth canal is inspected for lacerations.

Delivery Note

1. Note the age, gravida, para, and gestational age.
2. Time of birth, type of birth (spontaneous vaginal delivery), position (left occiput anterior).
3. Bulb suctioned, sex, weight, APGAR scores, nuchal cord, and number of cord vessels.
4. Placenta expressed spontaneously intact. Describe episiotomy degree and repair technique.
5. Note lacerations of cervix, vagina, rectum, perineum.
6. Estimated blood loss:
7. Disposition: Mother to recovery room in stable condition. Infant to nursery in stable condition.

Routine Postpartum Orders

Transfer: To recovery room, then postpartum ward when stable.
Vitals: Check vitals, bleeding, fundus q15min x 1 hr or until stable, then q4h.
Activity: Ambulate in 2 hours if stable
Nursing Orders: If unable to void, straight catheterize; sitz baths prn with 1:1000 Betadine prn, ice pack to perineum prn, record urine output.
Diet: Regular
IV Fluids: D5LR at 125 cc/h. Discontinue when stable and taking PO diet.
Medications:
　Oxytocin (Pitocin) 20 units in 1 L D5LR at 100 drops/minute or 10 U IM.
　FeSO4 325 mg PO bid-tid.
Symptomatic Medications:
　Acetaminophen/codeine (Tylenol #3) 1-2 tab PO q3-4h prn **OR**
　Oxycodone/acetaminophen (Percocet) 1 tab q6h prn pain.
　Milk of magnesia 30 mL PO q6h prn constipation.
　Docusate Sodium (Colace) 100 mg PO bid.
　Dulcolax suppository PR prn constipation.
　A and D cream or Lanolin prn if breast feeding.
　Breast binder or tight brazier and ice packs prn if not to breast feed.
Labs: Hemoglobin/hematocrit in AM. Give rubella vaccine if titer <1:10.

Perineal Lacerations and Episiotomies

I. **First-degree laceration**
　A. A first degree perineal laceration extends only through the vaginal and perineal skin.
　B. **Repair:** Place a single layer of interrupted 3-O chromic or Vicryl sutures about 1 cm apart.
II. **Second-degree laceration and repair of midline episiotomy**
　A. A second degree laceration extends deeply into the soft tissues of the perineum, down to, but not including, the external anal sphincter capsule. The disruption involves the bulbocavernosus and transverse perineal muscles.
　B. **Repair**
　　1. Proximate the deep tissues of the perineal body by placing 3-4 interrupted 2-O or 3-O chromic or Vicryl absorbable sutures. Reapproximate the superficial layers of the perineal body with a running suture extending to the bottom of the episiotomy.

   2. Identify the apex of the vaginal laceration. Suture the vaginal mucosa with running, interlocking, 3-O chromic or Vicryl absorbable suture.
   3. Close the perineal skin with a running, subcuticular suture. Tie off the suture and remove the needle.

III. Third-degree laceration
   A. This laceration extends through the perineum and through the anal sphincter.
   B. Repair
   1. Identify each severed end of the external anal sphincter capsule, and grasp each end with an Allis clamp.
   2. Proximate the capsule of the sphincter with 4 interrupted sutures of 2-O or 3-O Vicryl suture, making sure the sutures do not penetrate the rectal mucosa.
   3. Continue the repair as for a second degree laceration as above. Stool softeners and sitz baths are prescribed post-partum.

IV. Fourth-degree laceration
   A. The laceration extends through the perineum, anal sphincter, and extends through the rectal mucosa to expose the lumen of the rectum.
   B. Repair
   1. Irrigate the laceration with sterile saline solution. Identify the anatomy, including the apex of the rectal mucosal laceration.
   2. Approximate the rectal submucosa with a running suture using a 3-O chromic on a GI needle extending to the margin of the anal skin.
   3. Place a second layer of running suture to invert the first suture line, and take some tension from the first layer closure.
   4. Identify and grasp the torn edges of the external anal sphincter capsule with Allis clamps, and perform a repair as for a third-degree laceration. Close the remaining layers as for a second-degree laceration.
   5. A low-residue diet, stool softeners, and sitz baths are prescribed post-partum.

References: See page 290.

Fetal Heart Rate Monitoring

Intrapartum fetal heart rate (FHR) monitoring can detect fetal hypoxia, umbilical cord compression, tachycardia, and acidosis. Fetal heart rate monitoring can significantly reduce the risk of newborn seizures (relative risk 0.5).

I. Pathophysiology
   A. Uterine contractions decrease placental blood flow and result in intermittent episodes of decreased oxygen delivery.
   B. The fetus normally tolerates contractions without difficulty, but if the frequency, duration, or strength of contractions becomes excessive, fetal hypoxemia may result.

II. Fetal heart rate monitoring method
   A. Continuous FHR and contraction monitoring may be accomplished externally or internally. Internal FHR monitoring is accomplished with a spiral wire attached to the fetal scalp or other presenting part.
   B. Uterine contractions are monitored externally or internally. The paper speed is usually 3 cm/min.

III. Fetal heart rate patterns
   A. Fetal heart rate
   1. The FHR at term ranges from 120-160 bpm. The initial response of the FHR to intermittent hypoxia is deceleration, but tachycardia may develop if the hypoxia is prolonged and severe.
   2. Tachycardia may also be associated with maternal fever, intra-amniotic infection, and congenital heart disease.
   B. Fetal heart rate variability
   1. Decreasing fetal heart rate variability is a fetal response to hypoxia. Fetal sleep cycles or medications may also decrease the FHR variability.
   2. The development of decreased variability in the absence of decelera-

tions is unlikely to be due to hypoxia.

C. Accelerations

1. Accelerations are common periodic changes, which are usually associated with fetal movement.
2. These changes are reassuring and almost always confirm that the fetus is not acidotic.

D. Variable decelerations

1. Variable decelerations are characterized by slowing of the FHR with an abrupt onset and return. They are frequently followed by small accelerations of the FHR. These decelerations vary in depth, duration, and shape. Variable decelerations are associated with cord compression, and they usually coincide with the timing of the uterine contractions.
2. Variable decelerations are caused by umbilical cord compression, and they are the most common decelerations seen in labor. These decelerations are generally associated with a favorable outcome. Persistent, deep, and long lasting variable decelerations are nonreassuring.
3. Persistent variable decelerations to less than 70 bpm lasting more than 60 seconds are concerning.
4. Variable decelerations with a persistently slow return to baseline are nonreassuring because they reflect persistent hypoxia. Nonreassuring variable decelerations are associated with tachycardia, absence of accelerations, and loss of variability.

E. Late decelerations

1. Late decelerations are U-shaped with a gradual onset and gradual return. They are usually shallow (10-30 beats per minute), and they reach their nadir after the peak of the contraction.
2. Late decelerations occur when uterine contractions cause decreased fetal oxygenation. In milder cases, they can be a result of CNS hypoxia. In more severe cases, they may be the result of direct myocardial depression.
3. Late decelerations become deeper as the degree of hypoxia becomes more severe. Occasional or intermittent late decelerations are not uncommon during labor. When late decelerations become persistent, they are nonreassuring.

F. Early decelerations

1. Early decelerations are shallow and symmetrical with a pattern similar to that of late decelerations, but they reach their nadir at the same time as the peak of the contraction.
2. These decelerations occur in the active phase of labor and are benign changes caused by fetal head compression.

G. Prolonged decelerations are isolated, abrupt decreases in the FHR to levels below baseline, for at least 60-90 seconds.

1. These changes may be caused by fetal hypoxia.
2. The degree to which such decelerations are nonreassuring depends on their depth and duration, loss of variability, and the frequency and progression of recurrence.

IV. Management of nonreassuring patterns

A. Approach to nonreassuring patterns

1. Determine the etiology of the pattern.
2. Attempt to correct the pattern by correcting the primary problem or by instituting measures aimed at improving fetal oxygenation and placental perfusion.
3. If attempts to correct the pattern are not successful, a scalp or sound stimulation test or fetal scalp blood pH assessment should be considered.
4. The need for operative intervention should be assessed.

B. Late decelerations. Excessive uterine contractions, maternal hypotension, or maternal hypoxemia should be corrected.

C. Severe variable or prolonged decelerations

1. A pelvic examination is performed to rule out umbilical cord prolapse or rapid descent of the fetal head.
2. If no causes are found, umbilical cord compression is likely to be

responsible.

D. Measures that improve fetal oxygenation and placental perfusion

    1. Oxygen therapy. Maternal oxygenation may be increased by giving oxygen at a flow rate of 8-10 L/min with a tight-fitting face mask.

    2. Maternal position

        a. In the supine position, the vena cava and aortoiliac vessels are compressed by the gravid uterus. This results in decreased return of blood to the maternal heart, leading to a fall in uterine blood flow.

        b. **The lateral recumbent position** (either side) is best for maximizing cardiac output and uterine blood flow, and it is often associated with an improvement in the FHR.

    3. Oxytocin (Pitocin). If nonreassuring FHR changes occur in patients receiving oxytocin, the infusion should be discontinued. Restarting the infusion at a lower rate may be better tolerated.

    4. Intravenous hydration. If the mother is hypovolemic, intravenous hydration should be initiated.

    5. Amnioinfusion

        a. Variable decelerations that occur prior to fetal descent at 8-9 cm of dilatation are most frequently caused by oligohydramnios. Replacement of amniotic fluid with normal saline infused through an intrauterine pressure catheter decreases variable decelerations in patients with decreased amniotic fluid volume.

        b. Saline amnioinfusion also decreases newborn respiratory complications from meconium due to the dilutional effect of amnioinfusion.

        c. Continuous amnioinfusion begins with a loading dose of 10 mL/min for 1 hour, followed by a maintenance dose of 3 mL/min via a double-lumen uterine pressure catheter.

    6. Tocolytic agents

        a. If a nonreassuring FHR pattern results from excessive uterine contractions, uterine activity can be decreased with tocolytics.

        b. Terbutaline, 0.25 mg subcutaneously or 0.125-0.25 mg intravenously, will suppress contractions. Magnesium sulfate is also of value in providing rapid uterine relaxation.

        c. Even in the absence of excessive uterine contractions, newborn condition may be improved by tocolytic agents.

V. Management of persistent nonreassuring fetal heart rate patterns

    A. Persistent nonreassuring decelerations with normal FHR variability and absence of tachycardia generally indicate a lack of fetal acidosis.

    B. Persistent late decelerations or severe variable decelerations associated with absence of variability are nonreassuring and generally require prompt intervention unless they spontaneously resolve or can be corrected rapidly with conservative measures (oxygen, hydration, maternal repositioning). In the presence of nonreassuring decelerations, a fetal scalp electrode should be placed.

    C. Spontaneous accelerations of greater than 15 bpm, lasting at least 15 seconds indicate the absence of fetal acidosis. Fetal scalp stimulation or vibroacoustic stimulation can be used to induce accelerations. If the fetus fails to respond to stimulation in the presence of an otherwise nonreassuring pattern, there is a 50% chance of acidosis.

    D. In cases in which the FHR patterns are persistently nonreassuring, the fetus should be delivered by either cesarean section or rapid vaginal delivery.

Management of Variant Fetal Heart Rate Patterns

FHR Pattern	Diagnosis	Action
Normal rate normal variability, accelerations, no decelerations	Fetus is well oxygenated	None

FHR Pattern	Diagnosis	Action
Normal variability, accelerations, mild variant pattern (bradycardia, late decelerations, variable decelerations)	Fetus is still well oxygenated centrally	Conservative management. This is a variant pattern
Normal variability, ± accelerations, moderate-severe variant pattern (bradycardia, late decelerations, variable decelerations)	Fetus is still well oxygenated centrally, but the FHR suggests hypoxia	Continue conservative management. Consider amnioinfusion and/or stimulation testing. Prepare for rapid delivery if pattern worsens
Decreasing variability, ± accelerations, moderate-severe variant patterns (bradycardia, late decelerations, variable decelerations)	Fetus may be on the verge of decompensation	Deliver if spontaneous delivery is remote, or if stimulation supports diagnosis of decompensation. Normal response to stimulation may allow time to await a vaginal delivery
Absent variability, no accelerations, moderate/severe variant patterns (bradycardia, late decelerations, variable decelerations)	Evidence of actual or impending asphyxia	Deliver. Stimulation or in-utero management may be attempted if delivery is not delayed

References: See page 290.

Antepartum Fetal Surveillance

Antepartum fetal surveillance techniques are now routinely used to assess the risk of fetal death in pregnancies complicated by preexisting maternal conditions (eg, type 1 diabetes mellitus) as well as those in which complications have developed (eg, intrauterine growth restriction).

I. **Antepartum fetal surveillance techniques**
   A. **Fetal movement assessment ("kick counts")**
      1. A diminution in the maternal perception of fetal movement often but not invariably precedes fetal death, in some cases by several days.
      2. The woman lies on her side and counts distinct fetal movements. Perception of 10 distinct movements in a period of up to 2 hours is considered reassuring. Once 10 movements have been perceived, the count may be discontinued. In the absence of a reassuring count, further fetal assessment is recommended.
   B. **Contraction stress test**
      1. The CST is based on the response of the fetal heart rate to uterine contractions. It relies on the premise that fetal oxygenation will be transiently worsened by uterine contractions. In the suboptimally oxygenated fetus, the resultant intermittent worsening in oxygenation will, in turn, lead to the fetal heart rate pattern of late decelerations. Uterine contractions also may provoke or accentuate a pattern of variable decelerations caused by fetal umbilical cord compression, which in some cases is associated with oligohydramnios.
      2. With the patient in the lateral recumbent position, the fetal heart rate and uterine contractions are simultaneously recorded with an external fetal monitor. If at least three spontaneous contractions of 40 seconds' duration each or longer are present in a 10-minute period, no uterine

stimulation is necessary. If fewer than three contractions of at least 40 seconds' duration occur in 10 minutes, contractions are induced with either nipple stimulation or intravenous administration of dilute oxytocin. An intravenous infusion of dilute oxytocin may be initiated at a rate of 0.5 mU/min and doubled every 20 minutes until an adequate contraction pattern is achieved.

3. The CST is interpreted according to the presence or absence of late fetal heart rate decelerations, which are defined as decelerations that reach their nadir after the peak of the contraction and that usually persist beyond the end of the contraction. The results of the CST are categorized as follows:

   a. **Negative:** no late or significant variable decelerations
   b. **Positive:** late decelerations following 50% or more of contractions (even if the contraction frequency is fewer than three in 10 minutes)
   c. **Equivocal-suspicious:** intermittent late decelerations or significant variable decelerations
   d. **Equivocal-hyperstimulatory:** fetal heart rate decelerations that occur in the presence of contractions more frequent than every 2 minutes or lasting longer than 90 seconds
   e. **Unsatisfactory:** fewer than three contractions in 10 minutes or an uninterpretable tracing

4. **Relative contraindications to the CST:**

   a. Preterm labor or certain patients at high risk of pre-term labor
   b. Preterm membrane rupture
   c. History of extensive uterine surgery or classical cesarean delivery
   d. Known placenta previa

C. **Nonstress test**

1. The NST is based on the premise that the heart rate of the fetus that is not acidotic or neurologically depressed will temporarily accelerate with fetal movement. Heart rate reactivity is a good indicator of normal fetal autonomic function. Loss of reactivity is associated most commonly with a fetal sleep cycle but may result from any cause of central nervous system depression, including fetal acidosis.

2. With the patient in the lateral tilt position, the fetal heart rate is monitored. The tracing is observed for fetal heart rate accelerations that peak at least 15 beats per minute above the baseline and last 15 seconds from baseline to baseline. Acoustic stimulation of the nonacidotic fetus may elicit fetal heart rate accelerations.

3. The NST is considered reactive (normal) if there are two or more fetal heart rate accelerations (as defined previously) within a 20-minute period, with or without fetal movement discernible by the woman. A nonreactive NST is one that lacks sufficient fetal heart rate accelerations over a 40-minute period. The NST of the noncompromised preterm fetus is frequently nonreactive: from 24 to 28 weeks of gestation, up to 50% of NSTs may not be reactive, and from 28 to 32 weeks of gestation, 15% of NSTs are not reactive.

4. Variable decelerations may be observed in up to 50% of NSTs. If nonrepetitive and brief (<30 seconds), they indicate neither fetal compromise nor the need for obstetric intervention. Repetitive variable decelerations (at least 3 in 20 minutes), even if mild, are associated with an increased risk of cesarean delivery for a nonreassuring intrapartum fetal heart rate pattern. Fetal heart rate decelerations during an NST that persist for 1 minute or longer are associated with a markedly increased risk of both cesarean delivery for a nonreassuring fetal heart rate pattern and fetal demise.

D. **Biophysical profile**

1. The BPP consists of an NST combined with four observations made by ultrasonography. Thus, the BPP comprises five components:

   a. Nonstress test (which, if all four ultrasound components are normal, may be omitted without compromising the validity of the test results).
   b. Fetal breathing movements (one or more episodes of rhythmic fetal breathing movements of 30 seconds or more within 30 minutes).

        c. Fetal movement (three or more discrete body or limb movements within 30 minutes).

        d. Fetal tone (one or more episodes of extension of a fetal extremity with return to flexion, or opening or closing of a hand).

        e. Determination of the amniotic fluid volume (a single vertical pocket of amniotic fluid exceeding 2 cm is considered evidence of adequate amniotic fluid).

    2. Each of the five components is assigned a score of either 2 (normal or present as defined previously) or 0 (abnormal, absent, or insufficient). A composite score of 8 or 10 is normal, a score of 6 is considered equivocal, and a score of 4 or less is abnormal. Regardless of the composite score, in the presence of oligohydramnios (largest vertical pocket of amniotic fluid volume ≤2 cm), further evaluation is warranted.

Components of the Biophysical Profile

Parameter	Normal (score = 2)	Abnormal (score = 0)
Nonstress test	≥2 accelerations ≥15 beats per minute above baseline during test lasting ≥15 seconds in 20 minutes	<2 accelerations
Amniotic fluid volume	Amniotic fluid index >5 or at least 1 pocket measuring 2 cm x 2 cm in perpendicular planes	AFI <5 or no pocket >2 cm x 2 cm
Fetal breathing movement	Sustained FBM (≥30 seconds)	Absence of FBM or short gasps only <30 seconds total
Fetal body move-ments	≥3 episodes of either limb or trunk movement	<3 episodes during test
Fetal tone	Extremities in flexion at rest and ≥1 episode of extension of ex-tremity, hand or spine with return to flexion	Extension at rest or no return to flexion after movement

A total score of 8 to 10 is reassuring; a score of 6 is suspicious, and a score of 4 or less is ominous.
Amniotic fluid index = the sum of the largest vertical pocket in each of four quadrants on the maternal abdomen intersecting at the umbilicus.

  E. Modified biophysical profile combines the NST with the amniotic fluid index (AFI), which is the sum of measurements of the deepest cord-free amniotic fluid pocket in each of the abdominal quadrants, as an indicator of long-term placental function. The modified BPP is considered normal if the NST is reactive and the AFI is more than 5, and abnormal if either the NST is nonreactive or the AFI is 5 or less.

  F. Umbilical artery Doppler velocimetry

    1. Umbilical artery Doppler flow velocimetry is a technique of fetal surveillance based on the observation that flow velocity waveforms in the umbilical artery of normally growing fetuses differ from those of growth-restricted fetuses. The umbilical flow velocity waveform of normally growing fetuses is characterized by high-velocity diastolic flow, whereas with intrauterine growth restriction, there is diminution of umbilical artery diastolic flow. Abnormal flow velocity waveforms have been correlated with fetal hypoxia and acidosis and perinatal morbidity and mortality.

    2. No benefit has been demonstrated for umbilical artery velocimetry for conditions other than suspected intrauterine growth restriction, such as

postterm gestation, diabetes mellitus, systemic lupus erythematosus, or antiphospholipid syndrome. Doppler ultrasonography has not been shown to be of value as a screening test for detecting fetal compromise in the general obstetric population.

II. Clinical considerations and recommendations

A. Indications for antepartum fetal surveillance

1. Maternal conditions

    a. Antiphospholipid syndrome

    b. Hyperthyroidism (poorly controlled)

    c. Hemoglobinopathies (hemoglobin SS, SC, or S-thalassemia)

    d. Cyanotic heart disease

    e. Systemic lupus erythematosus

    f. Chronic renal disease

    g. Type 1 diabetes mellitus

    h. Hypertensive disorders

2. Pregnancy-related conditions

    a. Pregnancy-induced hypertension

    b. Decreased fetal movement

    c. Oligohydramnios

    d. Polyhydramnios

    e. Intrauterine growth restriction

    f. Postterm pregnancy

    g. Isoimmunization (moderate to severe)

    h. Previous fetal demise (unexplained or recurrent risk)

    i. Multiple gestation (with significant growth discrepancy)

B. Initiation of antepartum fetal surveillance at 32-34 weeks of gestation is appropriate for most at-risk patients. However, in pregnancies with multiple or particularly worrisome high-risk conditions (eg, chronic hypertension with suspected intrauterine growth restriction), testing might begin as early as 26-28 weeks of gestation.

C. Frequency of testing. If the maternal medical condition is stable and CST results are negative, the CST is typically repeated in 1 week. Other tests of fetal well-being (NST, BPP, or modified BPP) are typically repeated at weekly intervals, but in the presence of certain high-risk conditions, such as postterm pregnancy, type 1 diabetes, intrauterine growth restriction, or pregnancy-induced hypertension, NST, BPP, or modified BPP testing are performed twice weekly.

Guidelines for Antepartum Testing

Indication	Initiation	Frequency
Post-term pregnancy	41 weeks	Twice a week
Preterm rupture of the membranes	At onset	Daily
Bleeding	26 weeks or at onset	Twice a week
Oligohydramnios	26 weeks or at onset	Twice a week
Polyhydramnios	32 weeks	Weekly
Diabetes	32 weeks	Twice a week
Chronic or pregnancy-induced hypertension	28 weeks	Weekly. Increase to twice-weekly at 32 weeks.

Indication	Initiation	Frequency
Steroid-dependent or poorly controlled asthma	28 weeks	Weekly
Sickle cell disease	32 weeks (earlier if symptoms)	Weekly (more often if severe)
Impaired renal function	28 weeks	Weekly
Substance abuse	32 weeks	Weekly
Prior stillbirth	At 2 weeks before prior fetal death	Weekly
Multiple gestation	32 weeks	Weekly
Congenital anomaly	32 weeks	Weekly
Fetal growth restriction	26 weeks	Twice a week or at onset
Decreased fetal movement	At time of complaint	Once

D. Management of abnormal test results
1. Maternal reports of decreased fetal movement should be evaluated by an NST, CST, BPP, or modified BPP; these results, if normal, usually are sufficient to exclude imminent fetal jeopardy. A nonreactive NST or an abnormal modified BPP generally should be followed by additional testing (either a CST or a full BPP). In many circumstances, a positive CST result generally indicates that delivery is warranted. However, the combination of a nonreactive NST and a positive CST result is associated frequently with serious fetal malformation and justifies ultrasonographic investigation for anomalies whenever possible
2. A BPP score of 6 is considered equivocal; in the term fetus, this score generally should prompt delivery, whereas in the preterm fetus, it should result in a repeat BPP in 24 hours. In the interim, maternal corticosteroid administration should be considered for pregnancies of less than 34 weeks of gestation. Repeat equivocal scores should result either in delivery or continued intensive surveillance. A BPP score of 4 usually indicates that delivery is warranted.

References: See page 290.

Brief Postoperative Cesarean Section Note

Pre-op diagnosis:
   1. 23 year old G_1P_0, estimated gestational age = 40 weeks
   2. Dystocia
   3. Non-reassuring fetal tracing
Post-op diagnosis: Same as above
Procedure: Primary low segment transverse cesarean section
Attending Surgeon, Assistant:
Anesthesia: Epidural
Operative Findings: Weight and sex of infant, APGARs at 1 min and 5 min; normal uterus, tubes, ovaries.
Cord pH:
Specimens: Placenta, cord blood (type and Rh).

Estimated Blood Loss: 800 cc; no blood replaced.
Fluids, blood and urine output:
Drains: Foley to gravity.
Complications: None
Disposition: Patient sent to recovery room in stable condition.

Cesarean Section Operative Report

Preoperative Diagnosis:
    1. 23 year old G_1P_0, estimated gestational age = 40 weeks
    2. Dystocia
    3. Non-reassuring fetal tracing
Postoperative Diagnosis: Same as above
Title of Operation: Primary low segment transverse cesarean section
Surgeon:
Assistant:
Anesthesia: Epidural
Findings At Surgery: Male infant in occiput posterior presentation. Thin meconium with none below the cords, pediatrics present at delivery, APGAR's 6/8, weight 3980 g. Normal uterus, tubes, and ovaries.
Description of Operative Procedure:
    After assuring informed consent, the patient was taken to the operating room and spinal anesthesia was initiated. The patient was placed in the dorsal, supine position with left lateral tilt. The abdomen was prepped and draped in sterile fashion.
    A Pfannenstiel skin incision was made with a scalpel and carried through to the level of the fascia. The fascial incision was extended bilaterally with Mayo scissors. The fascial incision was then grasped with the Kocher clamps, elevated, and sharply and bluntly dissected superiorly and inferiorly from the rectus muscles.
    The rectus muscles were then separated in the midline, and the peritoneum was tented up, and entered sharply with Metzenbaum scissors. The peritoneal incision was extended superiorly and inferiorly with good visualization of the bladder.
    A bladder blade was then inserted, and the vesicouterine peritoneum was identified, grasped with the pick-ups, and entered sharply with the Metzenbaum scissors. This incision was then extended laterally, and a bladder flap was created. The bladder was retracted using the bladder blade. The lower uterine segment was incised in a transverse fashion with the scalpel, then extended bilaterally with bandage scissors. The bladder blade was removed, and the infants head was delivered atraumatically. The nose and mouth were suctioned and the cord clamped and cut. The infant was handed off to the pediatrician. Cord gases and cord blood were sent.
    The placenta was then removed manually, and the uterus was exteriorized, and cleared of all clots and debris. The uterine incision was repaired with 1-O chromic in a running locking fashion. A second layer of 1-O chromic was used to obtain excellent hemostasis. The bladder flap was repaired with a 3-O Vicryl in a running fashion. The cul-de-sac was cleared of clots and the uterus was returned to the abdomen. The peritoneum was closed with 3-0 Vicryl. The fascia was reapproximated with O Vicryl in a running fashion. The skin was closed with staples.
    The patient tolerated the procedure well. Needle and sponge counts were correct times two. Two grams of Ancef was given at cord clamp, and a sterile dressing was placed over the incision.
Estimated Blood Loss (EBL): 800 cc; no blood replaced (normal blood loss is 500-1000 cc).
Specimens: Placenta, cord pH, cord blood specimens.
Drains: Foley to gravity.
Fluids: Input - 2000 cc LR; Output - 300 cc clear urine.
Complications: None.
Disposition: The patient was taken to the recovery room then postpartum ward

in stable condition.

Postoperative Management after Cesarean Section

I. **Post Cesarean Section Orders**
   A. **Transfer:** to post partum ward when stable.
   B. **Vital signs:** q4h x 24 hours, I and O.
   C. **Activity:** Bed rest x 6-8 hours, then ambulate; if given spinal, keep patient flat on back x 8h. Incentive spirometer q1h while awake.
   D. **Diet:** NPO x 8h, then sips of water. Advance to clear liquids, then to regular diet as tolerated.
   E. **IV Fluids:** IV D5 LR or D5 ½ NS at 125 cc/h. Foley to gravity; discontinue after 12 hours. I and O catheterize prn.
   F. **Medications**
      1. Cefazolin (Ancef) 1 gm IVPB x one dose at time of cesarean section.
      2. Nalbuphine (Nubain) 5 to 10 mg SC or IV q2-3h **OR**
      3. Meperidine (Demerol) 50-75 mg IM q3-4h prn pain.
      4. Hydroxyzine (Vistaril) 25-50 mg IM q3-4h prn nausea.
      5. Prochlorperazine (Compazine) 10 mg IV q4-6h prn nausea **OR**
      6. Promethazine (Phenergan) 25-50 mg IV q3-4h prn nausea
   G. **Labs:** CBC in AM.

II. **Postoperative Day #1**
   A. Assess pain, lungs, cardiac status, fundal height, lochia, passing of flatus, bowel movement, distension, tenderness, bowel sounds, incision.
   B. Discontinue IV when taking adequate PO fluids.
   C. Discontinue Foley, and I and O catheterize prn.
   D. Ambulate tid with assistance; incentive spirometer q1h while awake.
   E. Check hematocrit, hemoglobin, Rh, and rubella status.
   F. **Medications**
      1. Acetaminophen/codeine (Tylenol #3) 1-2 PO q4-6h prn pain **OR**
      2. Oxycodone/acetaminophen (Percocet) 1 tab q6h prn pain.
      3. FeSO4 325 mg PO bid-tid.
      4. Multivitamin PO qd, Colace 100 mg PO bid. Mylicon 80 mg PO qid prn bloating.

III. **Postoperative Day #2**
   A. If passing gas and/or bowel movement, advance to regular diet.
   B. Laxatives: Dulcolax supp prn or Milk of magnesia 30 cc PO tid prn. Mylicon 80 mg PO qid prn bloating.

IV. **Postoperative Day #3**
   A. If transverse incision, remove staples and place steri-strips on day 3. If a vertical incision, remove staples on post op day 5.
   B. Discharge home on appropriate medications; follow up in 2 and 6 weeks.

Laparoscopic Bilateral Tubal Ligation Operative Report

Preoperative Diagnosis: Multiparous female desiring permanent sterilization.
Postoperative Diagnosis: Same as above
Title of Operation: Laparoscopic bilateral tubal ligation with Falope rings
Surgeon:
Assistant:
Anesthesia: General endotracheal
Findings At Surgery: Normal uterus, tubes, and ovaries.
Description of Operative Procedure
   After informed consent, the patient was taken to the operating room where general anesthesia was administered. The patient was examined under

anesthesia and found to have a normal uterus with normal adnexa. She was placed in the dorsal lithotomy position and prepped and draped in sterile fashion. A bivalve speculum was placed in the vagina, and the anterior lip of the cervix was grasped with a single toothed tenaculum. A uterine manipulator was placed into the endocervical canal and articulated with the tenaculum. The speculum was removed from the vagina.

An infraumbilical incision was made with a scalpel, then while tenting up on the abdomen, a Verres needle was admitted into the intraabdominal cavity. A saline drop test was performed and noted to be within normal limits. Pneumoperitoneum was attained with 4 liters of carbon dioxide. The Verres needle was removed, and a 10 mm trocar and sleeve were advanced into the intraabdominal cavity while tenting up on the abdomen. The laparoscope was inserted and proper location was confirmed. A second incision was made 2 cm above the symphysis pubis, and a 5 mm trocar and sleeve were inserted into the abdomen under laparoscopic visualization without complication.

A survey revealed normal pelvic and abdominal anatomy. A Falope ring applicator was advanced through the second trocar sleeve, and the left Fallopian tube was identified, followed out to the fimbriated end, and grasped 4 cm from the cornual region. The Falope ring was applied to a knuckle of tube and good blanching was noted at the site of application. No bleeding was observed from the mesosalpinx. The Falope ring applicator was reloaded, and a Falope ring was applied in a similar fashion to the opposite tube. Carbon dioxide was allowed to escape from the abdomen.

The instruments were removed, and the skin incisions were closed with #3-O Vicryl in a subcuticular fashion. The instruments were removed from the vagina, and excellent hemostasis was noted. The patient tolerated the procedure well, and sponge, lap and needle counts were correct times two. The patient was taken to the recovery room in stable condition.

Estimated Blood Loss (EBL): <10 cc
Specimens: None
Drains: Foley to gravity
Fluids: 1500 cc LR
Complications: None
Disposition: The patient was taken to the recovery room in stable condition.

Postpartum Tubal Ligation Operative Report

Preoperative Diagnosis: Multiparous female after vaginal delivery, desiring permanent sterilization.
Postoperative Diagnosis: Same as above
Title of Operation: Modified Pomeroy bilateral tubal ligation
Surgeon:
Assistant:
Anesthesia: Epidural
Findings At Surgery: Normal fallopian tubes bilaterally
Description of Operative Procedure:

After assuring informed consent, the patient was taken to the operating room and spinal anesthesia administered. A small, transverse, infraumbilical skin incision was made with a scalpel, and the incision was carried down through the underlying fascia until the peritoneum was identified and entered. The left fallopian tube was identified, brought into the incision and grasped with a Babcock clamp. The tube was then followed out to the fimbria. An avascular midsection of the fallopian tube was grasped with a Babcock clamp and brought into a knuckle. The tube was doubly ligated with an O-plain suture and transected. The specimen was sent to pathology. Excellent hemostasis was noted, and the tube was returned to the abdomen. The same procedure was performed on the opposite fallopian tube.

The fascia was then closed with O-Vicryl in a single layer. The skin was closed with 3-O Vicryl in a subcuticular fashion. The patient tolerated the procedure well. Needle and sponge counts were correct times 2.

Estimated Blood Loss (EBL): <20 cc

Specimens: Segments of right and left tubes
Drains: Foley to gravity
Fluids: Input - 500 cc LR; output - 300 cc clear urine
Complications: None
Disposition: The patient was taken to the recovery room in stable condition.
References: See page 290.

Prevention of D Isoimmunization

The morbidity and mortality of Rh hemolytic disease can be significantly reduced by identification of women at risk for isoimmunization and by administration of D immunoglobulin. Administration of D immunoglobulin [RhoGAM, Rho(D) immunoglobulin, RhIg] is very effective in the preventing isoimmunization to the D antigen.

I. **Prenatal testing**
   A. Routine prenatal laboratory evaluation includes ABO and D blood type determination and antibody screen.
   B. At 28-29 weeks of gestation woman who are D negative but not D isoimmunized should be retested for D antibody. If the test reveals that no D antibody is present, prophylactic D immunoglobulin [RhoGAM, Rho(D) immunoglobulin, RhIg] is indicated.
   C. If D antibody is present, D immunoglobulin will not be beneficial, and specialized management of the D isoimmunized pregnancy is undertaken to manage hemolytic disease of the fetus and hydrops fetalis.

II. **Routine administration of D immunoglobulin**
   A. **Abortion.** D sensitization may be caused by abortion. D sensitization occurs more frequently after induced abortion than after spontaneous abortion, and it occurs more frequently after late abortion than after early abortion. D sensitization occurs following induced abortion in 4-5% of susceptible women. All unsensitized, D-negative women who have an induced or spontaneous abortion should be treated with D immunoglobulin unless the father is known to be D negative.
   B. **Dosage** of D immunoglobulin is determined by the stage of gestation. If the abortion occurs before 13 weeks of gestation, 50 mcg of D immunoglobulin prevents sensitization. For abortions occurring at 13 weeks of gestation and later, 300-mcg is given.
   C. **Ectopic pregnancy** can cause D sensitization. All unsensitized, D-negative women who have an ectopic pregnancy should be given D immunoglobulin. The dosage is determined by the gestational age, as described above for abortion.
   D. **Amniocentesis**
      1. D isoimmunization can occur after amniocentesis. D immunoglobulin, 300 mcg, should be administered to unsensitized, D-negative, susceptible patients following first- and second-trimester amniocentesis.
      2. Following third-trimester amniocentesis, 300 mcg of D immunoglobulin should be administered. If amniocentesis is performed and delivery is planned within 48 hours, D immunoglobulin can be withheld until after delivery, when the newborn can be tested for D positivity. If the amniocentesis is expected to precede delivery by more than 48 hours, the patient should receive 300 mcg of D immunoglobulin at the time of amniocentesis.
   E. **Antepartum prophylaxis**
      1. Isoimmunized occurs in 1-2% of D-negative women during the antepartum period. D immunoglobulin, administered both during pregnancy and postpartum, can reduce the incidence of D isoimmunization to 0.3%.
      2. Antepartum prophylaxis is given at 28-29 weeks of gestation. Antibody-negative, Rh-negative gravidas should have a repeat assessment at 28 weeks. D immunoglobulin (RhoGAM, RhIg), 300 mcg, is given to D-

negative women. However, if the father of the fetus is known with certainty to be D negative, antepartum prophylaxis is not necessary.

F. Postpartum D immunoglobulin

1. D immunoglobulin is given to the D negative mother as soon after delivery as cord blood findings indicate that the baby is Rh positive.

2. A woman at risk who is inadvertently not given D immunoglobulin within 72 hours after delivery should still receive prophylaxis at any time up until two weeks after delivery. If prophylaxis is delayed, it may not be effective.

3. A quantitative Kleihauer-Betke analysis should be performed in situations in which significant maternal bleeding may have occurred (eg, after maternal abdominal trauma, abruptio placentae, external cephalic version). If the quantitative determination is thought to be more than 30 mL, D immune globulin should be given to the mother in multiples of one vial (300 mcg) for each 30 mL of estimated fetal whole blood in her circulation, unless the father of the baby is known to be D negative.

G. Abruptio placentae, placenta previa, cesarean delivery, intrauterine manipulation, or manual removal of the placenta may cause more than 30 mL of fetal-to-maternal bleeding. In these conditions, testing for excessive bleeding (Kleihauer-Betke test) or inadequate D immunoglobulin dosage (indirect Coombs test) is necessary.

References: See page 290.

Complications of Pregnancy

Nausea, Vomiting and Hyperemesis Gravidarum

At least three-fourths of all pregnant women experience some degree of nausea or vomiting. The clinical presentation may range from mild and self-limited discomfort to pernicious vomiting with dehydration, electrolyte disturbances, and prostration. Illness of this severity is called hyperemesis gravidarum.

I. **Evaluation**
   A. Gestational trophoblastic disease and several other conditions associated with pregnancy predispose women to excessive nausea and vomiting. An appropriate workup for these conditions may include:
      1. History and physical examination
      2. Complete blood count
      3. Urinalysis or urine culture, or both
      4. Serology for hepatitis A, B, and C
      5. Hepatic transaminases
      6. Ultrasound examination of the uterus

Conditions That May Predispose to Excessive Nausea and Vomiting

Viral gastroenteritis
Gestational trophoblastic disease
Hepatitis
Urinary tract infection
Multifetal gestation
Gallbladder disease
Migraine

   B. An assessment of hydration should be completed, and helpful laboratory studies include the following:
      1. Urine-specific gravity
      2. Urine acetone or ketones
      3. Serum acetone
      4. Serum electrolytes
   C. The appearance of acetone in the urine is nonspecific and may follow an overnight fast by a normal gravida. Large amounts of urine acetone or the presence of significant acetone in serum, however, suggest that the pregnant woman is obtaining much of her caloric requirement from lipolysis. This finding, in turn, suggests that she has exhausted glucose and glycogen stores and may benefit from IV therapy.
II. **Therapy**
   A. Instruct pregnant patients to eat frequent small meals and to avoid foods that do not appeal to them. The patient should eat small amounts of food that she is able to tolerate.
   B. In early pregnany, prenatal vitamin and iron pills often are associated with nausea and vomiting and should be avoided if such symptoms occur, although adequate folic acid intake (0.4 mg/day) needs to be assured.
   C. Patients with hyperemesis gravidarum may require hospitalization and IV hydration. The average woman with no severe electrolyte abnormalities should be given IV therapy with 0.5 normal saline in 5% dextrose with 20 mEq KCL in each liter to run continuously at 125 mL/hr. Women with persistent vomiting may develop hypokalemia and hypochloremic alkalosis. In such instances, additional potassium chloride may be required. The concentration of potassium chloride should not exceed 30 mEq/L. In rare instances, prolonged nausea and vomiting may require

total parenteral nutrition.
  D. Medications. The medications used include agents with antihistamine or phenothiazine characteristics, or both. Common drug regimens are:
    1. Promethazine (Phenergan), 12.5 to 25.0 mg every 6 hours po or rectally
    2. Hydroxyzine (Vistaril), 25 to 50 mg every 6 hours po or rectally
    3. Trimethobenzamide (Tigan), 200 mg every 6 hours po
    4. Prochlorperazine (Compazine), 5 to 10 mg orally every 6 hr or 10 mg IM every 4 hours, or 25 mg suppository per rectum twice a day.
References: See page 290.

Spontaneous Abortion

Abortion is defined as termination of pregnancy resulting in expulsion of an immature, nonviable fetus. A fetus of <20 weeks gestation or a fetus weighing <500 gm is considered an abortus. Spontaneous abortion occurs in 15% of all pregnancies.
I. **Threatened abortion** is defined as vaginal bleeding occurring in the first 20 weeks of pregnancy, without the passage of tissue or rupture of membranes.
  A. Symptoms of pregnancy (nausea, vomiting, fatigue, breast tenderness, urinary frequency) are usually present.
  B. Speculum exam reveals blood coming from the cervical os without amniotic fluid or tissue in the endocervical canal.
  C. The internal cervical os is closed, and the uterus is soft and enlarged appropriate for gestational age.
  D. Differential diagnosis
    1. **Benign and malignant lesions.** The cervix often bleeds from an ectropion of friable tissue. Hemostasis can be accomplished by applying pressure for several minutes with a large swab or by cautery with a silver nitrate stick. Atypical cervical lesions are evaluated with colposcopy and biopsy.
    2. **Disorders of pregnancy**
      a. Hydatidiform mole may present with early pregnancy bleeding, passage of grape-like vesicles, and a uterus that is enlarged in excess of that expected from dates. An absence of heart tones by Doppler after 12 weeks is characteristic. Hyperemesis, preeclampsia, or hyperthyroidism may be present. Ultrasonography confirms the diagnosis.
      b. Ectopic pregnancy should be excluded when first trimester bleeding is associated with pelvic pain. Orthostatic light-headedness, syncope or shoulder pain (from diaphragmatic irritation) may occur.
        (1) Abdominal tenderness is noted, and pelvic examination reveals cervical motion tenderness.
        (2) Serum beta-HCG is positive.
  E. Laboratory tests
    1. **Complete blood count.** The CBC will not reflect acute blood loss.
    2. **Quantitative serum beta-HCG level** may be positive in nonviable gestations since beta-HCG may persist in the serum for several weeks after fetal death.
    3. **Ultrasonography** should detect fetal heart motion by 7 weeks gestation or older. Failure to detect fetal heart motion after 9 weeks gestation should prompt consideration of curettage.
  F. Treatment of threatened abortion
    1. Bed rest with sedation and abstinence from intercourse.
    2. The patient should report increased bleeding (>normal menses), cramping, passage of tissue, or fever. Passed tissue should be saved for examination.
II. **Inevitable abortion** is defined as a threatened abortion with a dilated cervical os. Menstrual-like cramps usually occur.

A. **Differential diagnosis**
   1. **Incomplete abortion** is diagnosed when tissue has passed. Tissue may be visible in the vagina or endocervical canal.
   2. **Threatened abortion** is diagnosed when the internal os is closed and will not admit a fingertip.
   3. **Incompetent cervix** is characterized by dilatation of the cervix without cramps.
B. **Treatment of inevitable abortion**
   1. Surgical evacuation of the uterus is necessary.
   2. D immunoglobulin (RhoGAM) is administered to Rh-negative, unsensitized patients to prevent isoimmunization. Before 13 weeks gestation, the dosage is 50 mcg IM; at 13 weeks gestation, the dosage is 300 mcg IM.
III. **Incomplete abortion** is characterized by cramping, bleeding, passage of tissue, and a dilated internal os with tissue present in the vagina or endocervical canal. Profuse bleeding, orthostatic dizziness, syncope, and postural pulse and blood pressure changes may occur.
   A. **Laboratory evaluation**
      1. **Complete blood count.** CBC will not reflect acute blood loss.
      2. **Rh typing**
      3. **Blood typing and cress-matching.**
      4. **Karyotyping** of products of conception is completed if loss is recurrent.
   B. **Treatment**
      1. **Stabilization.** If the patient has signs and symptoms of heavy bleeding, at least 2 large-bore IV catheters (<16 gauge) are placed. Lactate Ringer's or normal saline with 40 U oxytocin/L is given IV at 200 mL/hour or greater.
      2. Products of conception are removed from the endocervical canal and uterus with a ring forceps. Immediate removal decreases bleeding. Curettage is performed after vital signs have stabilized.
      3. **Suction dilation and curettage**
         a. Analgesia consists of meperidine (Demerol), 35-50 mg IV over 3-5 minutes until the patient is drowsy.
         b. The patient is placed in the dorsal lithotomy position in stirrups, prepared, draped, and sedated.
         c. A weighted speculum is placed intravaginally, the vagina and cervix are cleansed, and a paracervical block is placed.
         d. Bimanual examination confirms uterine position and size, and uterine sounding confirms the direction of the endocervical canal.
         e. Mechanical dilatation is completed with dilators if necessary. Curettage is performed with an 8 mm suction curette, with a single-tooth tenaculum on the anterior lip of the cervix.
      4. **Post-curettage.** After curettage, a blood count is ordered. If the vital signs are stable for several hours, the patient is discharged with instructions to avoid coitus, douching, or the use of tampons for 2 weeks. Ferrous sulfate and ibuprofen are prescribed for pain.
      5. **Rh-negative**, unsensitized patients are given IM RhoGAM.
      6. **Methylergonovine (Methergine)**, 0.2 mg PO q4h for 6 doses, is given if there is continued moderate bleeding.
IV. **Complete abortion**
   A. A complete abortion is diagnosed when complete passage of products of conception has occurred. The uterus is well contracted, and the cervical os may be closed.
   B. **Differential diagnosis**
      1. **Incomplete abortion**
      2. **Ectopic pregnancy.** Products of conception should be examined grossly and submitted for pathologic examination. If no fetal tissue or villi are observed grossly, ectopic pregnancy must be excluded by ultrasound.
   C. **Management of complete abortion**
      1. Between 8 and 14 weeks, curettage is necessary because of the high probability that the abortion was incomplete.

      2. D immunoglobulin (RhoGAM) is administered to Rh-negative, unsensitized patients.

      3. Beta-HCG levels are obtained weekly until zero. Incomplete abortion is suspected if beta-HCG levels plateau or fail to reach zero within 4 weeks.

V. Missed abortion is diagnosed when products of conception are retained after the fetus has expired. If products are retained, a severe coagulopathy with bleeding often occurs.

    A. Missed abortion should be suspected when the pregnant uterus fails to grow as expected or when fetal heart tones disappear.

    B. Amenorrhea may persist, or intermittent vaginal bleeding, spotting, or brown discharge may be noted.

    C. Ultrasonography confirms the diagnosis.

    D. Management of missed abortion

      1. CBC with platelet count, fibrinogen level, partial thromboplastin time, and ABO blood typing and antibody screen are obtained.

      2. **Evacuation** of the uterus is completed after fetal death has been confirmed. Dilation and evacuation by suction curettage is appropriate when the uterus is less than 12-14 weeks gestational size.

      3. **D immunoglobulin (RhoGAM)** is administered to Rh-negative, unsensitized patients.

References: See page 290.

Antepartum Urinary Tract Infection

Four to 8% of pregnant women will develop asymptomatic bacteriuria, and 1-3% will develop symptomatic cystitis with dysuria. Pyelonephritis develops in 25-30% of women with untreated bacteriuria.

I. Asymptomatic bacteriuria is diagnosed by prenatal urine culture screening, and it is defined as a colony count $\geq 10^5$ organisms per milliliter. Patients with symptomatic cystitis should be treated with oral antibiotics without waiting for urine culture results.

    A. Approximately 80% of infections are caused by Escherichia coli; 10-15% are due to Klebsiella pneumonia or Proteus species; 5% or less are caused by group B streptococci, enterococci, or staphylococci.

    B. Antibiotic therapy

      1. Cystitis or asymptomatic bacteriuria is treated for 3 days. A repeat culture is completed after therapy.

      2. Nitrofurantoin monohydrate (Macrobid) 100 mg PO bid **OR**

      3. Nitrofurantoin (Macrodantin) 100 mg PO qid **OR**

      4. Amoxicillin 250-500 mg PO tid **OR**

      5. Cephalexin (Keflex) 250-500 mg PO qid.

II. Pyelonephritis

    A. In pregnancy, pyelonephritis can progress rapidly to septic shock and may cause preterm labor. Upper tract urinary infections are associated with an increased incidence of fetal prematurity. Pyelonephritis is characterized by fever, chills, nausea, uterine contractions, and dysuria.

    B. Physical exam usually reveals fever and costovertebral angle tenderness.

    C. The most common pathogens are Escherichia coli and Klebsiella pneumoniae.

    D. Patients should be hospitalized for intravenous antibiotics and fluids. Pyelonephritis is treated with an intravenous antibiotic regimen to which the infectious organism is sensitive for 7-10 days.

    E. Cefazolin (Ancef) 1-2 gm IVPB q8h **OR**

    F. Ampicillin 1 gm IVPB q4-6h **AND**

    G. Gentamicin 2 mg/kg IVPB then 1.5 mg/kg IV q8h **OR**

    H. Ampicillin/sulbactam (Unasyn) 1.5-3 gm IVPB q6h.

    I. Bedrest in the semi Fowler's position on the side opposite affected kidney may help to relieve the pain. Patients with continued fever and pain for more than 48 to 72 hours may have a resistant organism, obstruction, perinephric abscess, or an infected calculus or cyst.

J. **Oral antibiotics** are initiated once fever and pain have resolved for at least 24 hours.
   1. **Nitrofurantoin monohydrate (Macrobid)** 100 mg PO bid x 7-10 days, then 100 mg PO qhs **OR**
   2. **Nitrofurantoin (Macrodantin)** 100 mg PO qid x 7-10 days, then 100 mg PO qhs **OR**
   3. **Cephalexin (Keflex)** 500 mg PO qid x 7-10 days **OR**
   4. **Amoxicillin,** 250 mg tid; sulfisoxazole, 500 mg qid x 7-10 days
   5. **Contraindicated Antibiotics.** Sulfonamides should not be used within four weeks of delivery because kernicterus is a theoretical risk. Aminoglycosides should be used for only short periods because of fetal ototoxicity and nephrotoxicity.
   6. Nitrofurantoin and sulfonamides may cause hemolysis in patients with glucose 6-phosphate dehydrogenase deficiency.
   7. After successful therapy, cultures are rechecked monthly during pregnancy, and subsequent infections are treated. Antibiotic prophylaxis is recommended for women with two or more bladder infections or one episode of pyelonephritis during pregnancy. Reinfection is treated for 10 days, then low dose prophylaxis is initiated until 2 weeks postpartum. Prophylactic therapy includes nitrofurantoin (Macrodantin), 100 mg at bedtime or sulfisoxazole (Gantrisin) 0.5 gm bid.

References: See page 290.

Trauma During Pregnancy

Trauma is the leading cause of nonobstetric death in women of reproductive age. Six percent of all pregnancies are complicated by some type of trauma.

I. **Mechanism of injury**
A. **Blunt abdominal trauma**
   1. Blunt abdominal trauma secondary to motor vehicle accidents is the leading cause of nonobstetric-related fetal death during pregnancy, followed by falls and assaults. Uterine rupture or laceration, retroperitoneal hemorrhage, renal injury and upper abdominal injuries may also occur after blunt trauma.
   2. **Abruptio placentae** occurs in 40-50% of patients with major traumatic injuries and in up to 5% of patients with minor injuries.
   3. **Clinical findings in blunt abdominal trauma.** Vaginal bleeding, uterine tenderness, uterine contractions, fetal tachycardia, late decelerations, fetal acidosis, and fetal death.
   4. **Detection of abruptio placentae**. Beyond 20 weeks of gestation, external electronic monitoring can detect uterine contractile activity. The presence of vaginal bleeding and tetanic or hypertonic contractions is presumptive evidence of abruptio placentae.
   5. **Uterine rupture**
      a. Uterine rupture is an infrequent but life-threatening complication. It usually occurs after a direct abdominal impact.
      b. Findings of uterine rupture range from subtle (uterine tenderness, nonreassuring fetal heart rate pattern) to severe, with rapid onset of maternal hypovolemic shock and death.
   6. **Direct fetal injury** is an infrequent complication of blunt trauma.
      a. The fetus is more frequently injured as a result of hypoxia from blood loss or abruption.
      b. In the first trimester the uterus is well protected by the maternal pelvis; therefore, minor trauma usually does not usually cause miscarriage in the first trimester.
B. **Penetrating trauma**
   1. Penetrating abdominal trauma from gunshot and stab wounds during pregnancy has a poor prognosis.
   2. Perinatal mortality is 41-71%. Maternal mortality is less than 5%.

II. **Major trauma in pregnancy**
A. **Initial evaluation of major abdominal trauma** in pregnant patients does not differ from evaluation of abdominal trauma in a nonpregnant patient.
B. **Maintain airway, breathing, and circulatory volume.** Two large-bore (14-16-gauge) intravenous lines are placed.
C. **Oxygen** should be administered by mask or endotracheal intubation. Maternal oxygen saturation should be kept at >90% (an oxygen partial pressure [pO_2] of 60 mm Hg).
D. **Volume resuscitation**
   1. Crystalloid in the form of lactated Ringer's or normal saline should be given as a 3:1 replacement for the estimated blood loss over the first 30-60 minutes of acute resuscitation.
   2. O-negative packed red cells are preferred if emergent blood is needed before the patient's own blood type is known.
   3. A urinary catheter should be placed to measure urine output and observe for hematuria.
E. **Deflection of the uterus** off the inferior vena cava and abdominal aorta can be achieved by placing the patient in the lateral decubitus position. If the patient must remain supine, manual deflection of the uterus to the left and placement of a wedge under the patient's hip or backboard will tilt the patient.
F. **Secondary survey.** Following stabilization, a more detailed secondary survey of the patient, including fetal evaluation, is performed.
III. **Minor trauma in pregnancy**
A. **Clinical evaluation**
   1. Pregnant patients who sustain seemingly minimal trauma require an evaluation to exclude significant injuries. Common "minor" trauma include falls, especially in the third trimester, blows to the abdomen, and "fender benders" motor vehicle accidents.
   2. The patient should be questioned about seat belt use, loss of consciousness, pain, vaginal bleeding, rupture of membranes, and fetal movement.
   3. **Physical examination**
      a. Physical examination should focus on upper abdominal tenderness (liver or spleen damage), flank pain (renal trauma), uterine pain (placental abruption, uterine rupture), and pain over the symphysis pubis (pelvic fracture, bladder laceration, fetal skull fracture).
      b. A search for orthopedic injuries should be completed.
B. **Management of minor trauma**
   1. The minor trauma patient with a fetus that is less than 20 weeks gestation (not yet viable), with no significant injury can be safely discharged after documentation of fetal heart rate. Patients with potentially viable fetuses (over 20 weeks of gestation) require fetal monitoring, laboratory tests and ultrasonographic evaluation.
   2. A complete blood count, urinalysis (hematuria), blood type and screen (to check Rh status), and coagulation panel, including measurement of the INR, PTT, fibrinogen and fibrin split products, should be obtained. The coagulation panel is useful if any suspicion of abruption exists.
   3. **The Kleihauer-Betke (KB) test**
      a. This test detects fetal red blood cells in the maternal circulation. A KB stain should be obtained routinely for any pregnant trauma patient whose fetus is over 12 weeks.
      b. Regardless of the patient's blood type and Rh status, the KB test can help determine if fetomaternal hemorrhage has occurred.
      c. The KB test can also be used to determine the amount of Rho(D) immunoglobulin (RhoGAM) required in patients who are Rh-negative.
      d. A positive KB stain indicates uterine trauma, and any patient with a positive KB stain should receive at least 24 hours of continuous uterine and fetal monitoring and a coagulation panel.
   4. **Ultrasonography** is less sensitive for diagnosing abruption than is the finding of uterine contractions on external tocodynamometry. Absence of sonographic evidence of abruption does not completely exclude an abruption.
   5. Patients with abdominal pain, significant bruising, vaginal bleeding, rupture

of membranes, or uterine contractions should be admitted to the hospital for overnight observation and continuous fetal monitor.
6. Uterine contractions and vaginal bleeding are suggestive of abruption. Even if vaginal bleeding is absent, the presence of contractions is still a concern, since the uterus can contain up to 2 L of blood from a concealed abruption.
7. Trauma patients with no uterine contraction activity, usually do not have abruption, while patients with greater than one contraction per 10 minutes (6 per hour) have a 20% incidence of abruption.
References: See page 290.

Diabetes and Pregnancy

Pregnancies complicated with gestational diabetes have an increased risk of maternal and perinatal complications, long-term maternal morbidity, and morbidity to the offspring. The causes of perinatal morbidity are neonatal hypoglycemia, hyperbilirubinemia, hypocalcemia, polycythemia, macrosomia birth weight more than 9 lbs (or 4 kg), and with that the problem shoulder dystocia, an abnormal apgar score, and Erb's palsy.

Risk Factors for Gestational Diabetes
• Maternal age older than 30 years • Pregravid weight more than 90 kg • Family history of diabetes • Race • Multiparity • Macrosomia

I. **Diagnosis of gestational diabetes**
   A. The diagnosis of gestational diabetes is usually accomplished early in the third trimester of pregnancy. The one-hour glucola test is the screening test for gestational diabetes. Nonfasting women are given 50 grams of glucose in a flavored solution, and their blood is taken one hour after ingestion. If the blood sugar equals or exceeds 140 mg/dL, then women are asked to take a three-hour glucose tolerance test (GTT).
   B. For the three-hour GTT, women are advised to consume an unrestricted diet containing at least 150 grams of carbohydrates daily three days prior to testing. They are asked to fast for 10-14 hours prior to testing. All tests are performed in the morning. Blood is drawn fasting and at 1, 2, and 3 hours postingestion of a 100-gram glucose-containing solution. If any two (out of 4) or more results are abnormal, then they are diagnosed as having gestational diabetes.

Criteria for Gestational Diabetes	
Fasting	105 mg/dL
1 hour	190 mg/dL
2 hour	165 mg/dL
3 hour	145 mg/dL
Any two or more abnormal results are diagnostic of gestational diabetes.	

II. Management

A. Dietary management. The meal schedule should consist of three meals a day with one or two snacks interspersed as well as a snack after dinner. Initial diet should consist of an intake of 35 kcal/kg of ideal body weight for most nonunderweight, nonobese patients. Generally a diet consisting of complex carbohydrates (as opposed to simple sugars), soluble fiber, low in fat, while reduced in saturated fats, is recommended.

B. Exercise management Participation in aerobic activities three to four days per week for 15-30 minutes per session may be beneficial. Pulse should not exceed 70-80% of her maximal heart rate adjusted for her age (target heart rate = [220 - age] x 70%). This will be between 130-150 bpm.

C. Insulin. The criteria for insulin therapy are failure of dietary and exercise management. If the fasting blood sugar is greater than 95, if the one-hour postprandial blood sugar is equal to or greater than 140, or if the two-hour postprandial blood sugar is equal to or greater than 120, then the patient needs tighter control of the blood sugar. Human insulin is the drug of choice for treatment of gestational or pregestational diabetes. Insulin dosing of 0.7-1.0 U/kg, depending on the patient's week of gestation (longer gestation usually requiring the higher dose), is recommended. The patient may require a combination of long-acting NPH with regular insulin. Give 2/3 of total daily requirement in the AM; divide AM dose into 2/3 NPH and 1/3 regular. Give 1/3 of daily requirement in evening: ½ as NPH and ½ as regular insulin. Adjust doses by no more than 20% at a time.

D. Blood glucose monitoring. In gestational diabetes the blood sugar should be checked at least four times daily. The fasting blood sugar should not exceed 95 mg/dL and the two-hour postprandial blood sugar should not exceed 120 mg/dL.

Treatment Goals for Gestational Diabetes Mellitus		
Time	Blood Sugar	Blood Sugar
Fasting	95 mg/dL	< 5.3 mmol/L
1 hr postprandial	140 mg/dL	< 7.8 mmol/L
2 hr postprandial	120 mg/dL	< 6.7 mmol/L

E. Fetal surveillance

1. **Kick counts** are a simple, inexpensive way of measuring fetal well-being. Kick counts are usually done after a meal or snack. The patient lies on her left side and counts the number of fetal movements over a one-hour period. When she gets to 10 movements, she has accomplished a reassuring test of fetal well-being.

2. **Ultrasonography** is useful in diagnosing abnormalities in fetal growth (such as macrosomia, intrauterine growth retardation, or polyhydramnios). Scanning the crown rump length in the first trimester can confirm dates. Fetal ultrasonography used in the third trimester can give an estimated fetal weight and allow measurement of the abdominal circumference.

3. **A maternal serum alpha-fetal protein** level is important at 16-18 weeks because of the increased incidence of open neural tube defects in diabetic pregnancies.

4. **Nonstress testing** is also used after 32 weeks to evaluate fetal well-being of pregestational or gestational diabetic pregnancies. Two accelerations of the heart rate from the baseline over a 20-minute period of monitoring is a favorable response.

5. **Biophysical profiles** combine ultrasonography with nonstress testing. This allows evaluation of amniotic fluid volume as well as abnormalities in fetal growth or development. A score is derived from observing fetal

activity, tone, breathing, and amniotic fluid. A score of 8 or above is reassuring.

F. Labor and delivery

1. **Delivery** after 38 weeks increases the probability of the infant developing macrosomia. Unless the pregnancy is complicated by macrosomia, polyhydramnios, poor control of diabetes, or other obstetrical indications (such as pre-eclampsia or intrauterine growth retardation), delivery at term is recommended.

2. **Amniocentesis** is usually indicated if delivery is decided on prior to 38 weeks. A lecithin to sphingomyelin (L/S) ratio of 2 or greater along with the presence of phosphatidylglycerol is what is recommended as being indicative of lung maturity for elective delivery before 38 weeks. After 38 weeks, if the patient has good dates and had a first or second trimester ultrasound that confirms the gestational age, an amniocentesis does not need to be performed.

3. **Induction** is recommended if the patient does not spontaneously go into labor between 39 and 40 weeks. At 40 weeks if her cervix is unfavorable, prostaglandin agents may be necessary to ripen the cervix.

4. **Diabetes management during labor** requires good control of blood sugar while avoiding hypoglycemia. Many patients require no insulin during labor. Blood sugar should be checked every 1-2 hours during labor. Dextrose will need to be given intravenously if the patient's blood sugar falls below 70 mg/dL. Short-acting regular insulin may need to be given intravenously for blood sugars rising above 140 mg/dL (7.8 mmol/L). Plasma glucose should be maintained at 100 to 130 mg/dL.

G. Postpartum care. Insulin requirements decrease after the placenta has been delivered. If the patient was on an insulin infusion during labor the dose should be cut in half at this time. For patients with pregestational diabetes the pre-pregnancy insulin dose should be reinitiated after the patient is able to eat.

Low-dosage Constant Insulin Infusion for the Intrapartum Period		
Blood Glucose (mg/100 mL)	**Insulin Dosage (U/h)**	**Fluids (125 mL/h)**
<100	0	5%dextrose/Lactated Ringer's solution
100-140	1.0	5% dextrose/Lactated Ringer's solution
141-180	1.5	Normal saline
181-220	2.0	Normal saline
>220	2.5	Normal saline
Dilution is 25 U of regular insulin in 250 mL of normal saline, with 25 mL flushed through line, administered intravenously.		

H. Elective cesarean delivery

1. An estimated fetal weight of greater than 4500 g is an indication for cesarean delivery to avoid birth trauma.

2. Elective cesarean delivery is scheduled for early morning. The usual morning insulin dose is withheld, and glucose levels are monitored hourly. A 5% dextrose solution is initiated and an insulin infusion is initiated. After delivery, intravenous dextrose is continued, and glucose levels are checked every 4-6 hours. In the postpartum period, short-

acting insulin is administered if the glucose level rises above 200 mg/dL.
3. For patients with pregestational diabetes, once the patient begins a regular diet, subcutaneous insulin can be reinstituted at dosages substantially lower than those given in the third trimester. It is helpful if the pregestational dose is known.

References: See page 290.

Premature Rupture of Membranes

Premature rupture of membranes (PROM) is the most common diagnosis associated with preterm delivery. The incidence of this disorder to be 7-12%. In pregnancies of less than 37 weeks of gestation, preterm birth (and its sequelae) and infection are the major concerns after PROM.

I. Pathophysiology

A. **Premature rupture of membranes** is defined as rupture of membranes prior to the onset of labor.

B. **Preterm premature rupture of membranes** is defined as rupture of membranes prior to term.

C. **Prolonged rupture of membranes** consists of rupture of membranes for more than 24 hours.

D. **The latent period** is the time interval from rupture of membranes to the onset of regular contractions or labor.

E. Many cases of preterm PROM are caused by idiopathic weakening of the membranes, many of which are caused by subclinical infection. Other causes of PROM include hydramnios, incompetent cervix, abruptio placentae, and amniocentesis.

F. At term, about 8% of patients will present with ruptured membranes prior to the onset of labor.

II. Maternal and neonatal complications

A. Labor usually follows shortly after the occurrence of PROM. Ninety percent of term patients and 50% of preterm patients go into labor within 24 hours after rupture.

B. Patients who do not go into labor immediately are at increasing risk of infection as the duration of rupture increases. Chorioamnionitis, endometritis, sepsis, and neonatal infections may occur.

C. Perinatal risks with preterm PROM are primarily complications from immaturity, including respiratory distress syndrome, intraventricular hemorrhage, patent ductus arteriosus, and necrotizing enterocolitis.

D. Premature gestational age is a more significant cause of neonatal morbidity than is the duration of membrane rupture.

III. Diagnosis of premature rupture of membranes

A. Diagnosis is based on history, physical examination, and laboratory testing. The patient's history alone is correct in 90% of patients. Urinary leakage or excess vaginal discharge is sometimes mistaken for PROM.

B. **Sterile speculum exam** is the first step in confirming the suspicion of PROM. Digital examination should be avoided because it increases the risk of infection.

1. The general appearance of the cervix should be assessed visually, and prolapse of the umbilical cord or a fetal extremity should be excluded. Cultures for group B streptococcus, gonorrhea, and chlamydia are obtained.

2. A pool of fluid in the posterior vaginal fornix supports the diagnosis of PROM.

3. The presence of amniotic fluid is confirmed by nitrazine testing for an alkaline pH. Amniotic fluid causes nitrazine paper to turn dark blue because the pH is above 6.0-6.5. Nitrazine may be false-positive with contamination from blood, semen, or vaginitis.

4. If pooling and nitrazine are both non-confirmatory, a swab from the posterior fornix should be smeared on a slide, allowed to dry, and examined under a microscope for "ferning," indicating amniotic fluid.

5. Ultrasound examination for oligohydramnios is useful to confirm the diagnosis, but oligohydramnios may be caused by other disorders besides PROM.

IV. Assessment of premature rupture of membranes

A. The gestational age must be carefully assessed. Menstrual history, prenatal exams, and previous sonograms are reviewed. An ultrasound examination should be performed.

B. The patient should be evaluated for the presence of chorioamnionitis [fever (over 38°C), leukocytosis, maternal and fetal tachycardia, uterine tenderness, foul-smelling vaginal discharge].

C. The patient should be evaluated for labor, and a sterile speculum examination should assess cervical change.

D. The fetus should be evaluated with heart rate monitoring because PROM increases the risk of umbilical cord prolapse and fetal distress caused by oligohydramnios.

V. Management of premature rupture of membranes

A. Term patients

1. At 36 weeks and beyond, management of PROM consists of delivery. Patients in active labor should be allowed to progress.

2. Patients with chorioamnionitis, who are not in labor, should be immediately induced with oxytocin (Pitocin).

3. Patients who are not yet in active labor (in the absence of fetal distress, meconium, or clinical infection) may be discharged for 48 hours, and labor usually follows. If labor has not begun within a reasonable time after rupture of membranes, induction with oxytocin (Pitocin) is appropriate. Use of prostaglandin E2 is safe for cervical ripening.

B. Preterm patients

1. Preterm patients with PROM prior to 36 weeks are managed expectantly. Delivery is delayed for the patients who are not in labor, not infected, and without evidence of fetal distress.

2. Patients should be monitored for infection. Cultures for gonococci, Chlamydia, and group B streptococci are obtained. Symptoms, vital signs, uterine tenderness, odor of the lochia, and leukocyte counts are monitored.

3. Suspected occult chorioamnionitis is diagnosed by amniocentesis for Gram stain and culture, which will reveal gram positive cocci in chains.

4. Ultrasound examination should be performed to detect oligohydramnios.

5. **Antibiotic prophylaxis for group B Streptococcus**. Intrapartum chemoprophylaxis consists of penicillin G, 5 million units, then 2.5 million units IV every 4 hours until delivery. Ampicillin, 2 g initially and then 1 g IV every 4 hours until delivery, is an alternative. Clindamycin or erythromycin may be used for women allergic to penicillin.

6. Prolonged continuous fetal heart rate monitoring in the initial assessment should be followed by frequent fetal evaluation.

7. Premature labor is the most common outcome of preterm PROM. Tocolytic drugs are often used and corticosteroids are recommended to accelerate fetal pulmonary maturity.

8. Expectant management consists of in-hospital observation. Delivery is indicated for chorioamnionitis, irreversible fetal distress, or premature labor. Once gestation reaches 36 weeks, the patient may be managed as any other term patient with PROM. Another option is to evaluate the fetus at less than 36 weeks for pulmonary maturity and expedite delivery once maturity is documented by testing of amniotic fluid collected by amniocentesis or from the vagina. A positive phosphatidylglycerol test indicates fetal lung maturity.

C. Previable or preterm premature rupture of membranes

1. In patients in whom membranes rupture very early in pregnancy (eg, <25 weeks). There is a relatively low likelihood (<25%) that a surviving infant will be delivered, and infants that do survive will deliver very premature and suffer significant morbidity.

2. **Fetal deformation syndrome.** The fetus suffering from prolonged early oligohydramnios may develop pulmonary hypoplasia, facial deformation,

limb contractures, and deformity.
3. Termination of pregnancy is advisable if the gestational age is early. If the patient elects to continue the pregnancy, expectant management with pelvic rest at home is reasonable.

D. Chorioamnionitis
1. Chorioamnionitis requires delivery (usually vaginally), regardless of the gestational age.
2. **Antibiotic therapy**
   a. Ampicillin 2 gm IV q4-6h **AND**
   b. Gentamicin 100 mg (2 mg/kg) IV load, then 100 mg (1.5 mg/kg) IV q8h.

References: See page 290.

Preterm Labor

Preterm labor is the leading cause of perinatal morbidity and mortality in the United States. It usually results in preterm birth, a complication that affects 8 to 10 percent of births.

Risk Factors for Preterm Labor	
Previous preterm delivery Low socioeconomic status Non-white race Maternal age <18 years or >40 years Preterm premature rupture of the membranes Multiple gestation Maternal history of one or more spontaneous second-trimester abortions Maternal complications --Maternal behaviors --Smoking--Illicit drug use --Alcohol use --Lack of prenatal care Uterine causes --Myomata (particularly submucosal or subplacental) --Uterine septum --Bicornuate uterus --Cervical incompetence --Exposure to diethylstilbestrol (DES)	Infectious causes --Chorioamnionitis --Bacterial vaginosis --Asymptomatic bacteriuria --Acute pyelonephritis --Cervical/vaginal colonization Fetal causes --Intrauterine fetal death --Intrauterine growth retardation --Congenital anomalies Abnormal placentation Presence of a retained intrauterine device

I. **Risk factors for preterm labor.** Preterm labor is characterized by cervical effacement and/or dilatation, and increased uterine irritability that occurs before 37 weeks of gestation. Women with a history of previous preterm delivery carry the highest risk of recurrence, estimated to be between 17 and 37 percent.

Preterm Labor, Threatened or Actual

1. Initial assessment to determine whether patient is experiencing preterm labor
   a. Assess for the following:
      i. Uterine activity
      ii. Rupture of membranes
      iii. Vaginal bleeding
      iv. Presentation
      v. Cervical dilation and effacement
      vi. Station
   b. Reassess estimate of gestational age
2. Search for a precipitating factor/cause
3. Consider specific management strategies, which may include the following:
   a. Intravenous tocolytic therapy (decision should be influenced by gestational age, cause of preterm labor and contraindications)
   b. Corticosteroid therapy (eg, betamethasone, in a dosage of 12 mg IM every 24 hours for a total of two doses)
   c. Antibiotic therapy if specific infectious agent is identified or if preterm premature rupture of the membranes

II. Management of preterm labor
A. Tocolysis
1. Tocolytic therapy may offer some short-term benefit in the management of preterm labor. A delay in delivery can be used to administer corticosteroids to enhance pulmonary maturity and reduce the severity of fetal respiratory distress syndrome, and to reduce the risk of intraventricular hemorrhage. No study has convincingly demonstrated an improvement in survival or neonatal outcome with the use of tocolytic therapy alone.
2. Contraindications to tocolysis include nonreassuring fetal heart rate tracing, eclampsia or severe preeclampsia, fetal demise (singleton), chorioamnionitis, fetal maturity and maternal hemodynamic instability.
3. Tocolytic therapy is indicated for regular uterine contractions and cervical change (effacement or dilatation). Oral terbutaline (Bricanyl) following successful parenteral tocolysis is not associated with prolonged pregnancy or reduced incidence of recurrent preterm labor.

Tocolytic Therapy for the Management of Preterm Labor		
Medication	**Mechanism of action**	**Dosage**
Magnesium sulfate	Intracellular calcium antagonism	4 to 6 g loading dose; then 2 to 4 g IV every hour
Terbutaline (Bricanyl)	Beta$_2$-adrenergic receptor agonist sympathomimetic; decreases free intracellular calcium ions	0.25 to 0.5 mg SC every three to four hours
Ritodrine (Yutopar)	Same as terbutaline	0.05 to 0.35 mg per minute IV
Nifedipine (Procardia)	Calcium channel blocker	5 to 10 mg SL every 15 to 20 minutes (up to four times), then 10 to 20 mg orally every four to six hours
Indomethacin (Indocin)	Prostaglandin inhibitor	50- to 100-mg rectal suppository, then 25 to 50 mg orally every six hours

Complications Associated With the Use of Tocolytic Agents

Magnesium sulfate
- Pulmonary edema
- Profound hypotension
- Profound muscular paralysis
- Maternal tetany
- Cardiac arrest
- Respiratory depression

Beta-adrenergic agents
- Hypokalemia
- Hyperglycemia
- Hypotension
- Pulmonary edema
- Arrhythmias
- Cardiac insufficiency
- Myocardial ischemia
- Maternal death

Indomethacin (Indocin)
- Renal failure
- Hepatitis
- Gastrointestinal bleeding

Nifedipine (Procardia)
- Transient hypotension

B. **Corticosteroid therapy**
   1. Dexamethasone and betamethasone are the preferred corticosteroids for antenatal therapy. Corticosteroid therapy for fetal maturation reduces mortality, respiratory distress syndrome and intraventricular hemorrhage in infants between 24 and 34 weeks of gestation.
   2. In women with preterm premature rapture of membranes (PPROM), antenatal corticosteroid therapy reduces the risk of respiratory distress syndrome. In women with PPROM at less than 30 to 32 weeks of gestation, in the absence of clinical chorioamnionitis, antenatal corticosteroid use is recommended because of the high risk of intraventricular hemorrhage at this early gestational age.

Recommended Antepartum Corticosteroid Regimens for Fetal Maturation in Preterm Infants

Medication	Dosage
Betamethasone (Celestone)	12 mg IM every 24 hours for two doses
Dexamethasone	6 mg IM every 12 hours for four doses

C. **Antibiotic therapy**. Group B streptococcal disease continues to be a major cause of illness and death among newborn infants and has been associated with preterm labor. A gestational age of less than 37 weeks is one of the major risk factors for group B streptococcal disease; therefore, prophylaxis is recommended

Recommended Regimens for Intrapartum Antimicrobial Prophylaxis for Perinatal Group B Streptococcal Disease

Regimen	Dosage
Recommended	Penicillin G, 5 million U IV, then 2.5 million U IV every four hours until delivery
Alternative	Ampicillin, 2 g IV loading dose, then 1 g IV every four hours until delivery

Regimen	Dosage
In patients allergic to penicillin	
Recommended	Clindamycin (Cleocin), 900 mg IV every eight hours until delivery
Alternative	Erythromycin, 500 mg IV every six hours until delivery

    D. Bed rest. Although bed rest is often prescribed for women at high risk for preterm labor and delivery, there are no conclusive studies documenting its benefit. A recent meta-analysis found no benefit to bed rest in the prevention of preterm labor or delivery.

References: See page 290.

Bleeding in the Second Half of Pregnancy

Bleeding in the second half of pregnancy occurs in 4% of all pregnancies. In 50% of cases, vaginal bleeding is secondary to placental abruption or placenta previa.

I. **Clinical evaluation of bleeding second half of pregnancy**
   A. **History** of trauma or pain and the amount and character of the bleeding should be assessed.
   B. **Physical examination**
     1. Vital signs and pulse pressure are measured. Hypotension and tachycardia are signs of serious hypovolemia.
     2. Fetal heart rate pattern and uterine activity are assessed.
     3. Ultrasound examination of the uterus, placenta and fetus should be completed.
     4. Speculum and digital pelvic examination should not be done until placenta previa has been excluded.
   C. **Laboratory Evaluation**
     1. **Hemoglobin** and hematocrit.
     2. **INR, partial thromboplastin time, platelet count, fibrinogen level, and fibrin split products** are checked when placental abruption is suspected or if there has been significant hemorrhage.
     3. **A red-top tube** of blood is used to perform a bedside clot test.
     4. **Blood type** and cross-match.
     5. **Urinalysis** for hematuria and proteinuria.
     6. The **Apt test** is used to distinguish maternal or fetal source of bleeding. (Vaginal blood is mixed with an equal part 0.25% sodium hydroxide. Fetal blood remains red; maternal blood turns brown.)
     7. **Kleihauer-Betke test** of maternal blood is used to quantify fetal to maternal hemorrhage.
II. **Placental abruption (abruptio placentae)** is defined as complete or partial placental separation from the decidua basalis after 20 weeks gestation.
   A. Placental abruption occurs in 1 in 100 deliveries.
   B. **Factors associated with placental abruption**
     1. Preeclampsia and hypertensive disorders
     2. History of placental abruption
     3. High multiparity
     4. Increasing maternal age
     5. Trauma
     6. Cigarette smoking
     7. Illicit drug use (especially cocaine)
     8. Excessive alcohol consumption
     9. Preterm premature rupture of the membranes

10. Rapid uterine decompression after delivery of the first fetus in a twin gestation or rupture of membranes with polyhydramnios
11. Uterine leiomyomas

C. Diagnosis of placental abruption

1. Abruption is characterized by vaginal bleeding, abdominal pain, uterine tenderness, and uterine contractions.
   a. Vaginal bleeding is visible in 80%; bleeding is concealed in 20%.
   b. Pain is usually of sudden onset, constant, and localized to the uterus and lower back.
   c. Localized or generalized uterine tenderness and increased uterine tone are found with severe placental abruption.
   d. An increase in uterine size may occur with placental abruption when the bleeding is concealed. Concealed bleeding may be detected by serial measurements of abdominal girth and fundal height.
   e. Amniotic fluid may be bloody.
   f. Fetal monitoring may detect distress.
   g. Placental abruption may cause preterm labor.
2. **Uterine contractions** by tocodynamometry is the most sensitive indicator of abruption.
3. **Laboratory findings** include proteinuria and a consumptive coagulopathy, characterized by decreased fibrinogen, prothrombin, factors V and VIII, and platelets. Fibrin split products are elevated.
4. **Ultrasonography** has a sensitivity in detecting placental abruption of only 15%.

D. Management of placental abruption

1. **Mild placental abruption**
   a. If maternal stability and reassuring fetal surveillance are assured and the fetus is immature, close expectant observation with fetal monitoring is justified.
   b. Maternal hematologic parameters are monitored and abnormalities corrected.
   c. Tocolysis with magnesium sulfate is initiated if the fetus is immature.
2. **Moderate to severe placental abruption**
   a. Shock is aggressively managed.
   b. **Coagulopathy**
      (1) Blood is transfused to replace blood loss.
      (2) Clotting factors may be replaced using cryoprecipitate or fresh-frozen plasma. One unit of fresh-frozen plasma increases fibrinogen by 10 mg/dL. Cryoprecipitate contains 250 mg fibrinogen/unit; 4 gm (15-20 U) is an effective dose.
      (3) Platelet transfusion is indicated if the platelet count is less than 50,000/mcL. One unit of platelets raises the platelet count 5000-10,000/mcL; 4 to 6 U is the smallest useful dose.
   c. **Oxygen** should be administered and urine output monitored with a Foley catheter.
   d. Vaginal delivery is expedited in all but the mildest cases once the mother has been stabilized. Amniotomy and oxytocin (Pitocin) augmentation may be used. Cesarean section is indicated for fetal distress, severe abruption, or failed trial of labor.

III. **Placenta previa** occurs when any part of the placenta implants in the lower uterine segment. It is associated with a risk of serious maternal hemorrhage. Placenta previa occurs in 1 in 200 pregnancies. Ninety percent of placenta previas diagnosed in the second trimester resolve spontaneously.

A. **Total placenta previa** occurs when the internal cervical os is completely covered by placenta.
B. **Partial placenta previa** occurs when part of the cervical os is covered by placenta.
C. **Marginal placenta previa** occurs when the placental edge is located within 2 cm of the cervical os.
D. **Clinical evaluation**
   1. Placenta previa presents with a sudden onset of painless vaginal bleeding in the second or third trimester. The peak incidence occurs at

34 weeks. The initial bleeding usually resolves spontaneously and then recurs later in pregnancy.
   2. One fourth of patients present with bleeding and uterine contractions.
   E. **Ultrasonography** is accurate in diagnosing placenta previa.
   F. **Management of placenta previa**
      1. In a pregnancy ≥36 weeks with documented fetal lung maturity, the neonate should be immediately delivered by cesarean section.
      2. Low vertical uterine incision is probably safer in patients with an anterior placenta. Incisions through the placenta should be avoided.
      3. If severe hemorrhage jeopardizes the mother or fetus, cesarean section is indicated regardless of gestational age.
      4. Expectant management is appropriate for immature fetuses if bleeding is not excessive, maternal physical activity can be restricted, intercourse and douching can be prohibited, and the hemoglobin can be maintained at ≥10 mg/dL.
      5. Rh immunoglobulin is administered to Rh-negative-unsensitized patients.
      6. Delivery is indicated once fetal lung maturity has been documented.
      7. Tocolysis with magnesium sulfate may be used for immature fetuses.
IV. **Cervical bleeding**
   A. Cytologic sampling is necessary.
   B. Bleeding can be controlled with cauterization or packing.
   C. Bacterial and viral cultures are sometimes diagnostic.
V. **Cervical polyps**
   A. Bleeding is usually self-limited.
   B. Trauma should be avoided.
   C. Polypectomy may control bleeding and yield a histologic diagnosis.
VI. **Bloody show** is a frequent benign cause of late third trimester bleeding. It is characterized by blood-tinged mucus associated with cervical change.
References: See page 290.

Pregnancy-Induced Hypertension

Women with hypertension during pregnancy typically present with few or no symptoms. The incidence of hypertension during pregnancy is 6 to 8 percent.

I. **Pathophysiology**
   A. **Chronic hypertension** is defined as hypertension before the pregnancy or early in the pregnancy.
   B. **Pregnancy-induced hypertension** occurs in about 5 percent of pregnancies. ACOG defines preeclampsia as pregnancy-induced hypertension accompanied by renal involvement and proteinuria. Eclampsia is preeclampsia that progresses to seizures. The HELLP syndrome (hemolysis, elevated liver enzymes, low platelet count) is a subcategory of pregnancy-induced hypertension.
   C. Blood pressure normally declines during the first trimester and reaches a nadir at 20 weeks gestation. Usually, blood pressure returns to baseline by term. This decline in blood pressure is not seen in women with pregnancy-induced hypertension. Women with chronic hypertension may be normotensive during pregnancy until term.
II. **Risk factors**
   A. Nulliparous women have an increased risk for preeclampsia. Women who are multiparous with a single partner are at the lowest risk. Daughters and sisters of women with a history of pregnancy-induced hypertension have an increased risk for the condition. Preeclampsia is more common in women with chronic hypertension or chronic renal disease.
   B. A history of preeclampsia is a primary risk factor. Other risk factors include diabetes, antiphospholipid antibody syndrome and molar pregnancy.
III. **Diagnosis**
   A. ACOG defines hypertension in pregnancy as a sustained blood pressure

of 140 mm Hg systolic or 90 mm Hg diastolic or greater. The onset of signs and symptoms of pregnancy-induced hypertension is usually after 20 weeks gestation

B. The classic triad of preeclampsia consists of hypertension, edema and proteinuria. A single urinalysis positive for proteinuria correlates poorly with the true level of proteinuria. A 24-hour urine collection that shows more than 300 mg protein per 24 hours is significant.

C. Excessive weight gain and edema are almost universally seen in preeclampsia. However, edema is also extremely common in normal pregnancies during the third trimester. Generalized edema is more significant than dependent edema occurring only in the lower extremities. Weight gain of greater than 1 to 2 lb per week may indicate significant fluid retention. An increasing hematocrit, which reflects intravascular dehydration, also often occurs in preeclampsia.

D. Renal function tests are often abnormal in preeclampsia. In normal pregnancies, the uric acid level declines during pregnancy and then returns to baseline by term. A uric acid level of greater than 5.0 mg per dL may indicate preeclampsia. Creatinine levels decrease from a normal of 1.0 to 1.5 mg per dL to 0.8 mg per dL or less throughout normal pregnancy but are increased in preeclampsia. Decreased renal perfusion may be indicated by the presence of creatinine levels at term that are the same as normal prepregnancy levels.

E. As preeclampsia worsens and with the HELLP syndrome, liver function test results may become abnormal and platelet levels may significantly decrease. Abnormal liver function test results and low platelet levels reflect the severity of preeclampsia and the possibility of development of disseminated intravascular coagulation (DIC).

F. **Severe pregnancy-induced hypertension** is indicated by symptoms of headache, blurred vision or abdominal pain in combination with elevated blood pressure.

G. **Clinical evaluation** of pregnancy-induced hypertension should include symptoms of headache, visual disturbances and abdominal pain. The woman's blood pressure should be taken in a sitting position five minutes after she is seated. The physical examination should include evaluation of the heart, lungs and abdomen, and neurologic system. Signs of end-organ effects, weight gain and edema should be sought.

H. **Laboratory evaluation.** The urine should be tested for protein. A complete blood count with platelet count, urinalysis, creatinine level, uric acid, a 24-hour urine collection, creatinine clearance and liver function tests should be completed. A screen for early DIC, including fibrin-split products, prothrombin time and total fibrinogen, should be done.

I. **Fetal well-being** and placental function should be assessed with a BPP or an amniotic fluid index and NST. Severe pregnancy-induced hypertension can result in fetal growth restriction. An ultrasound to assess fetal weight and gestational age should verify adequate fetal growth.

IV. Treatment

A. Delivery of the fetus is the only cure for pregnancy-induced hypertension.

B. **Mild disease**

1. Women with mild elevations in blood pressure and proteinuria but no evidence of severe signs or symptoms may be safely observed without immediate treatment or delivery. Women with mild preeclampsia at term should be considered candidates for induction of labor. Mild elevations in blood pressure (<170 mmHg systolic or <105 mmHg diastolic) do not require treatment with antihypertensive medications.

2. **Initial evaluation** may take place in the hospital with fetal monitoring, 24-hour urine collection and monitoring for progression of disease. All women managed as outpatients should be instructed to contact the physician if any symptoms of severe pregnancy-induced hypertension appear. Follow-up should include tests for proteinuria, blood pressure assessment, home health care nursing and frequent clinic visits. Bi-weekly NSTs, amniotic fluid index assessments, BPPs and serial ultrasounds to document appropriate fetal growth are needed to ensure

fetal well-being.
3. **Nonstress testing.** The nonstress test is performed after 32 to 34 weeks, 2-3 times a week or more.
4. **Ultrasonic assessment.** A baseline study is completed at 18 to 24 weeks. Monitoring of fetal growth and amniotic fluid index is initiated at 30 to 32 weeks.
C. **Moderate to severe disease**
   1. Women with any of the signs and symptoms of severe pregnancy-induced hypertension require hospitalization. Induction of labor is usually indicated to facilitate prompt delivery. Women at greater than 34 weeks gestation are delivered immediately.
   2. Treatment for women at earlier gestations (28 to 34 weeks) consists of conservative observation or immediate delivery. Monitoring may include daily antenatal testing, initial invasive monitoring for fluid status, seizure prophylaxis with magnesium sulfate and administration of corticosteroids.

Clinical Manifestations of Severe Disease in Women with Pregnancy-Induced Hypertension

Blood pressure greater than 160 to 180 mm Hg systolic or greater than 110 mm Hg diastolic
Proteinuria greater than 5 g per 24 hours (normal: less than 300 mg per 24 hours)
Elevated serum creatinine
Grand mal seizures (eclampsia)
Pulmonary edema
Oliguria less than 500 mL per 24 hours
Microangiopathic hemolysis
Thrombocytopenia
Hepatocellular dysfunction (elevated ALT, AST)
Intrauterine growth restriction or oligohydramnios
Symptoms suggesting significant end-organ involvement (ie, headache, visual disturbances, epigastric or right upper-quadrant pain)

---

3. **Magnesium sulfate** is an effective treatment for prevention of seizures in preeclampsia. An intravenous loading dose of 4 g over 20 minutes is given, followed by a dosage regimen of 2 to 3 g per hour. Serum drug levels and side effects should be carefully monitored.
4. **Hypertension** should be treated when blood pressure increases to higher than 170 mm Hg systolic or 105 mm Hg diastolic. Treatment consists of intravenous hydralazine (Apresoline), 6.25 to 25.0 mg every four to six hours. Recent studies have also used oral labetalol (Normodyne, Trandate) , 600 mg PO qid, or oral nifedipine, 20 mg PO q4h. Maintaining the blood pressure between 140 and 150 mm Hg systolic and between 90 and 100 mm Hg diastolic decreases the risk of placental hypoperfusion.
5. **Betamethasone (Celestone)** is given to women with a pregnancy between 28 and 34 weeks gestation in order to improve fetal lung maturity and neonatal survival.

V. Intrapartum management of hypertension

A. **Intrapartum prevention of seizures**. **Magnesium sulfate** is administered to all patients with hypertension at term to prevent seizures when delivery is indicated. An intravenous loading bolus of 4 g IV over 20 minutes, followed by continuous infusion of 2 g/h. When symptomatic magnesium overdose is suspected (apnea, obtundation), it can be reversed by the intravenous administration of 10% calcium gluconate, 10 mL IV over 2 minutes. Magnesium prophylaxis must be continued in the immediate postpartum period, as the risk of seizures is highest in the intrapartum stage and during the first 24 hours following delivery.

B. **Intrapartum blood pressure control**
   1. When blood pressure exceeds 105 mmHg diastolic or 170 mmHg systolic blood pressure should be lowered with intravenous hydralazine.
   2. Hydralazine is given IV as a 5-10-mg bolus as often as every 20 minutes as necessary. The goal of treatment is a systolic of 140-150 mmHg and a diastolic of 90-100 mmHg.
   3. Labetalol, 20 mg, given IV as often as every 10 minutes to a maximum dose of 300 mg, is an acceptable alternative. Unresponsive blood pressure can occasionally require sodium nitroprusside, with central hemodynamic monitoring.

C. **Vaginal delivery** is generally preferable to cesarean delivery, even in patients with manifestations of severe disease. Cervical ripening with prostaglandin E_2 gel may be considered; however, a seriously ill patient with an unfavorable cervix should receive a cesarean section.

References: See page 290.

Herpes Simplex Virus Infections in Pregnancy

Two types of herpes simplex virus have been identified, herpes simplex virus type 1 (HSV-1) and herpes simplex virus type 2 (HSV-2). Initial contact with HSV usually occurs early in childhood and usually involves HSV-1. Herpes simplex virus type 1 causes most nongenital herpetic lesions: eg, herpes labialis, gingivostomatitis, and keratoconjunctivitis. The female genital tract can be infected with HSV-1 or HSV-2. Most genital infection is from HSV-2.

I. Incidence

A. Herpes simplex virus infection of the genital tract is one of the most common viral STDs. The greatest incidence of overt HSV-2 infection occurs in women in their late teens and early twenties. However, 30% of the female population in the United States have antibodies to HSV-2.

B. Newborns may become infected in the perinatal period from contact with infected maternal secretions. Most newborns acquire the virus from asymptomatic mothers without identified lesions.

II. Presentation of infection

A. **Primary infection**
   1. Initial genital infection due to herpes may be either asymptomatic or associated with severe symptoms. With symptomatic primary infection, lesions may occur on the vulva, vagina, or cervix, or on all three, between 2 and 14 days following exposure to infectious virus. The initial vesicles rupture and subsequently appear as shallow and eroded ulcers. Inguinal lymphadenopathy is common.
   2. Systemic symptoms (malaise, myalgia, and fever) may occur with primary herpetic infections. Local symptoms of pain, dysuria, and soreness of the vulva and vagina are common in both primary and recurrent infections. The lesions of primary infection tends to resolve within 3 weeks without therapy.

B. **Nonprimary first episode disease** is associated with fewer systemic manifestations, less pain, a briefer duration of viral shedding, and a more rapid resolution of the clinical lesions in the nonprimary infection. These episodes usually are thought to be the result of an initial HSV-2 infection in the presence of partially protective HSV-1 antibodies.

C. **Recurrences of genital HSV infection** can be symptomatic or subclinical. The ulcers tend to be limited in size, number, and duration. Local symptoms predominate over systemic symptoms, with many patients indicating increased vaginal discharge or pain. Shedding of the virus from the genital tract without symptoms or signs of clinical lesions (subclinical shedding) is episodic.

D. **Neonatal herpes.** Most neonatal HSV infection is the consequence of delivery of a neonate through an infected birth canal. There are three categories of neonatal disease: localized disease of the skin, eye, and mouth; central nervous system (CNS) disease with or without skin, eye, and mouth disease; or disseminated disease. Most infected neonates have localized skin, eye, and mouth disease, which generally is a mild illness. Localized disease may progress to encephalitis or disseminated disease. Skin, eye, and mouth disease is usually self-limited. CNS disease has a 15% mortality, and there is a 57% mortality with disseminated disease.

III. Transmission

A. **Sexual and direct contact.** Herpes simplex virus is transmitted via direct contact with an individual who is infected. Genital-to-genital contact or contact of the genital tract with an area that is infected with HSV, such as oral-to-genital contact, can result in transmission.

B. **Maternal-fetal transmission.** Vertical transmission rates at the time of vaginal delivery based on the type of maternal disease may be summarized as follows: primary HSV result in 50% transmission; nonprimary first-episode HSV result in 33% transmission; and recurrent HSV result in 0-3% transmission.

IV. Laboratory diagnosis

A. The standard and most sensitive test for detecting HSV from clinical specimens is isolation of the virus by cell culture. More sensitive techniques are increasingly available, such as polymerase chain reaction and hybridization methods.

B. Early primary and nonprimary first-episode ulcers yield the virus in 80% of patients, whereas ulcers from recurrent infections are less likely to be culture-positive; only 40% of crusted lesions contain recoverable virus. When testing for HSV, overt lesions that are not in the ulcerated state should be unroofed and the fluid sampled.

V. Medical management

A. **Medical management of women with primary HSV infection during pregnancy.** Antiviral therapy for primary infection is recommended for women with primary HSV infection during pregnancy to reduce viral shedding and enhance lesion healing. Primary infection during pregnancy constitutes a higher risk for vertical transmission than does recurrent infection. Suppressive therapy for the duration of the pregnancy should be considered to reduce the potential of continued viral shedding and the likelihood of recurrent episodes.

B. **Medical management of women with recurrent HSV infection during pregnancy.** Acyclovir should be considered after 36 weeks of gestation in women with recurrent genital herpes infection because it results in a significant decrease in clinical recurrences. The likelihood of cesarean deliveries performed for active infection is not reduced significantly by acyclovir.

C. **Acyclovir (Zovirax),** a class-C medication, has activity against HSV- 1 and HSV-2. In the treatment of primary genital herpes infections, oral acyclovir reduces viral shedding, reduces pain, and heals lesions faster when compared with a placebo. Acyclovir has been shown to be safe in pregnancy and has minimal side effects. Oral dosage is 400 mg tid.

D. **Valacyclovir (Valtrex) and famciclovir (Famvir)** are class-B medications. Their increased bio-availability means that they may require less frequent dosing to achieve the same therapeutic benefits as acyclovir. The U.S. Food and Drug Administration has approved both valacyclovir and famciclovir for the treatment of primary genital herpes, the treatment of episodes of recurrent disease, and the daily treatment for suppression of

outbreaks of recurrent genital herpes.
  E. Valacyclovir therapy, 500 mg once daily, is effective in suppressing recurrent genital herpes. Suppressive famciclovir therapy requires a 250 mg twice daily.
VI. **Cesarean delivery** is indicated for term pregnancies with active genital lesions or symptoms of vulvar pain or burning, which may indicate an impending outbreak.
VII. **Active HSV and preterm premature rupture of membranes**. In pregnancies remote from term, especially in women with recurrent disease, the pregnancy should be continued to gain benefit from time and glucocorticoids. Treatment with an antiviral agent is indicated.
References: See page 290.

Dystocia and Augmentation of Labor

I. **Normal labor**
  A. **First stage of labor**
    1. The first stage of labor consists of the period from the onset of labor until complete cervical dilation (10 cm). This stage is divided into the latent phase and the active phase.
    2. **Latent phase**
      a. During the latent phase, uterine contractions are infrequent and irregular and result in only modest discomfort. They result in gradual effacement and dilation of the cervix.
      b. A prolonged latent phase is one that exceeds 20 hours in the nullipara or one that exceeds 14 hours in the multipara.
    3. **Active phase**
      a. The active phase of labor occurs when the cervix reaches 3-4 cm of dilatation.
      b. The active phase of labor is characterized by an increased rate of cervical dilation and by descent of the presenting fetal part.
  B. **Second stage of labor**
    1. **The second stage of labor** consists of the period from complete cervical dilation (10 cm) until delivery of the infant. This stage is usually brief, averaging 20 minutes for parous women and 50 minutes for nulliparous women.
    2. The duration of the second stage of labor is unrelated to perinatal outcome in the absence of a nonreassuring fetal heart rate pattern as long as progress occurs.
II. **Abnormal labor**
  A. **Dystocia** is defined as difficult labor or childbirth resulting from abnormalities of the cervix and uterus, the fetus, the maternal pelvis, or a combination of these factors.
  B. **Cephalopelvic disproportion** is a disparity between the size of the maternal pelvis and the fetal head that precludes vaginal delivery. This condition can rarely be diagnosed in advance.
  C. **Slower-than-normal (protraction disorders) or complete cessation of progress (arrest disorder)** are disorders that can be diagnosed only after the parturient has entered the active phase of labor.
III. **Assessment of labor abnormalities**
  A. **Labor abnormalities caused by inadequate uterine contractility (powers)**. The minimal uterine contractile pattern of women in spontaneous labor consists of 3 to 5 contractions in a 10-minute period.
  B. **Labor abnormalities caused by fetal characteristics (passenger)**
    1. Assessment of the fetus consists of estimating fetal weight and position. Estimations of fetal size, even those obtained by ultrasonography, are frequently inaccurate.
    2. In the first stage of labor, the diagnosis of dystocia can not be made unless the active phase of labor and adequate uterine contractile forces have been present.

    3. Fetal anomalies such as hydrocephaly, encephalocele, and soft tissue tumors may obstruct labor. Fetal imaging should be considered when malpresentation or anomalies are suspected based on vaginal or abdominal examination or when the presenting fetal part is persistently high.

C. Labor abnormalities due to the pelvic passage (passage)
    1. Inefficient uterine action should be corrected before attributing dystocia to a pelvic problem.
    2. The bony pelvis is very rarely the factor that limits vaginal delivery of a fetus in cephalic presentation. Radiographic pelvimetry is of limited value in managing most cephalic presentations.
    3. Clinical pelvimetry can only be useful to qualitatively identify the general architectural features of the pelvis.

IV. Augmentation of labor
  A. Uterine hypocontractility should be augmented only after both the maternal pelvis and fetal presentation have been assessed.
  B. Contraindications to augmentation include placenta or vasa previa, umbilical cord prolapse, prior classical uterine incision, pelvic structural deformities, and invasive cervical cancer.
  C. Oxytocin (Pitocin)
    1. The goal of oxytocin administration is to stimulate uterine activity that is sufficient to produce cervical change and fetal descent while avoiding uterine hyperstimulation and fetal compromise.
    2. Minimally effective uterine activity is 3 contractions per 10 minutes averaging greater than 25 mm Hg above baseline. A maximum of 5 contractions in a 10-minute period with resultant cervical dilatation is considered adequate.
    3. Hyperstimulation is characterized by more than five contractions in 10 minutes, contractions lasting 2 minutes or more, or contractions of normal duration occurring within 1 minute of each other.
    4. Oxytocin is administered when a patient is progressing slowly through the latent phase of labor or has a protraction or an arrest disorder of labor, or when a hypotonic uterine contraction pattern is identified.
    5. A pelvic examination should be performed before initiation of oxytocin infusion.
    6. Oxytocin is usually diluted 10 units in 1 liter of normal saline IVPB.

Labor Stimulation with Oxytocin (Pitocin)				
Regimen	Starting Dose (mU/min)	Incremental Increase (mU/min)	Dosage Interval (min)	Maximum Dose (mU/min)
Low-Dose	0.5-1	1	30-40	20

    7. Management of oxytocin-induced hyperstimulation
      a. The most common adverse effect of hyperstimulation is fetal heart rate deceleration associated with uterine hyperstimulation. Stopping or decreasing the dose of oxytocin may correct the abnormal pattern.
      b. Additional measures may include changing the patient to the lateral decubitus position and administering oxygen or more intravenous fluid.
      c. If oxytocin-induced uterine hyperstimulation does not respond to conservative measures, intravenous terbutaline (0.125-0.25 mg) or magnesium sulfate (2-6 g in 10-20% dilution) may be used to stop uterine contractions.

References: See page 290.

Fetal Macrosomia

Excessive birth weight is associated with an increased risk of maternal and neonatal injury. Macrosomia is defined as a fetus with an estimated weight of more than 4,500 grams, regardless of gestational age.

I. **Diagnosis of macrosomia**
   A. Clinical estimates of fetal weight based on Leopold's maneuvers or fundal height measurements are often inaccurate.
   B. Diagnosis of macrosomia requires ultrasound evaluation; however, estimation of fetal weight based on ultrasound is associated with a large margin of error.
   C. Maternal weight, height, previous obstetric history, fundal height, and the presence of gestational diabetes should be evaluated.

II. **Factors influencing fetal weight**
   A. **Gestational age.** Post-term pregnancy is a risk factor for macrosomia. At 42 weeks and beyond, 2.5% of fetuses weigh more than 4,500 g. Ten to twenty percent of macrosomic infants are post-term fetuses.
   B. **Maternal weight.** Heavy women have a greater risk of giving birth to excessively large infants. Fifteen to 35% of women who deliver macrosomic fetuses weigh 90 kg or more.
   C. **Multiparity.** Macrosomic infants are 2-3 times more likely to be born to parous women.
   D. **Macrosomia in a prior infant.** The risk of delivering an infant weighing more than 4,500 g is increased if a prior infant weighed more than 4,000 g.
   E. **Maternal diabetes**
      1. Maternal diabetes increases the risk of fetal macrosomia and shoulder dystocia.
      2. Cesarean delivery is indicated when the estimated fetal weight exceeds 4,500 g.

III. **Morbidity and mortality**
   A. **Abnormalities of labor.** Macrosomic fetuses have a higher incidence of labor abnormalities and instrumental deliveries.
   B. **Maternal morbidity.** Macrosomic fetuses have a two- to threefold increased rate of cesarean delivery.
   C. **Birth injury**
      1. The incidence of birth injuries occurring during delivery of a macrosomic infant is much greater with vaginal than with cesarean birth. The most common injury is brachial plexus palsy, often caused by shoulder dystocia.
      2. The incidence of shoulder dystocia in infants weighing more than 4,500 g is 8-20%. Macrosomic infants also may sustain fractures of the clavicle or humerus.

IV. **Management of delivery**
   A. If the estimated fetal weight is greater than 4500 gm in the nondiabetic or greater than 4000 gm in the diabetic patient, delivery by cesarean section is indicated.
   B. **Management of shoulder dystocia**
      1. If a shoulder dystocia occurs, an assistant should provide suprapubic pressure to dislodge the impacted anterior fetal shoulder from the symphysis. McRobert maneuver (extreme hip flexion) should be done simultaneously.
      2. If the shoulder remains impacted anteriorly, an ample episiotomy should be cut and the posterior arm delivered.
      3. In almost all instances, one or both of these procedures will result in successful delivery. The Zavanelli maneuver consists of replacement of the fetal lead into the vaginal canal and delivery by emergency cesarean section.
      4. Fundal pressure is not recommended because it often results in further impaction of the shoulder against the symphysis.

References: See page 290.

Shoulder Dystocia

Shoulder dystocia, defined as failure of the shoulders to deliver following the head, is an obstetric emergency. The incidence varies from 0.6% to 1.4% of all vaginal deliveries. Up to 30% of shoulder dystocias can result in brachial plexus injury; many fewer sustain serious asphyxia or death. Most commonly, size discrepancy secondary to fetal macrosomia is associated with difficult shoulder delivery. Causal factors of macrosomia include maternal diabetes, postdates gestation, and obesity. The fetus of the diabetic gravida may also have disproportionately large shoulders and body size compared with the head.

I. Prediction
A. The diagnosis of shoulder dystocia is made after delivery of the head. The "turtle" sign is the retraction of the chin against the perineum or retraction of the head into the birth canal. This sign demonstrates that the shoulder girdle is resisting entry into the pelvic inlet, and possibly impaction of the anterior shoulder.
B. Macrosomia has the strongest association. ACOG defines macrosomia as an estimated fetal weight (EFW) greater than 4500 g.
C. Risk factors for macrosomia include maternal birth weight, prior macrosomia, preexisting diabetes, obesity, multiparity, advanced maternal age, and a prior shoulder dystocia. The recurrence rate has been reported to be 13.8%, nearly seven times the primary rate. Shoulder dystocia occurs in 5.1% of obese women. In the antepartum period, risk factors include gestational diabetes, excessive weight gain, short stature, macrosomia, and postterm pregnancy. Intrapartum factors include prolonged second stage of labor, abnormal first stage, arrest disorders, and instrumental (especially midforceps) delivery. Many shoulder dystocias will occur in the absence of any risk factors.

II. Management
A. Shoulder dystocia is a medical and possibly surgical emergency. Two assistants should be called for if not already present, as well as an anesthesiologist and pediatrician. A generous episiotomy should be cut. The following sequence is suggested:
   1. **McRoberts maneuver:** The legs are removed from the lithotomy position and flexed at the hips, with flexion of the knees against the abdomen. Two assistants are required. This maneuver may be performed prophylactically in anticipation of a difficult delivery.
   2. **Suprapubic pressure:** An assistant is requested to apply pressure downward, above the symphysis pubis. This can be done in a lateral direction to help dislodge the anterior shoulder from behind the pubic symphysis. It can also be performed in anticipation of a difficult delivery. Fundal pressure may increase the likelihood of uterine rupture and is contraindicated.
   3. **Rotational maneuvers:** The Woods' corkscrew maneuver consists of placing two fingers against the anterior aspect of the posterior shoulder. Gentle upward rotational pressure is applied so that the posterior shoulder girdle rotates anteriorly, allowing it to be delivered first. The Rubin maneuver is the reverse of Woods's maneuver. Two fingers are placed against the posterior aspect of the posterior (or anterior) shoulder and forward pressure applied. This results in adduction of the shoulders and displacement of the anterior shoulder from behind the symphysis pubis.
   4. **Posterior arm release:** The operator places a hand into the posterior vagina along the infant's back. The posterior arm is identified and followed to the elbow. The elbow is then swept across the chest, keeping the elbow flexed. The fetal forearm or hand is then grasped and the posterior arm delivered, followed by the anterior shoulder. If the fetus still remains undelivered, vaginal delivery should be abandoned and the Zavanelli maneuver performed followed by cesarean delivery.
   5. **Zavanelli maneuver:** The fetal head is replaced into the womb. Tocolysis is recommended to produce uterine relaxation. The maneuver

consists of rotation of the head to occiput anterior. The head is then flexed and pushed back into the vagina, followed abdominal delivery. Immediate preparations should be made for cesarean delivery.
6. If cephalic replacement fails, an emergency symphysiotomy should be performed. The urethra should be laterally displaced to minimize the risk of lower urinary tract injury.
B. The McRoberts maneuver alone will successfully alleviate the shoulder dystocia in 42% to 79% of cases. For those requiring additional maneuvers, vaginal delivery can be expected in more than 90%. Finally, favorable results have been reported for the Zavanelli maneuver in up to 90%.

References: See page 290.

Postdates Pregnancy

A term gestation is defined as one completed in 38 to 42 weeks. Pregnancy is considered prolonged or postdates when it exceeds 294 days or 42 weeks from the first day of the last menstrual period (LMP). About 10% of those pregnancies are postdates. The incidence of patients reaching the 42nd week is 3-12%.

I. **Morbidity and mortality**
   A. The rate of maternal, fetal, and neonatal complications increases with gestational age. The cesarean delivery rate more than doubles when passing the 42nd week compared with 40 weeks because of cephalopelvic disproportion resulting from larger infants and by fetal intolerance of labor.
   B. Neonatal complications from postdates pregnancies include placental insufficiency, birth trauma from macrosomia, meconium aspiration syndrome, and oligohydramnios.
II. **Diagnosis**
   A. The accurate diagnosis of postdates pregnancy can be made only by proper dating. The estimated date of confinement (EDC) is most accurately determined early in pregnancy. An EDC can be calculated by subtracting 3 months from the first day of the last menses and adding 7 days (Naegele's rule). Other clinical parameters that should be consistent with the EDC include maternal perception of fetal movements (quickening) at about 16 to 20 weeks; first auscultation of fetal heart tones with Doppler ultrasound by 12 weeks; uterine size at early examination (first trimester) consistent with dates; and, at 20 weeks, a fundal height 20 cm above the symphysis pubis or at the umbilicus.

Clinical Estimates of Gestational Age	
Parameter	**Gestational age (weeks)**
Positive urine hCG	5
Fetal heart tones by Doppler	11 to 12

Quickening
    Primigravida
    Multigravida
	
	20
	16

Fundal height at umbilicus	20

   B. In patients without reliable clinical data, ultrasound is beneficial. Ultrasonography is most accurate in early gestation. The crown-rump length becomes less accurate after 12 weeks in determining gestational age because the fetus begins to curve.
III. **Management of the postdates pregnancy**
   A. A postdates patient with a favorable cervix should receive induction of

labor. Only 8.2% of pregnancies at 42 weeks have a ripe cervix (Bishop score >6). Induction at 41 weeks with PGE_2 cervical ripening lowers the cesarean delivery rate.

B. Cervical ripening with prostaglandin
  1. Prostaglandin E_2 gel is a valuable tool for improving cervical ripeness and for increasing the likelihood of successful induction.
  2. Pre- and postapplication fetal monitoring are usually utilized. If the fetus has a nonreassuring heart rate tracing or there is excessive uterine activity, the use of PGE_2 gel is not advisable. The incidence of uterine hyperstimulation with PGE_2 gel, at approximately 5%, is comparable to that seen with oxytocin. Current PGE_2 modalities include the following:
     a. 2 to 3 mg of PGE_2 suspended in a gel placed intravaginally
     b. 0.5 mg of PGE_2 suspended in a gel placed intracervically (Prepidil)
     c. 10 mg of PGE_2 gel in a sustained-release tape (Cervidil)
     d. 25 μg of PGE_1 (one-fourth of tablet) placed intravaginally every 3 to 4 hours (misoprostol)

C. Stripping of membranes, starting at 38 weeks and repeated weekly may be an effective method of inducing labor in post-term women with a favorable cervix. Stripping of membranes is performed by placing a finger in the cervical os and circling 3 times in the plane between the fetal head and cervix.

D. Expectant management with antenatal surveillance
  1. Begin testing near the end of the 41st week of pregnancy. Antepartum testing consists of the nonstress test (NST) combined with the amniotic fluid index (AFI) twice weekly. The false-negative rate is 6.1/1000 (stillbirth within 1 week of a reassuring test) with twice weekly NSTs.
  2. The AFI involves measuring the deepest vertical fluid pocket in each uterine quadrant and summing the four together. Less than 5 cm is considered oligohydramnios, 5 to 8 cm borderline, and greater than 8 cm normal.

E. Fetal movement counting (kick counts). Fetal movement has been correlated with fetal health. It consist of having the mother lie on her side and count fetal movements. Perception of 10 distinct movements in a period of up to 2 hours is considered reassuring. After 10 movements have been perceived, the count may be discontinued.

F. Delivery is indicated if the amniotic fluid index is less than 5 cm, a nonreactive non-stress test is identified, or if decelerations are identified on the nonstress test.

G. Intrapartum management
  1. **Meconium staining** is more common in postdates pregnancies. If oligohydramnios is present, amnioinfusion dilutes meconium and decreases the number of infants with meconium below the vocal cords. Instillation of normal saline through an intrauterine pressure catheter may reduce variable decelerations.
  2. **Macrosomia** should be suspected in all postdates gestations. Fetal weight should be estimated prior to labor in all postdates pregnancies. Ultrasonographic weight predictions generally fall within 20% of the actual birth weight.
  3. **Management of suspected macrosomia.** The pediatrician and anesthesiologist should be notified so that they can prepare for delivery. Cesarean delivery should be considered in patients with an estimated fetal weight greater than 4500 g and a marginal pelvis, or someone with a previous difficult vaginal delivery with a similarly sized or larger infant.
  4. Intrapartum asphyxia is also more common in the postdates pregnancy. Therefore, close observation of the fetal heart rate tracing is necessary during labor. Variable decelerations representing cord compression are frequently seen in postdates pregnancies
  5. Cord compression can be treated with amnioinfusion, which can reduce variable decelerations. Late decelerations are more direct evidence of fetal hypoxia. If intermittent, late decelerations are managed conservatively with positioning and oxygen. If persistent late decelerations are associated with decreased variability or an elevated baseline fetal heart

rate, immediate evaluation or delivery is indicated. This additional evaluation can include observation for fetal heart acceleration following fetal scalp or acoustic stimulation, or a fetal scalp pH.

References: See page 290.

Induction of Labor

Induction of labor consists of stimulation of uterine contractions before the spontaneous onset of labor for the purpose of accomplishing delivery.

I. Indications and contraindications
 A. Common indications for induction of labor
   1. Pregnancy-induced hypertension
   2. Premature rupture of membranes
   3. Chorioamnionitis
   4. Suspected fetal jeopardy (eg, severe fetal growth restriction, isoimmunization)
   5. Maternal medical problems (eg, diabetes mellitus, renal disease)
   6. Fetal demise
   7. Postterm pregnancy
 B. Contraindications to labor induction or spontaneous labor
   1. Placenta previa or vasa previa
   2. Transverse fetal lie
   3. Prolapsed umbilical cord
   4. Prior classical uterine incision
 C. Obstetric conditions requiring special caution during induction
   1. Multifetal gestation
   2. Polyhydramnios
   3. Maternal cardiac disease
   4. Abnormal fetal heart rate patterns not requiring emergency delivery
   5. Grand multiparity
   6. Severe hypertension
   7. Breech presentation
   8. Presenting part above the pelvic inlet
 D. A trial of labor with induction is not contraindicated in women with one or more previous low transverse cesarean deliveries.
II. Requirements for induction
 A. Labor should be induced only after the mother and fetus have been examined and fetal maturity has been assured.
 B. Criteria for fetal maturity
   1. An ultrasound measurement of the crown-rump length, obtained at 6-11 weeks, supports a gestational age of 39 weeks or more.
   2. An ultrasound obtained at 12-20 weeks, confirms the gestational age of 39 weeks or more determined by history and physical examination.
   3. Fetal heart tones have been documented for 30 weeks by Doppler.
   4. 36 weeks have elapsed since a positive serum or urine pregnancy test was performed.
 C. If one or more of these criteria are not met, amniocentesis should be performed to document fetal maturity.
 D. A cervical examination should be performed immediately before cervical ripening or oxytocin (Pitocin) infusion.
III. Cervical ripening
 A. In a significant proportion of postdate pregnancies, the condition of the cervix is unfavorable, and cervical ripening is necessary.
 B. Prostaglandin E2
   1. Prostaglandin E2 vaginal gel may be prepared and administered for cervical ripening as 5 mg in 10 cc gel intravaginally q4h.
   2. Prostaglandin E2 gel is available in a 2.5-mL syringe which contains 0.5 mg of dinoprostone (Prepidil).
   3. A prostaglandin vaginal insert (Cervidil, 10 mg of dinoprostone) provides

a lower rate of release of medication (0.3 mg/h) than the gel. The vaginal insert has an advantage over the gel because it can be removed should hyperstimulation occur.

4. There is no difference in efficacy between vaginal or cervical routes. The vaginal route is much more comfortable for the patient.

5. The prostaglandin-induced cervical ripening process often induces labor that is similar to that of spontaneous labor. Prostaglandin E2 may enhance sensitivity to oxytocin (Pitocin).

6. Before initiating prostaglandin E2, a reassuring fetal heart rate tracing should be present, and there should be an the absence of regular uterine contractions (every 5 minutes or less). After prostaglandin E2 intravaginal gel is placed, the patient is continuously monitored for 2 hours, then discharged.

7. **Protocol for administration**
   a. The patient should remain recumbent for at least 30 minutes.
   b. Effects of prostaglandin E2 may be exaggerated with oxytocin (Pitocin); therefore, oxytocin induction should be delayed for 6-12 hours. If the patient continues to have uterine activity as a result of the prostaglandin E2 gel, oxytocin should be deferred or used in low doses.
   c. If there is insufficient cervical change with minimal uterine activity with one dose of prostaglandin E2, a second dose of prostaglandin E2 may be given 6-12 hours later.

8. **Side effects of prostaglandin E2**
   a. The rate of uterine hyperstimulation is 1% for the intracervical gel, usually beginning within 1 hour after the gel is applied. Pulling on the tail of the net surrounding the vaginal insert will usually reverse this effect.
   b. Terbutaline, 250 mg SC or IV will rapidly stop hyperstimulation.

IV. **Amniotomy**. Artificial rupture of membranes results in a reduction in the duration of labor. Before and after amniotomy the cervix should be palpated for the presence of an umbilical cord, and the fetal heart rate should be assessed and monitored.

V. **Oxytocin (Pitocin)**

A. Oxytocin administration stimulates uterine activity. No physiologic difference between oxytocin-stimulated labor and natural labor has been found.

B. **Administration**
   1. Oxytocin is diluted 10 units in 1 liter (10 mU/ mL) of normal saline solution. Starting dosage is 0.5-2 mU/min, with increases of 1-2 mU/min increments, every 30-60 minutes.
   2. A cervical dilation rate of 1 cm/h in the active phase indicates that labor is progressing sufficiently.

C. **Side effects**
   1. **Uterine hyperstimulation**
      a. The most common adverse effect of hyperstimulation is fetal heart rate deceleration. Decreasing the oxytocin dose rather than stopping it may correct the abnormal pattern. Uterine hyperstimulation or a resting tone above 20 mm Hg between contractions can lead to fetal hypoxia.
      b. Additional measures may include changing the patient to the lateral decubitus position, administering oxygen, or increasing intravenous fluid. When restarting the oxytocin, the dose should be lowered.
   2. Oxytocin does not cross the placenta; therefore, it has no direct effects on the fetus.
   3. Hypotension is seen only with rapid intravenous injection of oxytocin.

References: See page 290.

Postpartum Hemorrhage

Obstetric hemorrhage remains a leading causes of maternal mortality. Postpartum hemorrhage is defined as the loss of more than 500 mL of blood following delivery. However, the average blood loss in an uncomplicated vaginal delivery is about 500 mL, with 5% losing more than 1,000 mL.

I. Clinical evaluation of postpartum hemorrhage
   A. **Uterine atony** is the most common cause of postpartum hemorrhage. Conditions associated with uterine atony include an overdistended uterus (eg, polyhydramnios, multiple gestation), rapid or prolonged labor, macrosomia, high parity, and chorioamnionitis.
   B. **Conditions associated with bleeding from trauma** include forceps delivery, macrosomia, precipitous labor and delivery, and episiotomy.
   C. **Conditions associated with bleeding from coagulopathy and thrombocytopenia** include abruptio placentae, amniotic fluid embolism, preeclampsia, coagulation disorders, autoimmune thrombocytopenia, and anticoagulants.
   D. **Uterine rupture** is associated with previous uterine surgery, internal podalic version, breech extraction, multiple gestation, and abnormal fetal presentation. High parity is a risk factor for both uterine atony and rupture.
   E. **Uterine inversion** is detected by abdominal vaginal examination, which will reveal a uterus with an unusual shape after delivery.

II. Management of postpartum hemorrhage
   A. **Following delivery** of the placenta, the uterus should be palpated to determine whether atony is present. If atony is present, vigorous fundal massage should be administered. If bleeding continues despite uterine massage, it can often be controlled with bimanual uterine compression.
   B. **Genital tract lacerations** should be suspected in patients who have a firm uterus, but who continue to bleed. The cervix and vagina should be inspected to rule out lacerations. If no laceration is found but bleeding is still profuse, the uterus should be manually examined to exclude rupture.
   C. **The placenta and uterus should be examined** for retained placental fragments. Placenta accreta is usually manifest by failure of spontaneous placental separation.
   D. **Bleeding from non-genital areas** (venous puncture sites) suggests coagulopathy. Laboratory tests that confirm coagulopathy include INR, partial thromboplastin time, platelet count, fibrinogen, fibrin split products, and a clot retraction test.
   E. **Medical management of postpartum hemorrhage**
      1. **Oxytocin (Pitocin)** is usually given routinely immediately after delivery to stimulate uterine firmness and diminish blood loss. 20 units of oxytocin in 1,000 mL of normal saline or Ringer's lactate is administered at 100 drops/minute. Oxytocin should not be given as a rapid bolus injection because of the potential for circulatory collapse.
      2. If uterine massage and oxytocin are not effective in correcting uterine atony, methylergonovine (Methergine) 0.2 mg can be given IM, provided there is no hypertension. If hypertension is present, 15-methyl prostaglandin F2-alpha (Hemabate), one ampule (0.25 mg), can be given IM, with repeat injections every 20min, up to 4 doses; it is contraindicated in asthma.

Treatment of Postpartum Hemorrhage Secondary to Uterine Atony	
Drug	**Protocol**
Oxytocin	20 U in 1,000 mL of lactated Ringer's as IV infusion
Methylergonovine (Methergine)	0.2 mg IM
Prostaglandin (15 methyl PGF2-alpha [Prostin/15M])	0.25 mg as IM every 15-60 minutes as necessary

F. **Volume replacement**
   1. Patients with postpartum hemorrhage that is refractory to medical therapy require a second large-bore IV catheter. If the patient has had a major blood group determination and has a negative indirect Coombs test, type-specific blood may be given without waiting for a complete cross-match. Lactated Ringer's solution or normal saline is generously infused until blood can be replaced. Replacement consists of 3 mL of crystalloid solution per 1 mL of blood lost.
   2. A Foley catheter is placed, and urine output is maintained at greater than 30 mL/h.
G. **Surgical management of postpartum hemorrhage.** If medical therapy fails, ligation of the uterine or uteroovarian artery, infundibulopelvic vessels, or hypogastric arteries, or hysterectomy may be indicated.
H. **Management of uterine inversion**
   1. The inverted uterus should be immediately repositioned vaginally. Blood and/or fluids should be administered. If the placenta is still attached, it should not be removed until the uterus has been repositioned.
   2. Uterine relaxation can be achieved with a halogenated anesthetic agent. Terbutaline is also useful for relaxing the uterus.
   3. Following successful uterine repositioning and placental separation, oxytocin (Pitocin) is given to contract the uterus.

References: See page 290.

Uterine Infection

I. **Pathophysiology**
   A. The major predisposing clinical factor for pelvic infections is cesarean delivery The frequency and severity of infection are greater after abdominal delivery than after vaginal delivery. The incidence of infection after vaginal delivery is only 1-3%, whereas the incidence after abdominal delivery is 5-10 times greater. Those patients who undergo elective cesarean section (with no labor and no rupture of membranes) have lower infection rates than do those who undergo emergency or nonelective procedures (with labor, rupture of membranes, or both).
   B. Prolonged labor and premature ruptured membranes are the two most common risk factors associated with infection after cesarean birth. The number of vaginal examinations, socioeconomic status, and internal fetal monitoring have also been implicated.
   C. Endometritis is a polymicrobial infection, with a mixture of aerobes and anaerobes. Aerobes include gram-negative bacilli (eg, E coli) and gram-positive cocci (eg, group B streptococci). Anaerobic organisms have major roles in infection after cesarean birth; they are found in 80% of specimens. The most common isolated organism is Bacteroides.

II. **Clinical evaluation**
   A. The diagnosis of endometritis is based on the presence of fever and the absence of other causes of fever. Uterine tenderness, especially

parametrial, and purulent or foul-smelling lochia are common.
   B. Laboratory studies, with the exception of blood cultures, are usually not
   helpful.
III. **Treatment**
   A. Clindamycin-gentamicin most effective regimen, a combination that is
   curative in 85-95% of patients.
      a. Gentamicin 100 mg (2 mg/kg) IV load, then 100 mg (1.5 mg/kg) IV
      q8h.
      b. Clindamycin, 600-900 mg IV q8h.
   B. Treatment with ampicillin (2 gm IV q4-6h) and an aminoglycoside is less ef-
   fective in postcesarean endometritis. Good results have been reported with
   cefoxitin (1-2 gm IV q6h), cefoperazone (1-2 gm IV/IM q8h), cefotaxime,
   piperacillin, and cefotetan. Antibiotics containing a penicillin derivative and
   a beta-lactamase inhibitor are also effective.
   C. Treatment is continued until the patient has been afebrile for 24-48 hours.
   Further antibiotic therapy on an outpatient basis is generally not necessary.
   D. Causes of initial failure of antibiotic therapy include the presence of an
   abscess, resistant organisms, a wound infection, infection at other sites, or
   septic thrombophlebitis. Surgical drainage, especially for an abscess, may
   occasionally be necessary, although hysterectomy is rarely required.
References: See page 290.

Postpartum Fever Workup

History: Postpartum fever is ≥100.4 F (38 degrees C) on 2 occasions >6h apart
after the first postpartum day (during the first 10 days postpartum), or ≥101 on the
first postpartum day. Dysuria, abdominal pain, distention, breast pain, calf pain.
Predisposing Factors: Cesarean section, prolonged labor, premature rupture
of membranes, internal monitors, multiple vaginal exams, meconium, manual
placenta extraction, anemia, poor nutrition.
Physical Examination: Temperature, throat, chest, lung exams; breasts,
abdomen. Costovertebral angle tenderness, uterine tenderness, phlebitis, calf
tenderness; wound exam. Speculum exam.
Differential Diagnosis: UTI, upper respiratory infection, atelectasis, pneumonia,
wound infection, mastitis, episiotomy abscess; uterine infection, deep vein
thrombosis, pyelonephritis, pelvic abscess.
Labs: CBC, SMA7, blood C&S x 2, catheter UA, C&S. Endometrial Pipelle
sample or swab for gram stain, C&S; gonococcus, chlamydia; wound C&S, CXR.

References

References may be obtained at www.ccspublishing.com.

Commonly Used Formulas

A-a gradient = $[(P_B - PH_2O) FiO_2 - PCO_2/R] - PO_2$ arterial

$\qquad$ = $(713 \times FiO2 - pCO2/0.8) - pO2$ arterial

$P_B = 760$ mmHg; $PH_2O = 47$ mmHg; $R \approx 0.8$
normal Aa gradient <10-15 mmHg (room air)

Arterial oxygen capacity = (Hgb(gm)/100 mL) x 1.36 mL O2/gm Hgb

Arterial O2 content = 1.36(Hgb)(SaO2)+0.003(PaO2)= NL 20 vol%

O2 delivery = CO x arterial O2 content = NL 640-1000 mL O2/min

Cardiac output = HR x stroke volume

$$CO\ L/min = \frac{125\ mL\ O2/min/M^2}{8.5\,\{(1.36)(Hgb)(SaO2) - (1.36)(Hgb)(SvO2)\}} \times 100$$

Normal CO = 4-6 L/min

Na (mEq) deficit = 0.6 x (wt kg) x (desired [Na] - actual [Na])

$SVR = \dfrac{MAP - CVP}{CO_{L/min}} \times 80$ = NL 800-1200 dyne/sec/cm^2

$PVR = \dfrac{PA - PCWP}{CO_{L/min}} \times 80$ = NL 45-120 dyne/sec/cm^2

GFR mL/min = $\dfrac{(140 - age)\ x\ wt\ in\ kg}{\substack{72\ (males)\ x\ serum\ creatinine\ (mg/dL)\\85\ (females)\ x\ serum\ creatinine\ (mg/dL)}}$

Creatinine clearance = $\dfrac{U\ creatinine\ (mg/100\ mL)\ x\ U\ vol\ (mL)}{P\ creatinine\ (mg/100\ mL)\ x\ time\ (1440\ min\ for\ 24h)}$

Normal creatinine clearance = 100-125 mL/min(males), 85-105(females)

Body water deficit (L) = $\dfrac{0.6(weight\ kg)([measured\ serum\ Na]-140)}{140}$

Serum Osmolality = $2\ [Na] + \dfrac{BUN}{2.8} + \dfrac{Glucose}{18}$ = 270-290

Na (mEq) deficit = 0.6 x (wt kg)x(desired [Na] - actual [Na])

Fractional excreted Na = $\dfrac{U\ Na/\ Serum\ Na}{U\ creatinine/\ Serum\ creatinine} \times 100$ = NL<1%

Anion Gap = Na - (Cl + HCO3)

For each 100 mg/dL ↑ in glucose, Na+ ↓ by 1.6 mEq/L.

Corrected serum Ca$^+$ (mg/dL) = measured Ca mg/dL + 0.8 x (4 - albumin g/dL)

Predicted Maximal Heart Rate = 220 - age

Normal ECG Intervals (sec)

PR	0.12-0.20
QRS	0.06-0.08
Heart rate/min	**Q-T**
60	0.33-0.43
70	0.31-0.41
80	0.29-0.38
90	0.28-0.36
100	0.27-0.35

Total Parenteral Nutrition Equations:

Caloric Requirements: (Harris-Benedict Equations)
   Basal energy expenditure (BEE)
      Females: 655 + (9.6 x wt in kg) + (1.85 x ht in cm) - (4.7 x age)
      Males: 66 + (13.7 x wt in kg) + (5 x ht in cm) - (6.8 x age)

   A. BEE x 1.2 = Caloric requirement for minimally stressed patient
   B. BEE x 1.3 = Caloric requirement for moderately stressed patient (inflammatory bowel disease, cancer, surgery)
   C. BEE x 1.5 = Caloric requirement for severely stressed patient (major sepsis, burns, AIDS, liver disease)
   D. BEE x 1.7 = Caloric requirement for extremely stressed patient (traumatic burns >50%, open head trauma, multiple stress)

Protein Requirements:
   A. 0.8 gm protein/kg = Protein requirement for nonstressed patient.
   B. 1.0-1.5 gm protein/kg = Protein requirement for patients with decreased visceral protein states (hypoalbumiaemia), recent weight loss, or hypercatabolic states.
   C. >1.5 gm protein/kg = Protein requirement for patients with negative nitrogen balance receiving 1.5 gm protein/kg

Estimation of Ideal Body Weight:
   A. Females: 5 feet (allow 100 lbs) + 5 lbs for each inch over 5 feet
   B. Males: 5 feet (allow 106 lbs) + 6 lbs for each inch over 5 foot

Drug Levels of Commonly Used Medications

DRUG	THERAPEUTIC RANGE*
Amikacin	Peak 25-30; trough <10 mcg/mL
Amitriptyline	100-250 ng/mL
Carbamazepine	4-10 mcg/mL
Chloramphenicol	Peak 10-15; trough <5 mcg/mL
Desipramine	150-300 ng/mL
Digitoxin	10-30 ng/mL
Digoxin	0.8-2.0 ng/mL
Disopyramide	2-5 mcg/mL
Doxepin	75-200 ng/mL
Ethosuximide	40-100 mcg/mL
Flecainide	0.2-1.0 mcg/mL
Gentamicin	Peak 6.0-8.0; trough <2.0 mcg/mL
Imipramine	150-300 ng/mL
Lidocaine	2-5 mcg/mL
Lithium	0.5-1.4 mEq/L
Nortriptyline	50-150 ng/mL
Phenobarbital	10-30 mEq/mL
Phenytoin**	8-20 mcg/mL
Procainamide	4.0-8.0 mcg/mL
Quinidine	2.5-5.0 mcg/mL
Salicylate	15-25 mg/dL

Streptomycin	Peak 10-20; trough <5 mcg/mL
Theophylline	8-20 mcg/mL
Tocainide	4-10 mcg/mL
Valproic acid	50-100 mcg/mL
Vancomycin	Peak 30-40; trough <10 mcg/mL

* The therapeutic range of some drugs may vary depending on the reference lab used.
** Therapeutic range of phenytoin is 4-10 mcg/mL in presence of significant azotemia and/or hypoalbuminemia.

Pediatric and Obstetric Formulas

Normal urine output = 50 ml/kg/d
Oliguria = 0.5 ml/kg/h
Normal feedings = 5 oz/kg/d
Formula = 20 calories/ounce, 24 cal/oz, 27 cal/oz
Ounce = 30 cc
Caloric Needs = 100 cal/kg/d
Calories/Kg = cc of formula x 30 cc/oz x 20 calories/oz divided by weight.

Weight in Kg = pounds divided by 2.2
Weight in Kg = [age in years x 2] +10

Blood volume (ml) = 80 ml/kg x weight (kg)

Blood Products:
   10 cc/kg RBC will raise Hct 5%
   0.1 unit/kg platelets will raise platelet count, 25000/mm^3.
   1 U/kg of Factor VIII will raise level by 2%.

Naegele's Rule: LMP minus 3 months plus 7 days = Estimated date of confinement.

$$GFR = \frac{(140 - age) \times wt \text{ in Kg}}{85 \times serum \text{ Cr}}$$

Normal Cr clearance = 85-105

Index

Titles from Current Clinical Strategies Publishing

In All Medical Bookstores Worldwide

Family Medicine, 2002 Edition
Outpatient Medicine, 2001 Edition
History and Physical Examination, 2001-2002 Edition
Medicine, 2001 Edition
Pediatrics 5-Minute Reviews, 2001-2002 Edition
Anesthesiology, 2002-2003 Edition
Handbook of Psychiatric Drugs, 2001-2002 Edition
Gynecology and Obstetrics, 2002 Edition
Manual of HIV/AIDS Therapy, 2001 Edition
Treatment Guidelines for Medicine and Primary Care, 2002 Edition
Surgery, 2002 Edition
Pediatric Drug Reference, 2002 Edition
Critical Care Medicine, 2000 Edition
Psychiatry, 2002 Edition
Pediatrics, 2002 Edition
Physicians' Drug Manual, 2001 Edition
Pediatric History and Physical Examination, Fourth Edition

Palm, Pocket PC, Windows, Windows CE, Macintosh, and Softcover Book